The Exercising Female

The Exercising Female: Science and Its Application is the first book to provide students, researchers, and professionals with an evidence-based reference on the exceptional scientific issues associated with female participation in sport and exercise. Based on the latest research, and treating women as a unique population, the book seeks to critically evaluate current debates, present the science underpinning female sport and exercise performance, and inform applied practice for the exercising female.

Featuring contributions from leading scientists from around the world, and adopting a multidisciplinary approach – from exercise physiology, endocrinology, and biochemistry to psychology, biomechanics, and sociology – the book includes chapters on topics such as:

- Exercise and the menstrual cycle, contraception, pregnancy, motherhood, and menopause.
- Body image, exercise dependency, the psychology of sports performance, and homophobia in female sport.
- The Female Athlete Triad, bone health, musculoskeletal injury, and breast biomechanics.
- Nutritional requirements for the exercising female, immune function and exercise, and cardiovascular health.

Filling a considerable gap in book literature around the science of female sport and exercise, this is crucial reading for any student studying female sport and exercise science, researchers of female sport, and any coach, sport scientist, strength and conditioning coach, sport psychologist, physician, or physiotherapist working with female athletes.

Jacky Forsyth is an associate professor at Staffordshire University, UK. She is a prominent researcher and speaker in the area of women's exercise and health. Her research is centred on the interactive effect of ovarian hormones, exercise, and bone. One of her research priorities is to promote raise awareness, and to advance understanding of the key influences, which impact the exercising female. She is vice chair of the Women in Sport and Exercise Academic Network (WISEAN), the aim of which is 'To grow, strengthen, and promote research on women in sport and exercise, with the ultimate goal of optimising women's athletic success and their participation'. Jacky publishes regularly in peer-reviewed journals in her field.

Claire-Marie Roberts is a senior lecturer in Sport and Exercise Psychology at the University of the West of England, Bristol, UK, and a practising Sport Psychology consultant. Her experiences of working with athletes reflect her research interests. These include female-specific issues relating to career transitions in sport such as pregnancy and motherhood and the psychology of female sport performance. Claire-Marie is the chair of the WISEAN, a non-executive board director of UK Anti-Doping, and a member of the Women in Sport Research Action Group.

Routledge Research in Sport and Exercise Science

The *Routledge Research in Sport and Exercise Science* series is a showcase for cutting-edge research from across the sport and exercise sciences, including physiology, psychology, biomechanics, motor control, physical activity, and health, and every core sub-discipline. Featuring the work of established and emerging scientists and practitioners from around the world, and covering the theoretical, investigative, and applied dimensions of sport and exercise, this series is an important channel for new and groundbreaking research in the human movement sciences.

Available in this series:

The Athlete Apperception Technique
Manual and Materials for Sport and Clinical Psychologists
Petah M. Gibbs, Mark B. Andersen and Daryl B. Marchant

Complex Sport Analytics
Felix Lebed

The Science of Figure Skating
Edited by Jason D. Vescovi and Jaci L. VanHeest

The Science of Judo
Edited by Mike Callan

Modelling and Simulation in Sport and Exercise
Edited by Arnold Baca and Jürgen Perl

The Exercising Female
Science and Its Application
Edited by Jacky Forsyth and Claire-Marie Roberts

For more information about this series, please visit: www.routledge.com/sport/series/RRSES

The Exercising Female
Science and Its Application

Edited by Jacky Forsyth and
Claire-Marie Roberts

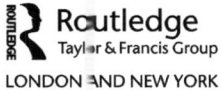
Routledge
Taylor & Francis Group

LONDON AND NEW YORK

First published 2019
by Routledge
2 Park Square, Milton Park, Abingdon, Oxon OX14 4RN

and by Routledge
605 Third Avenue, New York, NY 10017

First issued in paperback 2021

Routledge is an imprint of the Taylor & Francis Group, an informa business

British Library Cataloguing-in-Publication Data
A catalogue record for this book is available from the British Library

Library of Congress Cataloging-in-Publication Data
A catalog record has been requested for this book

ISBN 13: 978-0-367-61592-5 (pbk)
ISBN 13: 978-0-8153-9198-2 (hbk)
ISBN 13: 978-1-351-20027-1 (ebk)

DOI: 10.4324/9781351200271

Typeset in Garamond
by Wearset Ltd, Boldon, Tyne and Wear

Contents

Figures

Tables

Contributors

Dr Judith Allgrove, Kingston University, UK.

Miss Nicole C. Aurigemma, Pennsylvania State University, USA.

Professor Karen Birch, University of Leeds, UK.

Dr Tim Blackmore, University of Portsmouth, UK.

Dr Rachael Bullingham, University of Worcester, UK.

Dr Jenny Burbage, University of Portsmouth, UK.

Professor Amanda J. Daley, Loughborough University, UK.

Dr Glen Davison, University of Kent, UK.

Professor Mary Jane De Souza, Pennsylvania State University, USA.

Professor Joan M. Eckerson, Creighton University, USA.

Dr Kirsty J. Elliott-Sale, Nottingham Trent University, UK.

Dr Leah Ferguson, University of Saskatchewan, Canada.

Dr Jacky Forsyth, Staffordshire University, UK.

Miss Madeleine France, Liverpool John Moores University, UK.

Professor Sarah Grogan, Manchester Metropolitan University, UK.

Professor Heather A. Hausenblas, Jacksonville University, USA.

Dr Kirsty Marie Hicks, Northumbria University, UK.

Dr Karen Hind, Leeds Beckett University, UK.

Miss Brogan Horler, University of Portsmouth, UK.

Professor Helen Jones, Liverpool John Moores University, UK.

Dr Göran Kenttä, The Swedish School of Sport and Health Sciences GIH, Sweden.

Ms Kristen J. Koltun, Pennsylvania State University, USA.

Dr David A. Low, Liverpool John Moores University, UK.

Miss Gemma Lyall, University of Leeds, UK.

Dr Derek T. Y. Mann, Jacksonville University, USA.

Dr Amber Mosewich, University of Alberta, Canada.

Ms. Michelle Norris, University of Portsmouth, UK.

Dr Robin Pickering, Whitworth University, USA.

Dr Ruth V. Pritchett, University of Birmingham, UK.

Dr Claire-Marie Roberts, University of the West England, UK.

Miss Kaitlyn M. Ruffing, Pennsylvania State University, USA.

Miss Emly A. Southmayd, Pennsylvania State University, USA.

Professor Nancy I. Williams, Pennsylvania State University, USA.

Mrs Lindsay Woodford, University of the West England, UK.

Professor Mimi Zumwalt, Texas Tech University, USA.

Acknowledgements

Jacky Forsyth and Claire-Marie Roberts

We would both like to extend our heartfelt thanks to all the authors of each chapter, who contributed to the writing of this book. These authors put so much time and effort into ensuring that the content within each chapter was thoroughly researched and relevant, and we are both extremely grateful. Special thanks also go to Megan Smith, Rebecca Connor, and William Bailey at Routledge and Anastasia Said for their support and assistance in producing this book.

Mimi Zumwalt

I would like to dedicate Chapter 11 to significant females in my life: my mother Francoise and daughter Demi, both of whom I appreciate/love with all my heart! I also want to thank Mark Wellborn and Charles Henderson for their expert IT/AV assistance.

Abbreviations

3D	Three-dimensional
ACL	Anterior cruciate ligament
ACSM	American College of Sports Medicine
BCAA	Branched chain amino acids
BM	Body mass
BMD	Bone mineral density
BMI	Body mass index
BMR	Basal metabolic rate
CBT	Cognitive behavioural therapy
CHO	Carbohydrate
COLIA1	Collagen type I alpha 1
CRP	C-reactive protein
CVD	Cardiovascular disease
DCs	Dendritic cells
DMPA	Depot Medroxyprogesterone Acetate
DSM-5	Diagnostic and Statistical Manual, 5th edition
DT	Drive for thinness
DXA	Dual energy X-ray absorptiometry
EA	Energy availability
EAA	Essential amino acids
EEX	Energy expenditure from structured exercise
EI	Energy intake
eNOS	Endothelial nitric oxide synthase
EPOC	Excess post-exercise oxygen consumption
ERα	Oestrogen receptor-alpha
ERβ	Oestrogen receptor-beta
ET-1	Endothelin-1
FFA	Free-fatty acids
FFM	Fat-free mass
FHA	Functional hypothalamic amenorrhoea
FSH	Follicle-stimulating hormone
GABA	Gamma-aminobutyric acid
HDL-C	High-density lipoprotein cholesterol

HPA	Hypothalamic-pituitary-adrenal
HRT	Hormone replacement therapy
IDA	Iron-deficiency anaemia
IGF-1	Insulin-like growth factor-1
IL	Interleukin
IL-1ra	Interleukin receptor antagonist
IMTG	Intramuscular triglycerides
LBM	Lean body mass
LDL-C	Low-density lipoprotein cholesterol
LGBT	Lesbian, gay, bisexual, and transsexual
MPS	Muscle protein synthesis
MRI	Magnetic resonance imaging
NICE	National Institute for Health and Care Excellence
NK	Natural killer
NKCA	Natural killer cell cytotoxic activity
NO	Nitric oxide
OC	Oral contraceptive
OPG	Osteoprotegerin
OT	Overtraining syndrome
PEP	Prevent Injury and Enhance Performance
PND	Postnatal depression
pQCT	Peripheral quantitative computed tomography
PRO	Protein
RANK	Receptor Activator of Nuclear factor Kappa-B
RANKL	Receptor Activator of Nuclear factor Kappa-B Ligand
RBCs	Red blood cells
RCT	Randomised controlled trial
REE	Resting energy expenditure
RMR	Resting metabolic rate
ROS	Reactive oxygen species
SBP	Systolic blood pressure
SD	Standard deviation
sIgA	Secretory immunoglobulin
SOD	Superoxide dismutase
SOP	Self-oriented perfectionism
SPP	Socially-prescribed perfectionism
TDEE	Total daily energy expenditure
TEA	Thermic effect of activity
TEF	Thermic effect of food
TG	Triglycerides
TNFα	Tumour necrosis factor alpha
Triad	Female Athlete Triad
TT$_3$	Total triiodothyronine
URS	Upper respiratory symptoms
URTI	Upper respiratory tract infections

UVB	Ultraviolet B
$\dot{V}O_2max$	Maximal oxygen consumption
WHI	Women's Health Initiative
WHO	World Health Organization

1 Introduction to *The Exercising Female: Science and Its Application*

Jacky Forsyth and Claire-Marie Roberts

Trends in sport and exercise for females

At the recreational level, there is a general decline in rates of participation in sport and exercise through the female lifespan; sociocultural reasons can be used to explain this trend. However, recent efforts to engage women in sport and exercise worldwide have had a positive impact, and general participation trends are on the increase. Additionally, we are seeing a greater percentage of female athletes comprising national teams at multisport, major events such as the Olympic Games. The possible reasons for this increase include a change of mindset, where women are now rightly viewed as a unique population, with their own motivations and barriers to participation.

Despite this growth in women's participation in sport and exercise, research on the exercising female, and how a woman's body responds to exercise still falls short of that carried out on men. For instance, there is limited research on how variations in ovarian hormones can affect sports performance (Bruinvels et al., 2017), and females, as participants in research, are significantly under-represented in sport and exercise medicine (Costello, Bieuzen, & Bleakley, 2014). Training programmes, exercise regimes, dietary guidelines, psychological interventions, and injury prevention and rehabilitation programmes are therefore, largely based on research that has been carried out on men. It is important to keep studying and researching about females who exercise, since the research that has emerged in the last few decades, as explored in this book, has identified that women should be considered in isolation and not grouped with men, when conducting research, and when providing recommendations for training.

Sex discrimination, gender inequality, gender bias, and gender stereotyping in sport and exercise continue to exist, since, historically, sport has been a male-dominated, and male-controlled institution (Brown & Stone, 2016; Plaza, Boiché, Brunel, & Ruchaud, 2017; Shin, 2017). This sexual inequality is evidenced in the media portrayal of females in sport, where, as well as there being a lack of coverage on women's sport, a sports woman's physical attributes are often prioritised over their performance attributes (Musto, Cooky, & Messner, 2017; Walker & Bopp, 2010). Female professional athletes earn less than their male counterparts (Women's Sports Foundation, 2015), with no women featuring in the top 100 of Forbes' list of the world's highest-paid athletes for 2018 (Badenhausen, 2018). Males also outnumber females in sport- and exercise-related employment, especially in graduate-level jobs, senior roles, and in leadership positions (Hartmann-Tews & Pfister, 2005). For instance, there are far fewer female head athletic trainers (Mazerolle, Burton, & Raymond, 2015), sports physicians (Stern, Gateley, & Barrett, 2013), sport coaches/head coaches (Acosta & Carpenter, 2014; Norman, 2012; Walker & Bopp, 2010), and governance executives of organised sport (Burton, 2015; Koca & Öztürk, 2015; Pfister & Radtke, 2009) than there are male. From 87 subject-specific statues (ignoring anonymous and unknown figures) in the UK, there are only two that depict women, that of Mary Peters (athletics) and Dorothy Round (tennis) (Stride, Thomas, & Wilson, 2012). Of the 387 *in situ*, subject-specific football (soccer) statues around the world, only one (<1 per cent) is of a woman, a schoolgirl football enthusiast, who was killed in a drink-drive incident (Stride et al., 2012). There are, therefore, barriers to women's participation in exercise and sport that are a result of existing and historical social and cultural norms and behaviours (Koca & Öztürk, 2015; Walker & Sartore-Baldwin, 2013), which may also explain the limited scientific and medical research on the exercising female.

Aims and themes of the book

The 'exercising female'

The 'exercising female' is the term used in this book to encompass a wide range of women and girls who exercise, from the female, recreational exercise participant, to the elite female athlete. The book is, therefore, relevant to a wide audience including: students, researchers, and lecturers in sport, health, and exercise at both undergraduate and postgraduate level; practitioners and professionals working with women at recreational through to competitive performance level, such as coaches, strength and conditioning coaches, physiotherapists, sport psychologists, sports medics, physicians; and those involved in the governance of sport and exercise. The book is, of course, also relevant for exercising females, who wish to learn more about how to make the most of being a woman to achieve athletic success.

Understanding the exercising female can be advanced through science – the study of physiology, biomechanics, psychology, and nutrition. The focus of this book is, therefore, on these scientific issues facing the exercising female. There are two underpinning themes that run throughout each chapter: (1) the scientific issues that exercising females may encounter; and (2) how to make the most of being a woman to achieve athletic success. The second of these two themes is a unique perspective, since often there has been a tendency to examine women's performance relative to that of men, or to examine the issues that prevent women from performing as well as men.

In each chapter, the evidence base, and recent research developments are critically evaluated, and practical recommendations are made based on the two themes. Each chapter also includes a 'real-world' example (such as a quote, case study, experience, or short story) from an exercising female's perspective, which supports the points being made in the chapter. The overall aim of the book is, therefore, to provide scientific underpinning to inform applied practice for the exercising female.

The book starts with an examination of the issues facing the adolescent exercising female (*Chapter 2*). The adolescence is a particularly vulnerable time, since the exercising female is developing their sense of identity, and may be more susceptible to drop out from exercise, but also more susceptible to injury, overtraining, eating disorders, and mental health problems, especially if there is early sport specialisation. We then progress to the premenopausal exercising female. Women (in developed countries) have ~457 menstrual cycles in their lifetime, corresponding to 35.1 years of menstrual activity (Chavez-MacGregor, 2005). The menstrual cycle, and the associated changes in ovarian hormones (oestrogen and progesterone), therefore, pervades a woman's reproductive life, and these changes can impact the exercising female's physical and mental health and their exercise performance. In *Chapter 3*, menstrual disturbances as a result of insufficient energy availability are examined, and whether performance is affected by the menstrual cycle is critically evaluated. Since exercising females may use hormonal contraception to counteract the perceived negative symptoms associated with having a menstrual cycle, the different types and effects of these synthetic hormones on exercise performance is debated in *Chapter 4*.

Due to having unique metabolic and physiological needs, the exercising female requires optimal energy intake, in terms of macronutrients, micronutrients (especially calcium, iron, magnesium, and zinc), and hydration. These nutritional requirements, as well as dietary strategies to enhance performance, are discussed in *Chapter 5*. Since having low energy availability is seen to be the driving force behind the development of the Female Athlete Triad, in *Chapter 6*, this syndrome is reviewed, highlighting the physiology and prevalence of each component (low energy availability, menstrual disturbances, and poor bone health), and critically considering recommendations for prevention and treatment. Further discussion of bone health, as the clinical sequelae to the Triad is included in *Chapter 7*. An examination of the physiological processes of bone remodelling, with particular reference to oestrogen, is also presented in this chapter, as well as exercise strategies to improve bone health.

Although the Female Athlete Triad is often described in terms of physiology, psychological factors are important to consider as determinants. Sport-related and societal pressure can, for instance, lead to body dissatisfaction in the exercising female, which could stimulate eating disorders. The effects of subcultural and societal expectations on body image are analysed in *Chapter 8*, along with a consideration of the most effective interventions to promote positive body image. Indeed, concerns with body image may drive the exercising female to turn to maladaptive excessive exercise behaviours leading to exercise addiction, where the sole purpose of engaging and adhering to exercise is to lose weight. Exercise addiction, however, can also be primary, rather than secondary (as a result of the eating disorder). Primary exercise addiction, including causes and treatment, is discussed in *Chapter 9*.

Females, largely as a result of oestrogen, are not particularly susceptible to viral infections, but do have an increased risk of autoimmune disease. In *Chapter 10*, the relationship between exercise, immune function, and infection risk of the exercising female is examined. Consequently, recommendations on how to minimise immune system changes and infection risk to preserve exercise performance and health are provided. Additionally, exercising females, by nature of their physiology, are exposed to a high risk of musculoskeletal injury, especially anterior cruciate ligament (ACL) injury when exercising or playing sport. In *Chapter 11*, the epidemiology and aetiology of this increased injury risk in females is examined, and alternative methods of exercise training to help prevent injury are presented. Female-specific considerations in sport and exercise are extended in *Chapter 12*, where research into breast health and biomechanics is provided. This information is particularly pertinent as excessive breast motion during exercise, caused by a lack of appropriate breast support, can be a barrier to exercise participation.

Historical social and cultural norms and behaviours may, in part, be responsible for the unique psychology of the exercising female's performance. In *Chapter 13*, female-specific sources of competitive anxiety, sport and exercise confidence, and relationship conflict in teams are examined, and recommendations for effective working with exercising females are provided. The investigation of the inner workings of female sport teams also gives an opportunity to consider the 'coming out' process of lesbian athletes. In *Chapter 14*, an account of the different climates of homophobia are provided, from that of hostility in the 1980s through to more inclusive climates of today, which have implications for exercise participation and performance.

Although there are many benefits to exercising while pregnant, the associated changes to the physiological and anatomical systems of the body, as well as the presenting psychosocial challenges, have consequences for health, sport and exercise performance. In *Chapter 15*, a review of the anatomy and physiology of pregnancy is given, and guidelines for safe and effective sport and exercise participation during this time are provided. After childbirth, postnatal (or postpartum) depression may affect up to 20 per cent of women at some point during the perinatal period (Schmied et al., 2013). This serious and debilitating psychiatric disorder can have long-term effects on both the mother and child. *Chapter 16* contains a summary of the effectiveness of exercise for the relief of postnatal depression, and includes the viewpoints expressed by women who have engaged in exercise to successfully relieve their symptoms. The mechanistic causes and the practicalities of exercise as an intervention are also explored. Moreover, motherhood, for an elite or recreational athlete, has the propensity to be both facilitative and constraining for the exercising female. Issues, such as the postponement of motherhood in pursuit of an athletic career, the meticulous planning of conception to coincide with the competitive schedules, and the challenges of a return to sport are examined in *Chapter 17*.

When exercising females reach the end of their athletic career, it is widely accepted that this can be one of the most challenging transitions to negotiate. Females are more likely to initiate the termination of their athletic career of their own volition, citing a multitude of reasons including starting a family, or due to the higher injury rate in female athletes. In *Chapter 18*, the gender specificity of athletic career termination in female athletes is explored, and a critical evaluation of relevant topics is provided.

Finally, as the exercising female progresses through her lifecycle, the menopausal state is one in which the individual will spend a large portion of time. In the menopause, oestrogen deficiency predisposes her to an increased risk of cardiovascular disease. In *Chapter 19*, the role of oestrogen in maintaining cardiovascular health is explained alongside the role of exercise in restoring cardiovascular health even when oestrogen levels are low. The menopause itself is examined in detail in *Chapter 20*, with an explanation of the symptoms and a presentation of evidence of how certain exercise during the menopause transition and beyond can enhance cardiovascular and metabolic health and well-being.

Summary

Despite increases in exercise and sport participation for females worldwide, the research governing the exercising female is far from ideal, possibly being perpetuated by social and cultural norms, where sport is perceived to be a male domain. Through the specific content within each chapter of this book, our scientific and critical research knowledge and understanding of the exercising female can be advanced, and an appreciation of the recommendations to improve athletic success for the exercising female gained.

References

Acosta, R. V., & Carpenter, L. J. (2014). *Women in intercollegiate sport. A longitudinal, national study. Thirty-seven year update. 1977–2014.* Retrieved from www.acosta-carpenter.org.

Badenhausen, K. (2018). *The world's 100 highest-paid athletes 2018: Behind the numbers.* Retrieved from www.forbes.com/sites/kurtbadenhausen/2018/06/05/the-worlds-100-highest-paid-athletes-2018-behind-the-numbers/#6f61699e4dd0.

Brown, C. S., & Stone, E. A. (2016). Gender stereotypes and discrimination: How sexism impacts development. *Advances in Child Development and Behavior, 50,* 105–133. http://doi.org/10.1016/BS.ACDB.2015.11.001.

Bruinvels, G., Burden, R. J., McGregor, A. J., Ackerman, K. E., Dooley, M., Richards, T., & Pedlar, C. (2017). Sport, exercise and the menstrual cycle: Where is the research? *British Journal of Sports Medicine, 51*(6), 487–488. http://doi.org/10.1136/bjsports-2016-096279.

Burton, L. J. (2015). Underrepresentation of women in sport leadership: A review of research. *Sport Management Review, 18*(2), 155–165. http://doi.org/10.1016/j.smr.2014.02.004.

Chavez-MacGregor, M. (2005). Postmenopausal breast cancer risk and cumulative number of menstrual cycle. *Cancer Epidemiology Biomarkers & Prevention, 14*(4), 799–804. http://doi.org/10.1158/1055-9965.EPI-04-0465.

Costello, J. T., Bieuzen, F., & Bleakley, C. M. (2014). Where are all the female participants in Sports and Exercise Medicine research? *European Journal of Sport Science, 14*(8), 847–851. http://doi.org/10.1080/17461391.2014.911354.

Koca, C., & Öztürk, P. (2015). Gendered perceptions about female managers in Turkish sport organizations. *European Sport Management Quarterly, 15*(3), 381–406. http://doi.org/10.1080/16184742.2015.1040046.

Mazerolle, S. M., Burton, L., & Raymond, J. (2015). The experiences of female athletic trainers in the role of the head athletic trainer. *Journal of Athletic Training, 50*(1), 71–81. http://doi.org/10.4085/1062-6050-49.3.50.

Musto, M., Cooky, C., & Messner, M. A. (2017). 'From fizzle to sizzle!' Televised sports news and the production of gender-bland sexism. *Gender & Society, 31*(5), 573–596. http://doi.org/10.1177/0891243217726056.

Norman, L. (2012). Developing female coaches: strategies from women themselves. *Asia-Pacific Journal of Health, Sport and Physical Education, 3*(3), 227–238. http://doi.org/10.1080/18377122.2012.721725.

Pfister, G., & Radtke, S. (2009). Sport, women, and leadership: Results of a project on executives in German sports organizations. *European Journal of Sport Science, 9*(4), 229–243. http://doi.org/10.1080/17461390902818286.

Plaza, M., Boiché, J., Brunel, L., & Ruchaud, F. (2017). Sport = male … but not all sports: Investigating the gender stereotypes of sport activities at the explicit and implicit levels. *Sex Roles, 76*(3–4), 202–217. http://doi.org/10.1007/s11199-016-0650-x.

Schmied, V., Johnson, M., Naidoo, N., Austin, M.-P., Matthey, S., Kemp, L., … Yeo, A. (2013). Maternal mental health in Australia and New Zealand: A review of longitudinal studies. *Women and Birth, 26*(3), 167–178. http://doi.org/10.1016/j.wombi.2013.02.006.

Shin, P. S. (2017). Sex and gender segregation in competitive sport: Internal and external normative perspectives. *Law and Contemporary Problems, 80*, 47–61.

Stern, N. G., Gateley, A., & Barrett, J. R. (2013). Is there perceived gender disparity for women practicing sports medicine? *Advancing Women in Leadership, 33*, 48–51.

Stride, C. B., Thomas, F. E., & Wilson, J. P. (2012). The sporting statues project.

Walker, N. A., & Bopp, T. (2010). The underrepresentation of women in the male-dominated sport workplace: Perspectives of female coaches. *Journal of Workplace Rights, 15*(1), 47–64. http://doi.org/10.2190/WR.15.1.d.

Walker, N. A., & Sartore-Baldwin, M. L. (2013). Hegemonic masculinity and the institutionalized bias toward women in men's collegiate basketball: What do men think? *Journal of Sport Management, 27*(4), 303–315. http://doi.org/10.1123/jsm.27.4.303.

Women's Sports Foundation. (2015). *Pay inequity in athletics.* Retrieved from www.womenssportsfoundation.org/research/article-and-report/elite-athletes/pay-inequity/

2 The adolescent exercising female

Lindsay Woodford

Introduction

Adolescence is the unique period of life between childhood and adulthood, and its definition has been a topic of much debate. It encompasses elements of biological growth and major social role transitions, both of which have changed in the past century. Arguably, the transition period from childhood to adulthood now occupies a larger portion of the life course than ever before; rather than age 10–19 years, a definition of 10–24 years has been suggested to correspond more closely with adolescent development (Sawyer, Azzopardi, Wickremarathne, & Patton, 2018). The primary developmental task of late adolescence is to establish a sense of self-identity (Erikson, 1959), whereby young people begin to define who they are through the goals, values, and beliefs that they find personally expressive and to which they commit. For females, adolescence is a crucial stage of development that incorporates menarche, bringing about a profound change in physiology. Any personal challenges experienced in adolescence may impact the female's mental health and personal well-being. It is during this developmental phase that a steep decline in the frequency and intensity of physical activity, exercise, and sport occurs. This change is attributable to a number of factors including sociocultural norms, problems with body image, fear of judgement, and a number of competing interests (Sport England, 2016). For the adolescent exercising female then, this developmental stage is likely to be critical as the sport and exercise domain brings with it a number of additional challenges, yet it may also mediate the stress and pressure of this stage, in this phase of the lifecycle.

Aims of the chapter

The aims of the chapter are as follows:

1   To consider the key issues facing adolescent exercising females.
2   To provide practical recommendations to help exercising females negotiate these challenges.

3   To present a real-world example of the work of a sport and exercise psychologist with an adolescent female athlete.

Identity formation

Engaging in exploratory behaviours (e.g., standing up to peers and potential health risk behaviours such as substance abuse and risky sexual activity) provide an opportunity for individuals to make informed decisions about their personal values, interests, and skills. Furthermore, it encourages them to feel confident in their abilities to be successful in their adult life and to develop coping strategies to tackle future challenges (Brewer & Petitpas, 2017). However, if an adolescent female athlete puts the majority of her time and energy into sport participation and does not engage in essential exploratory behaviour, the process of her identity formation is hindered. Athletes, who make firm commitments to sport as their primary source of identity during late adolescence, have been described as being in a state of identity foreclosure (Pearson & Petitpas, 1990). Adolescent female athletes are at an increased risk of identity foreclosure due to the influence of situational factors such as recognition for athletic achievements, extensive time demands of participation, and emphasis on conformity and compliance rather than independence and autonomy in the sporting environment (Petitpas & France, 2010). It has been reported that identity foreclosure is higher in athletes than their non-athlete peers due to the role of athletic identity (Linnemeyer & Brown, 2010).

Athletic identity refers to the sport-related component of self-identity and is defined as, 'the degree to which an individual identifies with the athlete role' (Brewer, Van Raalte, & Linder, 1993, p. 37). The maintenance of a strong athletic identity in exercising females has been documented to impact negatively on mainstream education, overcomplicate rehabilitation from injury, and lead to outcomes such as burnout, poor psychological adjustment to sport transitions, and substance abuse. Ronkainen, Kavoura, and Ryba (2016) reviewed the literature on athletic identity and concluded that, 'athletic identity can be a positive source of meaning and self-esteem but is also highly problematic for wellbeing when sport is not going well, or the career is abruptly terminated' (p. 57). Associations between athletic identity and substance abuse, such as excessive alcohol consumption (Grossbard et al., 2009) and the willingness to take performance-enhancing drugs (Hale & Waalkes, 1994) have been documented in several studies. Furthermore, adolescent female athletes who identify strongly with the athletic role are also more likely to incur an injury (McKay, Campbell, Meeuwisse, & Emery, 2013), experience poor psychological adjustment to that injury (Manuel et al., 2002), and to continue to play while injured (Weinberg, Vernau, & Horn, 2013). This pattern of behaviour may cause long-term complications, which could negatively affect the exercising female's ability to participate in sport in the future. It is important, therefore, to be able to recognise those adolescent exercising females whose identity foreclosure may be putting them at risk psychologically and physically.

Early sport specialisation

Adolescent exercising females, who are identified socially as an athlete, may have a higher level of athletic identity, driven by early sport specialisation. Acrobatic and artistic sports such as gymnastics, diving, and figure skating are considered 'early specialisation' sports, as the athletes often reach the peak of their career at a young age. Other sports such as athletics, cycling, rowing, and most team-orientated sports are considered 'late specialisation', as peak performance is achieved in late adolescence or early adulthood. The essential feature of early specialisation sport programmes is a high volume of deliberate practice; it is based on the proposition that it takes a notional average of 10,000 hr to achieve domain-specific expertise (Eriksson, Krampe, & Tech-Römer, 1993). It is important to note, however, that the 10,000-hr rule is under debate, with other scholars believing it takes fewer hours to achieve elite sport performance (e.g., Soberlak & Côté, 2003). In a review of the literature on this topic, Smucny, Parikh, and Pandya (2015), reported that: (a) early single sport specialisation has *not* been shown to improve future athletic performance, and may be detrimental to the adolescent female athlete both physically and emotionally; (b) the adolescent female growth spurt (around age 12) is a particularly vulnerable period of time for the adolescent athlete with repetitive microtrauma placing the body at risk structurally and, therefore, at an increased risk of injury; and (c) athletes who specialise at a young age may also be at an increased risk of burnout and long-term health effects that continue into adulthood. In light of the research findings, it is recommended that adolescent female athletes participate in and sample a variety of sports in order to excel in their sporting career in early adulthood. This early diversification leads to a longer sport career, promotes positive psychosocial development, intrinsic regulation, and intrinsic motivation through involvement in enjoyable activities. Ultimately, early diversification leads to the development of the physical, cognitive, social, emotional, and motor skills needed for the investment in the adolescent females' selection of principal sport(s) of interest.

Peer groups

Peer groups serve as a key facilitator for the development of the adolescent exercising female's identity. They can shape how females value and commit to sport and exercise versus other activities, as well as influence day-to-day experiences and outcomes in the sporting environment. It has been suggested that adolescent females assign a greater importance than males to socialising, and this may impact on their decision to participate in sport and exercise. In comparison to their relationships with adults, adolescents have a much greater balance of power in their relationships with one another and ascribe more importance to their peers as a source of influence and validation during this period of their lives (Smith & d'Arripe-Longueville, 2014). Furthermore, contextual sports factors such as team positions/roles (e.g., central playing positions and captaincy) and different ability levels can influence positions of power among peers. Practitioners and coaches working with adolescent female athletes need to be aware of such contextual factors, as they can influence peer relationships and the overall youth sport experience (Smith, 2007). For example, coaches could help members of the group identify their individual roles and responsibilities in order to acknowledge the unique contributions of each person. In addition, a rotating captaincy system could be introduced to allow each member of the team to develop her leadership skills and ensure a more equal balance of power.

Injury

Female adolescent athletes who strongly identify with the athletic role are at an increased risk of incurring an injury (McKay, Campbell, Meeuwisse, & Emery, 2013), training while in pain (Weinberg et al., 2013), and experiencing psychological distress after sustaining an injury (Manuel et al., 2002). While adolescent athletes high in athletic identity are more likely to adhere to a rehabilitation programme (Brewer et al., 1993), they are also more likely to push themselves too hard too soon (Podlog et al., 2013). However, the adolescent female athlete, who has experienced an injury, often decreases their athletic identity, especially when rehabilitation has not been progressing well (Brewer, Cornelius, Stephan, & Van Raalte, 2010). This is likely to be a possible coping mechanism to protect them from the threat of not being able to participate at the level they aspired to in their sport.

Several factors make the experience of injury particularly challenging for adolescent female athletes such as immature coping strategies, lack of a functional support system, and high/exclusive athletic identity (Brewer, 2001). Subsequently, they may experience negative responses to injury such as depression, anxiety, decreased self-esteem, tension, and concerns regarding re-injury and return to play (Brewer, 2001). Given the high injury rates associated with participation in adolescent sport and the negative consequences of becoming injured, it is imperative that strategies for prevention and support during rehabilitation are developed.

While there have been different conceptual approaches to psychologically-based injury prevention programmes, they all target stress management techniques (e.g., goal setting, relaxation) and self-reflection. For example, mindfulness is a concept that has recently been introduced in injury prevention programmes. It has been described as, 'openhearted, moment-to-moment, non-judgmental awareness' (Kabet-Zinn, 2005, p. 54). Mindfulness practice has been shown in a number of studies to positively influence athletes' stress responses (e.g., Cozolino, 2010) and their appraisal of stressful situations (e.g., Weinstein, Brown, & Ryan, 2009). Mindfulness training has also been shown to improve adolescent female athletes' decision-making capacity, which may reduce impulsive behaviours and decrease injury risk (i.e., the athlete acts without first thinking of the consequences).

Recommendations to support injured female adolescent athletes during their rehabilitation process focus on developing strategies to deal with negative emotions and building strong support networks. Negative emotional reactions are common in adolescent injured athletes; for example, feelings of depression, anger, and frustration may distract the athlete from adherence to their rehabilitation programme. Interventions that help reduce negative emotional reactions, such as educating the injured athlete about rehabilitation expectations (Johnson, Carlsson, Hinic, & Lindwall, 2003) and formulating realistic goal setting plans (Santi & Pietrantoni, 2013), can help adolescent athletes feel more confident and positive about the rehabilitation process. Causes of musculoskeletal injury for the exercising female are covered in Chapter 11.

Overtraining

Female adolescent athletes are particularly vulnerable to overtraining, as common social practices in sport place value on training and competing, despite underlying health problems such as injury or illness. Overtraining is often accompanied by the excessive use of painkillers, disregard of medical advice, and hiding pain from coaches and teammates (Thiel, Mayer, & Digel, 2010). Playing injured can have short-term implications for the adolescent exercising female such as exacerbated medical conditions, and long-term consequences such as chronic overuse injuries, irreversible physical damage, and recurring traumatic injuries (Kujala, Orava, Parkkari, Kaprio, & Sarna, 2003).

It is not uncommon for high-performance female adolescent athletes to push themselves too far in training and experience extreme fatigue on a regular basis. This imbalance between training load and recovery has been described as overtraining syndrome (OT), whereby the athlete experiences persistent fatigue and underperformance that is often associated with frequent infections and depression, which occurs following hard training and competition. OT is often diagnosed when the symptoms do not resolve themselves despite 2 weeks' rest and there is no other identifiable medical cause (Budgett, 1998). In female adolescent athletes, the symptoms of OT may contribute to delayed menarche (e.g., Frisch et al., 1981) or the onset of the Female Athlete Triad (see Chapter 6 for a review) and are often exacerbated by the occurrence of athletic amenorrhoea.

Stress, emotions, and coping

Competitive sport presents a myriad of stressors for female adolescent athletes which include: high training demands; injury and fear of injury;

interpersonal conflict with coaches, teammates, officials, and opponents; parental and coach pressure to perform; personal performance expectations; performance errors; poor equipment and training facilities; an overemphasis on winning; sport organisation politics, coupled with conflict between sport and education (Crocker, Tamminen, & Gaudreau, 2015); and social commitments (Nicholls & Polman, 2007). Adolescence is also a period characterised by physical and cognitive maturation, changing social roles and obligations, increased curiosity about romantic relationships, growing peer relationships and increasing independence from parental control (Seiffge-Krenke, 2011). These events trigger a range of positive and negative cognitions, emotions, and behaviours. Therefore, it is imperative that adolescent athletes have effective stress and emotional control strategies if they are to manage the challenges presented. The research literature reports a clear relationship between coping, emotions, and well-being in adolescent athletes; therefore, coping skills' training is paramount (see Chapter 13 for a review of coping strategies).

Eating disorders

Female adolescents experience greater concerns with weight than women (Taylor et al., 1998) and have been identified as an at-risk group for eating disorders (Lewinsohn, Striegel-Moore, & Seely, 2000). Unhealthy eating behaviours are influenced by abnormal attitudes associated with maintaining or changing one's body weight (Holm-Denoma, Scaringi, Gordon, Van Orden, & Joiner, 2009). Behaviours exhibited often include self-inflicted vomiting, pathological food restriction, the use of laxatives/diuretics for weight loss, and the use of anabolic steroids to gain lean muscle mass (Fortes & Ferreira, 2011). In sport and exercise, it has been reported that, for aesthetic female athletes, a thin attractive body and an optimisation of body weight are crucial to successful performance (Mountjoy, 2008). Problems have, therefore, been identified in sports such as gymnastics, figure skating, synchronised swimming, diving, and activities such as dance (Bryne & McLean, 2002). Adolescent female athletes are confronted with body image pressures at various levels, 'ranging from the performance related pressures reinforced by coaches, parents and peers to those inherent in the judging criteria that give physically attractive athletes the winning edge' (Davis, 1997, p. 162).

There is a general consensus that eating disorders are a multifaceted issue (Banas, Januszkiewicz-Grabias, & Radziwillowicz, 2001), and several psychological variables such as self-esteem and body-esteem have been suggested to contribute in the case of adolescent female athletes (Mendelson, McLaren, Gauvin, & Steiger, 2002). Self-esteem is concerned with how a person values, approves, or appreciates herself. Body-esteem is a narrower concept of self-worth and refers to how a person feels about her body image. It is suggested that how adolescent female athletes feel about their body rather than their actual weight plays a more critical role in predicting eating disorder symptoms (Ferrand, Champely, & Filaire, 2009).

Prevention is the key to addressing the problem of eating disorders in adolescent female athletes and education is the first step. It would also be beneficial to understand how adolescent athletes interpret and respond to direct pressures, such as comments concerning weight loss and indirect pressure such as attitudes towards thinness and acceptance of unhealthy eating behaviours, in order to help them develop coping strategies. For this reason, more research in this area is recommended. For an in-depth review of issues with body image, see Chapter 8, and for a review of nutritional needs for the exercising female (including eating disorders), see Chapter 5.

Dropout

Despite the well-established links between exercise and physical and psychological health, alarming levels of decline in physical activity have been observed in recent years. In particular, the attrition rates for female adolescents are much higher than for males and they tend to withdraw from athletic participation at an earlier age (Kirshnit, Ham, & Richards, 1989). By age 14, only 1 in 10 girls are doing enough physical activity to benefit their health, compared with roughly twice the number of boys of the same age (National Health Service, 2009). However, in a large-scale survey conducted by the Women's Sport and Fitness Foundation (2011), it was reported that 74 per cent of adolescent females wanted to do more physical activity. Barriers to their sport participation were identified as lack of choice, overly competitive environments, confidence, body image, boys, and sport being undervalued in the context of an adolescent female's life.

Peer relationships have been suggested to play a vital role in female adolescents' continuation in sport and physical activity. Slater and Tiggemann (2010) identified peer-related issues to account for the gender disparity in sport participation attrition rates, such as it not being 'cool' or feminine to play sport, socialising as being more important, and concerns over body image and sporting attire. They recommended the following strategies for improving female adolescent girls' exercise participation rates: make the same number of sporting opportunities for girls as boys; offer more single sex sporting practices; offer informal and inclusive activities where the emphasis is on fun and fitness as opposed to skills and competition; help girls feel more comfortable and less on display in sporting attire; and encourage social sporting opportunities that are not regarded as competitive or serious. Perhaps the most difficult facet, but one of the most important in adolescent females' decision-making, is to change the perception that it is unfeminine or uncool for girls to play sport. This idea could be delivered via messages at school or at a global social policy level via the promotion of positive athletic female role models, such as seen in the recent Sport England 'This Girl Can' campaign (Sport England, 2016).

The prominent task of adolescence is the development of self-identity, and sport and exercise plays a mediating role in this process. In this chapter, an overview of some of the key issues faced by adolescent exercising females has been provided, such as: early sport specialisation; the influence of peer groups; psychological adjustment to injury; overtraining; stress, emotions, and coping; common mental health disorders; and dropout. Recommendations for practice have been provided to help athletes, coaches, parents, and athlete-support personnel to negotiate this often-challenging developmental period.

Real-world example

Hannah is a 13-year-old sports scholar at a fee-paying boarding school in the UK. She is part of the national junior performance squad in netball, and her goal is to be a professional netball player. She has very high expectations of herself and a strong work ethic. Since starting at her new school, she has found it difficult to make friends and to 'fit in'. She has little time to socialise due to her athletic and academic obligations, and is frustrated with her peer group's lack of sporting commitment and their preoccupation with body image, boys, drinking, and smoking.

Despite being a successful athlete, she feels her coach gives all his attention to the other sports scholars to 'keep them on the rails' and that she receives very little feedback and support. She desperately wants an athletic role model to aspire to, but cannot identify one at school. Hannah's mother referred her to a sport psychologist to help her address some of her problems, in the hope that it would enhance her athletic performance and her enjoyment at school.

Hannah's case study describes a typical example of the identity-formation challenges often experienced by adolescent female athletes, and she presents with a plethora of stressors such as high training demands, interpersonal conflicts with her coach and teammates, high personal performance expectations, and conflict between sport, academic, and social commitments. Adolescent female athletes, who develop a high athletic identity, are at risk of identity foreclosure; therefore, the first area of concern I explored during my work with Hannah focused on an exploration of her sense of self. We began by engaging in discussions on the role sport plays in her life, and, while acknowledging her outstanding athletic achievements and her continued commitment to her athletic goals, I helped her identify other aspects of her life that were important. These aspects included developing friendships, exploring romantic relationships, and playing the piano.

Hannah discussed the issue of identifying an athletic role model, and we considered how instead she might utilise support from a range of different people. We reflected on the accompanying strengths and weaknesses associated; for example, her teammates, while sharing her commitment to the athletic role, could not help her engage in typical adolescent, exploratory behaviour due to situational factors such as recognition for athletic achievement, time demands, of participation, and the emphasis on conformity and compliance. On the other hand, peers from her boarding house, while not being able to empathise with her athletic commitments, could help her explore her sense of independence and autonomy outside of the sporting environment.

Through this process of disclosure, feedback, and awareness building, it is hoped that Hannah will be protected against identity foreclosure due to her exploration of multiple selves. In future sessions we could begin developing effective stress and emotional control strategies to help her manage the challenges that being a female adolescent athlete might present.

Summary

Adolescence is a challenging period of growth and development in the exercising female's life and one in which sport and exercise can play an influential role. In this chapter, some of the most important psychological topics and considerations as they relate to adolescent exercising females have been considered. These topics have included: identity; early sport specialisation; peer groups; injury; overtraining; stress, emotions, and coping; eating disorders; and dropout. The coverage of the critical psychological considerations will help support adolescent exercising females to enjoy their sport and exercise experiences and to reach their individual potential.

References

Banas, A. Januszkiewicz-Grabias, A., & Radziwillowicz, P. (2001). Multifactorial aspects of eating disorders. *Archives of Psychiatry and Psychotherapy, 3*, 43–52.

Brewer, B. W. (2001). Psychology of sport injury rehabilitation. In R. N. Singer, H. A. Hausenblas, & C. M. Janelle (Eds.), *Handbook of sport psychology* (2nd ed., pp. 787–809). New York: Norton.

Brewer, B. W., Cornelius, A. E., Stephan, Y., & Van Raalte, J. L. (2010). Self-protective changes in athletic identity following ACL reconstruction. *Psychology of Sport and Exercise, 11*, 1–5. https://doi.org/10.1016/j.psychsport.2009.09.005.

Brewer, B. W., & Petitpas, A. J. (2017). Athletic identity foreclosure. *Current Opinion in Psychology, 16*, 118–122. https://doi.org/10.1016/j.copsyc.2017.05.004.

Brewer, B. W., Van Raalte, J. L., & Linder, D. E. (1993). Athletic identity: Hercules' muscles or Achilles heel? *International Journal of Sport Psychology, 24*, 237–254.

Budgett, R. (1990). Overtraining syndrome. *British Journal of Sports Medicine, 24*, 231–236.

Byrne, S. & McLean, N. (2002). Elite athletes: Effects of the pressure to be thin. *Journal of Science and Medicine in Sport, 5*, 80–94.

Cozolino, L. (2010). *The neuroscience of psychotherapy: Healing the social brain* (2nd ed.). New York: Norton.

Crocker, P. R. E., Tamminen, K. A., & Gaudreau, P. (2015). Coping in sport. In S. Hanton & S. D. Mellalieu (Eds.), *Contemporary advances in sport psychology: A review* (pp. 28–67). Abingdon, UK: Routledge.

Davis, C. (1997). Body image, exercise, and dieting behaviors. In K. Fox (Ed.), *The physical self from motivation to well-being* (pp. 143–174). Champaign, IL: Human Kinetics.

Ericsson, K. A., Krampe, R., & Tesch-Romer, C. (1993). The role of deliberate practice in the acquisition of expert performance. *Psychological Review, 100,* 363–406.

Erikson, E. H. (1959). Identity and the life cycle: Selected papers. *Psychological Issues, 1,* 1–171.

Ferrand, C., Champely, S., & Filaire, E. (2009). The role of body-esteem in predicting disordered eating symptoms: A comparison of French aesthetic athletes and non-athletic females. *Psychology of Sport and Exercise, 10,* 373–380. https://doi.org/10.1016/j.psychsport.2008.11.003.

Fortes, L. S., & Ferreira, M. E. C. (2011). Comparison of body dissatisfaction and inappropriate eating behavior in adolescent athletes of different sports. *Brazilian Journal of Physical Education in Sport, 25,* 707–716. https://doi.org/10.1111/sms.12098.

Frisch R., Gotz-Welbergen, A. V., McArthur, J. W., Albright, T., Witschi, J., Bullen, B., … Hermann, H. (1981). Delayed menarche and amenorrhea of college athletes in relation to age of onset of training. *Journal of the American Medical Association, 246,* 1559–1563.

Grossbard, J. R., Geisner, I. M., Mastroleo, N. R., Kilmer, J. R., Turrisi, R., & Larimer, M. E. (2009). Athletic identity, descriptive norms and drinking among athletes transitioning to college. *Addictive Behaviours, 34,* 352–359. https://doi.org/10.1016/j.addbeh.2008.11.011.

Holm-Denoma, J. M., Scaringi. V., Gordon, K. H., Van Orden, K. A., & Joiner, T. E. (2009). Eating disorder symptoms among undergraduate varsity athletes, club athletes, independent exercisers and non exercises. *International Journal of Eating Disorders, 12,* 47–53. https://doi.org/10.1002/eat.20560.

Johnson, U., Carlsson, B., Hinic, H., & Lindwall, M. (2003). Psychological reactions to injury among competitive athletes, youth athletes and exercisers compared to a non-injured reference group. In G. Patriksson (Ed.), *Aktuell Beteendvetenskaplig Idrottsforskning.* SVEBIsårsbok, 2003 (pp. 37–48). Lund, Sweden: SVEBI.

Kabet-Zinn, J. (2005). *Coming to our senses: Healing ourselves and the world through mindfulness.* New York: Hyperion.

Kirshnit, C. E., Ham, M., & Richards, M. H. (1989). The sporting life: Athletic activities during early adolescence. *Journal of Youth and Adolescence, 18,* 601–615. https://doi.org/10.1007/BF02139076.

Kujala, U.M., Orava, S., Parkkari, J., Kaprio, J., & Sarna. S. (2003). Sports career-related musculoskeletal injuries: Long-term health effects on former athletes. *Sports Medicine, 33,* 869–875.

Lewinsohn, P. M., Striegel-Moore, R. H., & Seely, J. H. (2000). Epidemiology and natural course of eating disorders in young women from adolescence to young adulthood. *Journal of the American Academy of Child and Adolescent Psychiatry, 39,* 1284–1292. https://doi.org/10.1097/00004583-200010000-00016.

Linnemeyer, R. M., & Brown, C. (2010). Career maturity and foreclosure in student-athletes, fine arts students, and general college students. *Journal of Career Development, 37,* 616–634. https://doi.org/10.1177/0894845309357049.

Manuel, J. C., Shilt, J. S., Curl, W. W., Smith, J. A., DuRant, R. H., Lester, L., & Sinal, S. H. (2002). Coping with sports injuries: An examination of the adolescent athlete. *Journal of Adolescent Health, 31,* 391–393. https://doi.org/10.1016/S1054-139X(02)00400-7.

McKay, C., Campbell, T., Meeuwisse, W., & Emery, C. (2013). The role of psychosocial risk factors for injury in elite youth ice-hockey. *Clinical Journal of Sport Medicine, 23*, 216–221. https://doi.org/10.1097/JSM.0b013e31826a86c9.

Mountjoy, M. (2008). Weight control strategies of Olympic athletes striving for leanness: What can be done to make sport a safer environment? *Clinical Journal of Sport Medicine, 18*, 2–4. https://doi.org/10.1097/JSM.0b013e3181635664.

National Health Service. (2009). *Health survey for England – 2008: Physical activity and fitness*. Retrieved from https://digital.nhs.uk/data-and-information/publications/statistical/health-survey-for-england/health-survey-for-england-2008-physical-activity-and-fitness.

Nicholls, A. R., & Polman, R. C. (2007). Stressors, coping and coping effectiveness among players from the England under 18 rugby union team. *Journal of Sport Behaviour, 30*, 119–218.

Pearson, R , & Petitpas, A. J. (1990). Transitions of athletes: Developmental and preventative perspectives. *Journal of Counselling Development, 69*, 7–10.

Petitpas, A J., & France, T. (2010). Identity foreclosure in sport. In S. J. Hanrahan & M. B. Andersen (Eds.), *Routledge handbook of applied sport psychology: A comprehensive guide for students and practitioners* (pp. 471–480). Abingdon, UK: Routledge.

Podlog, L. Gao, Z., Kenow, L., Kleinert, J., Granquist, M., Newton, M., & Hannon, J. (2013). Injury rehabilitation overadherence: Preliminary scale validation and relationships with athletic identity and self-presentation concerns. *Journal of Athletic Training, 48*, 372–381. https://doi.org/10.4085/1062-6050-48.2.20.

Ronkainen N. J., Kavoura, A., & Ryba, T. V. (2016). A meta study of athletic identity research in sport psychology: Current status and future directions. *International Review of Sport Psychology, 9*, 45–64. https://doi.org/10.1080/1750984X.2015.1095414.

Santi, G., & Pietrantoni, L. (2013). Psychology of sport injury rehabilitation: A review of models and interventions. *Journal of Human Sport and Exercise, 8*, 1029–1044. https://doi.org/10.4100/jhse.2013.84.13.

Sawyer, S., Azzopardi, P., Wickremarathne, D., & Patton, G. (2018). The age of adolescence. *The Lancet Child & Adolescent Health, 2*(3), 223–228. https://doi.org/10.1016/S2352-4642(18)30022-1.

Seiffge-Krenke, I. (2011). Coping with relationship stressors: A decade review. *Journal of Research on Adolescence, 21*, 196–210. https://doi.org/10.1111/j.1532-7795.2010.00723.x.

Slater, A., & Tiggemann, M. (2010). 'Uncool to do sport': A focus group study of adolescent girls' reasons for withdrawing from physical activity. *Psychology of Sport and Exercise, 11*, 619–626. https://doi.org/10.1016/j.psychsport.2010.07.006.

Smith, A. L. (2007). Youth peer relationships in sport. In S. Jowett & D. Lavallee (Eds.), *Social psychology in sport* (pp. 41–54). Champaign, IL: Human Kinetics.

Smith, A. L., & d'Arripe-Longueville, F. (2014). Peer relationships and the youth sport experience. In A. G. Papaioannou & D. Hackford (Eds.), *Routledge companion to sport and exercise psychology: Global perspectives and fundamental concepts* (pp. 199–212). New York: Routledge.

Smucny, M., Parikh, S. N., & Pandya N. K. (2015). Consequences of single sport specialization in the pediatric and adolescent athlete. *The Orthopaedic Clinics of North America, 46*(2), 249–258. https://doi.org/10.1016/j.ocl.2014.11.004.

Soberlak, P., & Côté, J. (2003). The developmental activities of elite ice hockey players. *Journal of Applied Sport Psychology, 15*, 41–49. https://doi.org/10.1080/10413200305401.

Sport England. (2016). *This girl can.* Retrieved from www.sportengland.org/our-work/women/this-girl-can/.

Taylor, C. B., Sharpe, T., Shisslak, C., Bryson, S., Estes, L. S., Gray, N., ... Killen, J. D. (1998). Factors associated with weight concerns in adolescent girls. *International Journal of Eating Disorders, 24*, 31–42. https://doi.org/10.1002/(SICI)1098-108X(199807)24:131::AID-EAT33.0.CO;2-1.

Thiel, A., Mayer, J., & Digel, H. (2010). *Gesundheit im Spitzensport. Ein sozialwissenschaftliche Analyse (Health in elite sports. An analysis from a social sciences perspective).* Schorndorf, Germany: Hofmann.

Weinberg, R. S., Vernau, D. & Horn, T. S. (2013). Playing through pain and injury: Psychosocial considerations. *Journal of Clinical Sport Psychology, 7*, 41–59. https://doi.org/10.1123/jcsp. 7.1.41.

Weinstein, N., Brown, K. W., & Ryan, R. M. (2009). A multi-method examination of the effects of mindfulness on stress attribution, coping, and emotional well-being. *Journal of Research in Personality, 43*, 374–385. https://doi.org/10.1016/j.jrp. 2008.12.008.

Women's Sport & Fitness Foundation. (2011). *Changing the game for girls.* Retrieved from www.womeninsport.org/wp-content/uploads/2015/04/Changing-the-Game-for-Girls-Policy-Report.pdf.

3 The menstrual cycle and the exercising female

Implications for health and performance

Nancy I. Williams and Kaitlyn M. Ruffing

Introduction

The menstrual cycle and its association with physical activity in women has been a topic of interest for centuries. In the latter part of the 19th century, women who were menstruating were advised to, 'treat themselves as invalids once a month, curtailing both physical and mental activity ... lest they succumb to accidents, disease, and loss of fertility' (Vertinsky, 1987, p. 7). The notion that physical activity and/or exercise should be avoided in order to maintain fertility was widely believed. Interestingly, the suppressive effects of an abruptly increased training on the menstrual cycle were documented in the seminal trial by Bullen and colleagues (1985), where up to 10 miles of running per day in untrained women resulted in a high proportion of menstrual disturbances including the loss of ovulation, luteal phase defects, and irregular menstrual cycle lengths. This study raised the question as to whether physical exercise was indeed too 'stressful' for women's bodies.

Decades of research now suggest that there is no suppressive effect of exercise per se on the menstrual cycle in women apart from its impact on the amount of energy available for vital bodily processes (Loucks & Thuma, 2003; Williams, Helmreich, Parfitt, Caston-Balderrama, & Cameron, 2001; Williams et al., 2015). Although the health-related benefits of physical activity are well understood, there are numerous clinical sequelae associated with sustained exercise-related menstrual disruption i.e., amenorrhoea or the absences of menses for at least 90 days (De Souza & Williams, 2004). Amenorrhoea is a component of the Female Athlete Triad i.e., interrelated conditions of low energy availability with or without disordered eating, menstrual disturbances, and bone loss (Torstveit & Sundgot-Borgen, 2005); for a review of the Female Athlete Triad, see Chapter 6, energy availability, Chapter 5, and for bone health, see Chapter 7. The clinical and physiological conditions associated with the Triad are well described and include clinical eating disorders and disordered eating, osteopaenia, transient infertility, dyslipidaemia, impaired endothelial function (Friday, Drinkwater, Bruemmer, Chesnut, & Chait, 1993; Hoch et al., 2007; O'Donnell & De Souza, 2004), and performance-related issues such as stress fractures (Barrow & Saha, 1988;

Bennell, Matheson, Meeuwisse, & Brukner, 1999; Brukner & Bennell, 1997), fatigue, and decrements in competitive performance (Vanheest, Rodgers, Mahoney, & De Souza, 2014).

While it is important to understand how an active lifestyle can disrupt the menstrual cycle, and thus impact health, it is also important to understand how the menstrual cycle may affect the physiological systems responsible for athletic performance and human functioning. Whether or not athletic performance, injury risk, and/or physiological systems change across the menstrual cycle is a topic of great interest to athletes and coaches, as is the question of whether hormonal contraceptives affect athletic performance.

Aims of the chapter

The aims of the chapter are as follows:

1   To examine the impact of exercise on the menstrual cycle and the associated impact on health.
2   To examine the role of the menstrual cycle and reproductive hormones in exercise performance.
3   To consider these unique perspectives in order to increase one's understanding of the complexities of the underlying research and of where knowledge gaps exist.

Effects of exercise on the menstrual cycle

In the general population, clinical disorders of menstruation per se are marked by irregularities in menstrual bleeding accompanied by a variety of endocrine abnormalities (Gray, 2013). These disorders range from dysmenorrhoea to hypothalamic amenorrhoea and can impact a significant proportion of adolescent and premenopausal women (Berga, 1997). In relation to exercise, however, a more specific set of disruptions have been well characterised (De Souza & Williams, 2004; Gibbs, Williams, & De Souza, 2013). It should not be assumed that menstrual abnormalities in an exercising female are associated with exercise until other physiological and/or psychological causes can be ruled out (Nattiv et al., 2007; Practice Committee of the American Society for Reproductive Medicine, 2004). A spectrum of exercise-related disturbances that progress in severity (De Souza & Williams, 2004) are characterised by irregular patterns of menstrual bleeding and significant changes in the ovarian secretion of oestradiol and progesterone that are caused by centrally mediated disruptions in pituitary gland synthesis and secretion of follicle-stimulating hormone and luteinising hormone (Gordon, 2010).

The most severe menstrual disturbance is the complete suppression of reproductive axis activity i.e., exercise-related functional hypothalamic amenorrhoea. Amenorrhoea occurs when there is an absence of menses for at least 3 months. Oestradiol and progesterone concentrations reflect ovarian quiescence and are low and unchanging. More subclinical menstrual disturbances that are also 'functional' and 'hypothalamic' include oligomenorrhoea, anovulation, and luteal phase deficiency. Oligomenorrhoea refers to irregular cycle lengths ranging from 36 to 90 days. Anovulatory cycles are associated with menstrual bleeding that occurs due to uterine stimulation by folliculogenesis-related oestradiol production, which occurs, but does not result in the development of a dominant follicle and ovulation (Mihm, Gangooly, & Muttukrishna, 2011). These cycles are associated with variable oestradiol concentrations and very low progesterone in accordance with the absence of a corpus luteum. Luteal phase defects in exercising females occur when the length of the luteal phase is short (<10 days) and/or there is an inadequate production of progesterone from the corpus luteum (Beitins, McArthur, Turnbull, Skrinar, & Bullen, 1991). Luteal phase disturbances may be precursors to more severe disturbances (Bullen et al., 1985), and are associated with suboptimal fertility (Devoto et al., 2009). Prevalence rates of exercise-related menstrual disturbances depend on the particular sport or activity but have been estimated as luteal phase defects (29 per cent), anovulation (20 per cent), oligomenorrhoea (7 per cent), and amenorrhoea (37 per cent) (De Souza et al., 2010).

Moreover, both low energy availability and the hypo-oestrogenic environment associated with amenorrhoea play a causal role in bone loss (De Souza et al., 2008; De Souza & Williams, 2005; Ihle & Loucks, 2004). Although recent reports have focused on the general physiological effects of chronic low energy availability (Mountjoy et al., 2014), the most clinically relevant sequelae are its effects on the menstrual cycle and reproductive hormones, and on the skeleton. Equally concerning is the fact that the pathway to low energy availability can include severe clinical eating disorders. Other documented physiological consequences include dyslipidaemia, impaired endothelial function (Friday et al., 1993; Hoch et al., 2007; O'Donnell & De Souza, 2004), fatigue, and decrements in competitive performance (Vanheest et al., 2014), but the prevalence of these effects and their clinical relevance has not been established. Much progress has been made in our understanding of the underlying behaviours and physiology of these conditions (Gibbs et al., 2013; Nichols, Rauh, Lawson, Ji, & Barkai, 2006; Sundgot-Borgen & Torstveit, 2004), as well as the creation and use of practical recommendations for prevention, screening, treatment, and return to play (De Souza et al., 2014; De Souza et al., 2014; Nattiv et al., 2007; Tenforde et al., 2017).

The importance of energy availability as an underlying cause of exercise-related menstrual disturbances is well established (Lieberman, De Souza, Wagstaff, & Williams, 2017; Loucks, Kiens, & Wright, 2011), but challenges remain with respect to quantifying energy availability in a field setting. Moreover, the impact of low energy availability and disrupted menstrual function on athletic performance has been inadequately explored (Vanheest et al., 2014). More recently, researchers are focusing on male athletes

(Tenforde, Barrack, Nattiv, & Fredericson, 2016), on athletes with dis-abilities, and athletes with varied racial backgrounds (Mountjoy et al., 2014; Muia, Wright, Onywera, & Kuria, 2016). Other work considers the role of psychogenic stress (Marcus, Loucks, & Berga, 2001) and gynaecological age (Loucks, 2006) as contributors to an individual's susceptibility to exercise-related menstrual disturbances.

Effects of the menstrual cycle on exercise performance

Researchers have suggested that physiological responses and athletic per-formance vary across the various phases of the menstrual cycle. Studies exam-ining maximal oxygen consumption ($\dot{V}O_2$max) have shown no change across the cycle despite one early study suggesting a drop in $\dot{V}O_2$max in the luteal phase (Brutsaert et al., 2002; Gordon et al., 2017; Lebrun, McKenzie, Prior, & Taunton, 1995; Smith, Brown, Murphy, & Harms, 2015; Vaiksaar et al., 2011). Another measurement to consider, physical working capacity or PWC, has been shown to decrease in the luteal phase, but limitations in the methods could affect the validity of these results (Doskin, Kozeeva, Lisit-skaya, & Shokina, 1979). Few studies have investigated cardiovascular per-formance variables such as stroke volume, heart rate, or cardiac output across the menstrual cycle phases. A recent study reported significant differences in stroke volume at different percentages of $\dot{V}O_2$max, however, the results were scattered and did not point to an overall difference between phases (Gordon et al., 2017). Another study found myocardial performance index, a variable that shows systolic and diastolic function, to increase in the luteal phase (Zengin et al., 2007). Apart from $\dot{V}O_2$max, the findings regarding the effects of the menstrual cycle on cardiovascular function per se are not consistent enough to make broad claims about endurance performance. However, insofar as $\dot{V}O_2$max is a determinant of endurance performance, the lack of a consistent finding regarding menstrual phase effects on this variable suggest that endurance performance does not vary across the cycle.

The effects of menstrual cycle phase on anaerobic performance should be considered as well because of the oestrogen's multiple effects on muscle during anaerobic performance. Oestrogen has been shown to increase glucose uptake in skeletal muscle during sprinting, but progesterone inhibits this action (Lebrun et al., 1995; Oosthuyse & Bosch, 2010; Phillips, Sanderson, Birch, Bruce, & Woledge, 1996; Tsampoukos, Peckham, James, & Nevill, 2010). In addition, there is a protective function of oestrogen in exercise-induced muscle damage, and, therefore, a quickened return to baseline strength with the recovery of exercise-induced muscle damage, which is likely due to the oestrogen's ability to increase satellite cell activation and proliferation (Minahan, Joyce, Bulmer, Cronin, & Sabapathy, 2015). Another protective function of oestrogen is impairment of the inflammatory cascade by suppressing neutrophil and macrophage synthesis (Chaffin et al., 2011). Despite the latter findings, there is little agreement regarding the effects of menstrual cycle phase on overall anaerobic performance and strength, with no recent reviews synthesising this area of research. Possible reasons for the inconsistent findings are that studies used different methods to test anaerobic, sprint, or strength performance and many found no difference across the menstrual cycle phases (Constantini, Dubnov, & Lebrun, 2005). To test strength, studies often used handgrip strength and found that strength did not significantly differ across the cycle (Elliott, Cable, Reilly, & Diver, 2003; Fridén, Hirschberg, & Saartok, 2003). Several found that power output did not change throughout the cycle using jumping power or a non-motorised treadmill (Julian, Hecksteden, Fullagar, & Meyer, 2017; Tsampoukos et al., 2010). Others investigated that sprint endurance did not differ between the phases using a cycling or running sprint test (Julian et al., 2017; Wiecek, Szymura Maciejczyk, Cempla, & Szygula, 2016). However, some investigations contradicted this and found that handgrip strength was highest and fatigue was lowest in the follicular phase when oestrogen concentration was high and progesterone concentration was low (Pallavi, De Souza, & Shivaprakash, 2017; Phillips et al., 1996; Sarwar, Niclos, & Rutherford, 1996).

A review of the many original studies leaves considerably more questions than answers regarding the effects of the menstrual cycle on direct measures of athletic performance. Regarding sports performance, a 2014 study demonstrated that eumenorrhoeic women dropped more time in a 400-m swim over a 12-week period than ovarian-suppressed women (Vanheest et al., 2014). This is an intriguing finding that needs to be replicated. In general, recommendations for performance-focused studies include accurate quantification of menstrual status and reproductive hormones and controlling for extraneous factors such as training status of participants, environmental influences, and/or including an appropriate sample size. Importantly, studies need to replicate the appropriate competitive and environmental conditions to test performance and, as such, this research is best done in an applied setting. Current research provides insufficient support for alterations in training or competition strategies based on hormonal or menstrual status.

There are many limitations that need to be considered regarding the latter studies. A major issue in over half of the reports is the use of self-reporting for determination of menstrual cycle phase. Other factors were seldom controlled, such as training status, body composition effects, environmental conditions, and the validity of the performance measures.

Real-world examples

Two case studies of exercising women with amenorrhoea of short (3 months') and long (11 months') duration were reported by Mallinson and colleagues (2013). These cases illustrate the individual differences that can exist in the ability of women to recover menses when low energy availability is reversed. Both women were enrolled in a randomised controlled trial to test whether increasing food intake could restore menstrual cyclicity and improve bone density over a one-year time span. Participant one was 19 years of age, with a body mass index (BMI) of 20.4kg/m^2. She was a recreationally active college student who participated in running, weightlifting, downhill skiing, and other sports. She exercised about 9 h per week. She had been amenorrhoeic for 11 months. She had increased her calorific intake by an average of 338 kcal/day and increased her body weight by about 2.5 kg when she resumed menses after 74 days of the intervention. Near the conclusion of the year-long intervention to increase calorific intake, she had increased her body weight by 3.3 kg and her per cent body fat to 21 per cent, and her circulating triiodothyronine had increased by 39 per cent. Her menstrual periods were irregular in length, and she had a total of six periods over the course of the year. While her menstrual status and energy status definitely improved, it is likely that continued increases in body weight and body fat would have been associated with the development of more regular, ovulatory menstrual cycles.

Participant two was 24 years of age, her BMI was 19.7kg/m^2, and her body fat percentage was 23 per cent. She exercised about 7 h per week and had not had a menstrual period for three months. She had a history of extended periods of amenorrhoea. She displayed scores in the range for eating disorder patients on subscales of the Eating Disorder Inventory-2 including high scores for perfectionism, social anxiety, and reservations about trusting others (Garner, Olmstead, & Polivy, 1983). By increasing her caloric intake by about 27 per cent over her initial levels to about 1838 kcal/day, she gained 2.8 kg over 12 months, and her BMI and fat mass increased. Metabolic hormones such as leptin and triiodothyronine increased by 280 per cent and 32 per cent, respectively, and ghrelin decreased by 12 per cent, indicating a reversal of low energy availability. Menses resumed after only 23 days of increased calorific intake, but then stopped again for 122 days. Regular menstrual periods developed after 145 days into the intervention. She resumed regular cycles for the remaining part of the year although these cycles were characterised by frequent anovulation and luteal phase defects.

Both of these case studies illustrate that menses can be restored when dietary intake is increased independently of modifications in exercise energy expenditure. This finding is important to know, because many women may not want to alter their training to restore menstrual health. Although body weight and body fat were increased in both women, these increases ranged from 2–3 kg of body weight, which is not substantial. It is important to note that bone mineral density did not improve in either participant, but there were some indications that bone metabolism were improving. It is possible that a time period of increased energy availability lasting longer than 12 months may be necessary for favourable changes in bone to occur.

Summary

Research has advanced our understanding of the importance of healthy menstrual cycles in the context of overall health and the optimal physiological function of numerous bodily systems. Exercise improves health and physical performance but as a behaviour, excessive exercise can contribute to a state of low energy availability, if dietary intake is not adjusted to offset the calorific costs of training. Practical recommendations to avoid low energy availability are available, but more research will help to define specific dietary strategies that take into account the unique aspects of the sport or type and timing of training. Individual characteristics such as race, age, genetics, and suscepti-bility to life stressors should be more thoroughly explored relative to the risk of exercise-related menstrual dysfunction. The effects of the menstrual cycle on physical performance have been explored and remain unclear. While some emerging research demonstrates that amenorrhoea may be associated with performance declines, more research that employs rigorous control and quantification of menstrual status and reproductive hormones is necessary to make definitive conclusions.

References

Barrow, G. W., & Saha, S. (1988). Menstrual irregularity and stress-fractures in col-legiate female distance runners. *American Journal of Sports Medicine, 16*(3), 209–216. https://doi.org/10.1177/036354658801600302.

Beitins, I. Z., McArthur, J. W., Turnbull, B. A., Skrinar, G. S., & Bullen, B. A. (1991). Exercise induces two types of human luteal dysfunction: confirmation by urinary free progesterone. *Journal of Clinical Endocrinology and Metabolism, 72*(6), 1350–1358. https://doi.org/10.1210/jcem-72-6-1350.

Bennell, K., Matheson, G., Meeuwisse, W., & Brukner, P. (1999). Risk factors for stress fractures. *Sports Medicine, 28*(2), 91–122.

Berga, S. L. (1997). Behaviorally induced reproductive compromise in women and men. *Seminars in Reproductive Endocrinology, 15*(1), 47–53. https://doi.org/10.1055/s-2008-1067967.

Brukner, P., & Bennell, K. (1997). Stress fractures in female athletes. Diagnosis, management and rehabilitation. *Sports Medicine, 24*(6), 419–429. https://doi.org/10.2165/00007256-199724060-00006.

Brutsaert, T. D., Spielvogel, H., Caceres, E., Araoz, M., Chatterton, R. T., & Vitz-thum, V. J. (2002). Effect of menstrual cycle phase on exercise performance of high-altitude native women at 3600 m. *Journal of Experimental Biology, 205*(Pt 2), 233–239.

Bullen, B. A., Skrinar, G. S., Beitins, I. Z., von Mering, G., Turnbull, B. A., & McArthur, J. W. (1985). Induction of menstrual disorders by strenuous exercise in untrained women. *New England Journal of Medicine, 312*(21), 1349–1353. https://doi.org/10.1056/nejm198505233122103.

Chaffin, M. E., Berg, K. E., Meendering, J. R., Llewellyn, T. L., French, J. A., & Davis, J. E. (2011). Interleukin-6 and delayed onset muscle soreness do not vary during the menstrual cycle. *Research Quarterly for Exercise and Sport, 82*(4), 693–701. https://doi.org/10.1080/02701367.2011.10599806.

Constantini, N. W., Dubnov, G., & Lebrun, C. M. (2005). The menstrual cycle and sport performance. *Clinics in Sports Medicine, 24*(2), e51–82, xiii–xiv. https://doi.org/10.1016/j.csm.2005.01.003.

De Souza, M. J., Nattiv, A., Joy, E., Misra, M., Williams, N. I., Mallinson, R. J., … American Bone Health, A. (2014b). 2014 Female Athlete Triad Coalition consensus statement on treatment and return to play of the female athlete triad: 1st International Conference held in San Francisco, CA, May 2012, and 2nd International Conference held in Indianapolis, Indiana, May 2013. *Clinical Journal of Sport Medicine, 24*(2), 96–119. https://doi.org/10.1097/JSM.0000000000000085.

De Souza, M. J., Toombs, R. J., Scheid, J. L., O'Donnell, E., West, S. L., & Williams, N. I. (2010). High prevalence of subtle and severe menstrual disturbances in exercising women: Confirmation using daily hormone measures. *Human Reproduction, 25*(2), 491–503. https://doi.org/10.1093/humrep/dep411.

De Souza, M. J., West, S. L., Jamal, S. A., Hawker, G. A., Gundberg, C. M., & Williams, N. I. (2008). The presence of both an energy deficiency and estrogen deficiency exacerbate alterations of bone metabolism in exercising women. *Bone, 43*(1), 140–148. https://doi.org/10.1016/j.bone.2008.03.013.

De Souza, M. J., & Williams, N. I. (2004). Physiological aspects and clinical sequelae of energy deficiency and hypoestrogenism in exercising women. *Human Reproduction Update, 10*(5), 433–448. https://doi.org/10.1093/humupd/dmh033.

De Souza, M. J., & Williams, N. I. (2005). Beyond hypoestrogenism in amenorrheic athletes: Energy deficiency as a contributing factor for bone loss. *Current Sports Medicine Reports, 4*(1), 38–44.

De Souza, M. J., Williams, N. I., Nattiv, A., Joy, E., Misra, M., Loucks, A. B., … McComb, J. (2014). Misunderstanding the female athlete triad: Refuting the IOC consensus statement on Relative Energy Deficiency in Sport (RED-S). *British Journal of Sports Medicine, 48*(20), 1461–1465. https://doi.org/doi:10.1136/bjsports-2014-093958.

Devoto, L., Fuentes, A., Kohen, P., Cespedes, P., Palomino, A., Pommer, R., … Strauss, J. F., 3rd. (2009). The human corpus luteum: Life cycle and function in natural cycles. *Fertility and Sterility, 92*(3), 1067–1079. https://doi.org/10.1016/j.fertnstert.2008.07.1745.

Doskin, V. A., Kozeeva, T. V., Lisitskaya, T. S., & Shokina, E. V. (1979). Changes in working capacity of female athletes in different phases of the menstrual cycle. *Human Physiology, 5*(2), 144–149.

Elliott, K. J., Cable, N. T., Reilly, T., & Diver, M. J. (2003). Effect of menstrual cycle phase on the concentration of bioavailable 17-beta oestradiol and testosterone and muscle strength. *Clinical Science (London), 105*(6), 663–669. https://doi.org/10.1042/CS20020360.

Friday, K. E., Drinkwater, B. L., Bruemmer, B., Chesnut, C., 3rd, & Chait, A. (1993). Elevated plasma low-density lipoprotein and high-density lipoprotein cholesterol levels in amenorrheic athletes: Effects of endogenous hormone status and nutrient intake. *Journal of Clinical Endocrinology and Metabolism, 77*(6), 1605–1609. https://doi.org/10.1210/jcem.77.6.8263148.

Fridén, C., Hirschberg, A. L., & Saartok, T. (2003). Muscle strength and endurance do not significantly vary across 3 phases of the menstrual cycle in moderately active premenopausal women. *Clinical Journal of Sport Medicine, 13*(4), 238–241.

Garner, D. M., Olmstead, M. P., & Polivy, J. (1983). Development and validation of a multidimensional eating disorder inventory for anorexia nervosa and bulimia. *International Journal of Eating Disorders, 2*(2), 15–34. doi:10.1002/1098-108x(198321)2:2<15::aid-eat2260020203>3.0.co;2-6.

Gibbs, J. C., Williams, N. I., & De Souza, M. J. (2013). Prevalence of individual and combined components of the female athlete triad. *Medicine & Science in Sports & Exercise, 45*(5), 985–996. https://doi.org/10.1249/MSS.0b013e31827e1bdc.

Gordon, C. M. (2010). Clinical practice. Functional hypothalamic amenorrhea. *New England Journal of Medicine, 363*(4), 365–371. https://doi.org/10.1056/NEJMcp0912024.

Gordon, D., Scruton, A., Barnes, R., Baker, J., Prado, L., & Merzbach, V. (2017). The effects of menstrual cycle phase on the incidence of plateau at $\dot{V}O_2$max and associated cardiorespiratory dynamics. *Clinical Physiology and Functional Imaging.* https://doi.org/10.1111/cpf.12469.

Gray, S. H. (2013). Menstrual disorders. *Pediatrics in Review, 34*(1), 6–17. https://doi.org/10.1542/pir.34-1-6.

Hoch, A. Z., Jurva, J. W., Staton, M. A., Thielke, R., Hoffmann, R. G., Pajewski, N., & Gutterman, D. D. (2007). Athletic amenorrhea and endothelial dysfunction. *Wisconsin Medical Journal, 106*(6), 301–306.

Ihle, R., & Loucks, A. B. (2004). Dose-response relationships between energy availability and bone turnover in young exercising women. *Journal of Bone & Mineral Research, 19*(8), 1231–1240. https://doi.org/10.1359/jbmr.040410.

Julian, R., Hecksteden, A., Fullagar, H. H., & Meyer, T. (2017). The effects of menstrual cycle phase on physical performance in female soccer players. *PLoS One, 12*(3), e0173951. https://doi.org/10.1371/journal.pone.0173951.

Lebrun, C. M., McKenzie, D. C., Prior, J. C., & Taunton, J. E. (1995). Effects of menstrual cycle phase on athletic performance. *Medicine & Science in Sports & Exercise, 27*(3), 437–444.

Lieberman, J. L., De Souza, M. J., Wagstaff, D. A., & Williams, N. I. (2017). Menstrual disruption with exercise is not linked to an energy availability threshold. *Medicine & Science in Sports & Exercise, 50*(3), 551–561. https://doi.org/10.1249/MSS.0000000000001451.

Loucks, A. B. (2006). The response of luteinizing hormone pulsatility to 5 days of low energy availability disappears by 14 years of gynecological age. *Journal of Clinical Endocrinology & Metabolism, 91*(8), 3158–3164. https://doi.org/10.1210/jc.2005-0570.

Loucks, A. B., Kiens, B., & Wright, H. H. (2011). Energy availability in athletes. *Journal of Sports Science, 29*(Suppl 1), S7–S15. https://doi.org/10.1080/02640414.2011.588958.

Loucks, A. B., & Thuma, J. R. (2003). Luteinizing hormone pulsatility is disrupted at a threshold of energy availability in regularly menstruating women. *Journal of Clinical Endocrinology & Metabolism, 88*(1), 297–311. https://doi.org/10.1210/jc.2002-020369.

Mallinson, R. J., Williams, N. I., Olmsted, M. P., Scheid, J. L., Riddle, E. S., & De Souza, M. J. (2013). A case report of recovery of menstrual function following a nutritional intervention in two exercising women with amenorrhea of varying duration. *Journal of the International Society of Sports Nutrition, 10*, 34. https://doi.org/10.1186/1550-2783-10-34.

Marcus, M. D., Loucks, T. L., & Berga, S. L. (2001). Psychological correlates of functional hypothalamic amenorrhea. *Fertility & Sterility, 76*(2), 310–316.

Mihm, M., Gangooly, S., & Muttukrishna, S. (2011). The normal menstrual cycle in women. *Animal Reproduction Science, 124*(3–4), 229–236. https://doi.org/10.1016/j.anireprosci.2010.08.030.

Minahan, C., Joyce, S., Bulmer, A. C., Cronin, N., & Sabapathy, S. (2015). The influence of estradiol on muscle damage and leg strength after intense eccentric exercise. *European Journal of Applied Physiology, 115*(7), 1493–1500. https://doi.org/10.1007/s00421-015-3133-9.

Mountjoy, M., Sundgot-Borgen, J., Burke, L., Carter, S., Constantini, N., Lebrun, C., … Ljungqvist, A. (2014). The IOC consensus statement: Beyond the Female Athlete Triad – Relative Energy Deficiency in Sport (RED-S). *British Journal of Sports Medicine, 48*(7), 491–497. https://doi.org/10.1136/bjsports-2014-093502.

Muia, E. N., Wright, H. H., Onywera, V. O., & Kuria, E. N. (2016). Adolescent elite Kenyan runners are at risk for energy deficiency, menstrual dysfunction and disordered eating. *Journal of Sports Science, 34*(7), 598–606. https://doi.org/10.1080/02640414.2015.1065340.

Nattiv, A., Loucks, A. B., Manore, M. M., Sanborn, C. F., Sundgot-Borgen, J., & Warren, M. P. (2007). American College of Sports Medicine position stand. The female athlete triad. *Medicine & Science in Sports & Exercise, 39*(10), 1867–1882. https://doi.org/10.1249/mss.0b013e318149f111.

Nichols, J. F., Rauh, M. J., Lawson, M. J., Ji, M., & Barkai, H. S. (2006). Prevalence of the female athlete triad syndrome among high school athletes. *Archives of Pediatric & Adolescent Medicine, 160*(2), 137–142. https://doi.org/10.1001/archpedi.160.2.137.

O'Donnell, E., & De Souza, M. J. (2004). The cardiovascular effects of chronic hypoestrogenism in amenorrhoeic athletes: A critical review. *Sports Medicine, 34*(9), 601–627. https://doi.org/10.2165/00007256-200434090-00004.

Oosthuyse, T., & Bosch, A. N. (2010). The effect of the menstrual cycle on exercise metabolism: implications for exercise performance in eumenorrhoeic women. *Sports Medicine, 40*(3), 207–227. https://doi.org/10.2165/11317090-000000000-00000.

Pallavi, L. C., D Souza, U. J., & Shivaprakash, G. (2017). Assessment of musculoskeletal strength and levels of fatigue during different phases of menstrual cycle in young adults. *Journal of Clinical & Diagnostic Research, 11*(2), CC11–CC13. https://doi.org/10.7860/JCDR/2017/24316.9408.

Phillips, S. K., Sanderson, A. G., Birch, K., Bruce, S. A., & Woledge, R. C. (1996). Changes in maximal voluntary force of human adductor pollicis muscle during the menstrual cycle. *Journal of Physiology, 496(Pt 2)*, 551–557.

Practice Committee of the American Society for Reproductive Medicine. (2004). Current evaluation of amenorrhea. *Fertility & Sterility, 82*(Suppl 1), S33–S39. https://doi.org/10.1016/j.fertnstert.2004.07.001.

Sarwar, R., Niclos, B. B., & Rutherford, O. M. (1996). Changes in muscle strength, relaxation rate and fatiguability during the human menstrual cycle. *Journal of Physiology, 493*(Pt 1), 267–272.

Smith, J. R., Brown, K. R., Murphy, J. D., & Harms, C. A. (2015). Does menstrual cycle phase affect lung diffusion capacity during exercise? *Respiratory Physiology & Neurobiology, 205*, 99–104. https://doi.org/10.1016/j.resp.2014.10.014.

Sundgot-Borgen, J., & Torstveit, M. K. (2004). Prevalence of eating disorders in elite athletes is higher than in the general population. *Clinical Journal of Sport Medicine, 14*(1), 25–32.

Tenforde, A. S., Barrack, M. T., Nattiv, A., & Fredericson, M. (2016). Parallels with the Female Athlete Triad in male athletes. *Sports Medicine, 46*(2), 171–182. https://doi.org/10.1007/s40279-015-0411-y.

Tenforde, A. S., Carlson, J. L., Chang, A., Sainani, K. L., Shultz, R., Kim, J. H., … Fredericson, M. (2017). Association of the Female Athlete Triad risk assessment stratification to the development of bone stress injuries in collegiate athletes. *American Journal of Sports Medicine, 45*(2), 302–310. https://doi.org/10.1177/0363546516676262.

Torstveit, M. K., & Sundgot-Borgen, J. (2005). The female athlete triad: Are elite athletes at increased risk? *Medicine & Science in Sports & Exercise, 37*(2), 184–193. https://doi.org/10.1249/01.MSS.0000152677.60545.3A.

Tsampoukos, A., Peckham, E. A., James, R., & Nevill, M. E. (2010). Effect of menstrual cycle phase on sprinting performance. *European Journal of Applied Physiology, 109*(4), 659–667. https://doi.org/10.1007/s00421-010-1384-z.

Vaiksaar, S., Jürimäe, J., Mäestu, J., Purge, P., Kalytka, S., Shakhlina, L., & Jürimäe, T. (2011). No effect of menstrual cycle phase and oral contraceptive use on endurance performance in rowers. *Journal of Strength & Conditioning Research, 25*(6), 1571–1578. https://doi.org/10.1519/JSC.0b013e3181df7fd2.

Vanheest, J. L., Rodgers, C. D., Mahoney, C. E., & De Souza, M. J. (2014). Ovarian suppression impairs sport performance in junior elite female swimmers. *Medicine & Science in Sports & Exercise, 46*(1), 156–166. https://doi.org/10.1249/MSS.0b013e3182a32b72.

Wiecek, M., Szymura, J., Maciejczyk, M., Cempla, J., & Szygula, Z. (2016). Effect of sex and menstrual cycle in women on starting speed, anaerobic endurance and muscle power. *Physiology International, 103*(1), 127–132. https://doi.org/10.1556/036.103.2016.1.13.

Williams, N. I., Helmreich, D. L., Parfitt, D. B., Caston-Balderrama, A., & Cameron, J. L. (2001). Evidence for a causal role of low energy availability in the induction of menstrual cycle disturbances during strenuous exercise training. *Journal of Clinical Endocrinology and Metabolism, 86*(11), 5184–5193. https://doi.org/10.1210/jcem.86.11.8024.

Williams, N. I., Leidy, H. J., Hill, B. R., Lieberman, J. L., Legro, R. S., & De Souza, M. J. (2015). Magnitude of daily energy deficit predicts frequency but not severity of menstrual disturbances associated with exercise and caloric restriction. *American Journal of Physiology-Endocrinology Metabolism, 308*(1), E29–E39. https://doi.org/10.1152/ajpendo.00386.2013.

Zengin, E., Tokac, M., Duzenli, M. A., Soylu, A., Aygul, N., & Ozdemir, K. (2007). Influence of menstrual cycle on cardiac performance. *Maturitas, 58*(1), 70–74. https://doi.org/10.1016/j.maturitas.2007.06.002.

4 Hormonal-based contraception and the exercising female

Kirsty J. Elliott-Sale and Kirsty Marie Hicks

Introduction

Not all exercising females have a textbook 28-day menstrual cycle. Hormonal contraceptives alter the naturally occurring ovarian cycle by changing the internal hormonal milieu and preventing pregnancy. While hormonal contraceptive users do not have to contend with the effects of menstrual cycle phase on performance, they still encounter challenges and benefits associated with hormonal contraceptive use. In this chapter, the different types of hormonal contraceptives are explained and their effects, both positive and negative, discussed on aspects of exercise performance in various types of exercising females, from recreationally active women to elite athletes. Practical guidance on hormonal use, based on the literature, is also given.

Aims of the chapter

The aims of the chapter are as follows:

1   To describe the different types of hormonal contraceptives.
2   To show the prevalence of hormonal contraceptive use in females.
3   To determine the role of hormonal contraceptives in an exercise setting.
4   To evaluate the effects of hormonal contraceptives on athletic performance.

Hormonal contraceptives

Hormonal contraceptives are designed to substantially reduce the risk of pregnancy (to less than one pregnancy per 100 couples per year), by preventing ovulation and follicular development and reducing sperm mobility and the endometrial lining. They provide exogenous oestrogens and progestins, which act on the hypothalamic-pituitary-ovarian axis by negative feedback on luteinising hormone, follicle-stimulating hormone, and gonadotropin-releasing hormone. As a result of this negative feedback loop, concentrations of endogenous oestrogen and progesterone are downregulated. Since the legal introduction of the first birth control pill in the 1960s, the term 'hormonal contraceptives' has come to define a wide range of brands (e.g., Microgynon®, Mirena®, and Depo-Provera®), preparations/types (e.g., combined, mono-/bi-/tri-phasic, progesterone-only), and delivery methods (e.g., oral pills, injections implants, and patches), although the bioequivalence between products is similar. The range of delivery methods, aside from oral ingestion, has expanded rapidly since the 2000s, and these alternative types of hormonal contraceptives account for 27 per cent of contraceptive use in the general population (Cea-Soriano, García Rodríguez, Machlitt, & Wallander, 2014) and, using the UK as an example, 22 per cent usage in elite athletes (Martin, Sale, Cooper, & Elliott-Sale, 2017). Despite the expansion and development of parenteral hormonal contraceptives, the oral contraceptive (OC) is the most common form of reversible contraceptive used, accounting for 73 per cent of contraceptive use in the general population (Cea-Soriano et al., 2014) and 78 per cent of contraceptive use in elite athletes (Martin et al., 2017). Data from Sweden (Brynhildsen et al., 1997) and Norway (Torstveit & Sundgot-Borgen, 2005) have shown 46 per cent and 42 per cent usage, respectively, of OCs in athletes. Limited data exist on the current prevalence of different types of hormonal contraceptives in athletes in other countries.

Oral contraceptives

Since their introduction, OCs have been reformulated four times to reflect different 'generations', based on the type of progestin used. In the majority of cases, the oestrogen is ethinyl oestradiol, although some older formulations contain mestranol, which has different pharmacokinetic properties. First-generation pills had high concentrations of oestrogen and progestin (e.g., norethynodrel, norethindrone, lynestrenol, and ethynodiol diacetate), while second-generation pills have lower concentrations of oestrogen and progestin (e.g., levonorgestrel, and norethisterone). Although first-generation pills are no longer available, second-generation pills are still commonly used and are considered to have the lowest risk of blood clots. Third-generation pills contain the progestins norgestimate, desogestrel, gestodene, and cyproterone acetate, and fourth-generation pills use the progestin drospirenone. The lower, more moderate, doses of oestrogen used since the introduction of second-generation pills have resulted in fewer side effects, such as fluid retention, weight gain, headaches, nausea, breast tenderness, and a decreased risk of blood clots.

OCs differ in terms of oestrogenic and progestogenic content (low-dose ≤0.02 mg and high dose ≥0.02 mg, and up to 0.05 mg and 0.1–3.0 mg, respectively) and the androgenicity and potency of progesterone (0.26–2.1 mg and 0.33–1.5 mg, respectively), and are available in either single (progesterone-only) or combined (oestrogen and progestin) regimes. Potency refers to the capacity of the progestin to exert its desired effects, and androgenicity refers to the capability of the progestin to exert masculine characteristics. Combined pills are available in mono-, bi-, and tri-phasic schedules, wherein the timing of different doses of synthetic hormones are released: Monophasic pills (e.g., Yasmin®) deliver the same amount of oestrogen and progestin every day; biphasic pills (e.g., Ortho-Novum®) deliver the same amount of oestrogen throughout the cycle; however, the oestrogen to progestin ratio is lower in the first half of the cycle (allowing the endometrium to thicken) and higher in the second half (allowing the endometrium to shed); triphasic pills (e.g., Logynon®) have constant or varying oestrogen concentrations and changeable progestin during the course of the cycle.

Oral contraceptives were initially designed to replicate the standardised 28-day menstrual cycle, with the pill-free (or placebo) and pill-taking days equalling 28 days; however, OCs mask normal hormonal changes during the menstrual cycle, and for monophasic pills, the bleed experienced during the pill-free days is not the same as that caused by the break-up of the endometrium during a eumenorrhoeic cycle (i.e., a normal menstrual cycle lasting between 21 and 35 days). While most OCs are packaged as 21-day (with 7 pill-free days) or 28-day (with 7 placebo pills) regimens, there are 24-day monophasic pills and extended-cycle OCs that last more than 28 days by skipping the inactive pills and continuing with the active pills.

Progesterone-only pills offer a suitable alternative to combined hormonal contraceptives when oestrogens are contraindicated. Bleeding has been shown to become irregular, lighter, more frequent, longer, or to cease completely with progesterone-only pill use. The desogestrel progesterone-only pill must be taken within 12 hr of the same time each day and the traditional progesterone-only pill must be taken within 3 hr of the same time each day; there is no break between pill packets (28 pills) for either of these progesterone-only pill types.

Parenteral hormonal contraceptives

The implant (e.g., Nexplanon®) is a long-term contraceptive that provides up to three years of continuous birth control. The implant is a small, thin, and flexible arm implant that delivers a low-dose, steady-state concentration of progestin, which thickens the mucus of the cervix and changes the lining of the womb, thus preventing pregnancy. Contraindications of the implant include more or less frequent menstruation and spotting. The contraceptive injection (e.g., Depo-Provera® and Sayana Press®) works in the same way as the implant and is effective for between eight and 13 weeks depending on the brand. Unlike the implant, which is easily removed and quickly reversible, the injection cannot be removed from the body. Menstruation may become irregular or cease, which may continue for up to 1 year following treatment. Progestogen-only, intra-uterine systems (e.g., Mirena®, Jaydess®, and Levosert®) release levonorgestrel directly into the uterine cavity and are also used to treat primary menorrhagia (heavy menstruation). Progestogen-only, intra-uterine systems may be preferable to copper, intra-uterine devices for exercising females, as they reduce dysmenorrhoea (pain associated with menstruation) and blood loss. The vaginal ring (e.g., NuvaRing®) is a small, soft, plastic ring that is placed inside the vagina, where it remains for 21 days and is removed for 7 days before a new ring is inserted. It contains both oestrogen and progestin and can ease premenstrual symptoms and cause bleeding to become lighter and less painful. Due to the invasive nature of the implant, injection, and vaginal ring, exercising females may prefer the contraceptive patch (e.g., Evra®), which delivers oestrogen and progestin through the skin and acts in the same way as the combined OC pill. Each patch lasts for one week, and three consecutive weeks of use are followed by a patch-free week, which may or may not result in a withdrawal bleed. The patch has been associated with more regular, lighter, and less painful periods, as well as alleviation from premenstrual symptoms, such as abdominal bloating, abdominal pain, sore breasts, headaches, and acne.

The role of contraceptives

Outside of contraceptive purposes, many exercising females use hormonal contraceptives to treat the symptoms of dysmenorrhoea, although the research evidence to support this use is conflicting. Wong, Farquhar, Roberts and Proctor (2009) concluded that, in women with dysmenorrhoea, OC use (both low and medium dose oestrogen) did not result in significant pain improvement. In contrast, Davis, Westhoff, O'Connell, and Gallagher (2005) showed that dysmenorrhoea-associated pain was relieved in adolescents using a low-dose OC compared with a placebo. Similarly, Milsom and Andersch (1984) showed that the severity and prevalence of dysmenorrhoea were significantly reduced in progestin-dominated OC users compared to non-OC or intra-uterine device users. Regardless of this contradictory evidence, hormonal contraceptives are still prescribed to reduce dysmenorrhoea.

The OC has also been used to treat amenorrhoea; however, the preparation (e.g., natural versus synthetic oestrogens; combination of oestrogen, progesterone, and testosterone) of exogenous hormones in OCs is often not comparable to hormone replacement therapy, which is commonly used to treat bone disorders in postmenopausal women. Moreover, the re-instigation of a 'bleed' with OC use is not the same as normal menstruation, thus the prescription of OCs may not be an effective treatment for amenorrhoea.

In a survey of 430 elite, UK-based, female athletes (Martin et al., 2017), 70 per cent of athletes reported a history of hormonal contraceptive use, with 50 per cent reporting current hormonal contraceptive use and 51 per cent reporting non-use, showing the prevalence of hormonal contraceptive use in an exercising female population. Of the current hormonal contraceptive users, 68.5 per cent used combined hormonal contraceptives and 30 per cent used progestin-only preparations (2 per cent used unspecified types). OCs were the most commonly used and accounted for 78 per cent of total hormonal contraceptive use. Hormonal contraceptive users self-reported 18 physical, negative side effects (e.g., weight gain and irregular periods), as well as negative changes to mood. Nineteen physical positive side effects (e.g., reduced period pain, cramps, and bloating) were also self-reported, alongside improved mood, reduced premenstrual tension, the ability to predict and change cycle date, and the elimination of the need to remember to take it. These data show the diversity of physical, emotional, and practical responses of athletes to hormonal contraceptive use, which need to be considered and monitored, alongside their subsequent effects on performance.

Although the athletes in the above study reported by Martin and colleagues (2017) recognised a number of physical, emotional, and practical benefits of hormonal contraceptives, the ability to manipulate menstruation was regarded as the main (57 per cent) positive side effect. In contrast, when deciding which hormonal contraceptive to use, ease of use (19 per cent), the timing of consumption (6 per cent), and the invasive nature of the delivery method (5 per cent) were considered most, with the ability to predict or change the cycle and to stop periods accounting for a combined total of 7 per cent. These findings suggest that athletes are choosing hormonal contraceptives for reasons other than the ability to manipulate bleeding, despite valuing this the most. In the future, athletes and practitioners must offset the reasons for choosing a particular hormonal contraceptive with the positive and negative side effects experienced, and with the effects of hormonal contraceptive use on performance and health. The study by Martin and colleagues (2017) only included UK-based athletes; the prevalence of hormonal contraceptive use may vary in other countries due to cultural/religious differences, the availability of particular contraceptives, economic issues, or education.

Manipulation of the menstrual cycle, through use of hormonal contraceptives, is not a recent idea and is not always limited to the exercising female; in 1976 it was noted that the popularity of the combined pill could be attributed to the predictable onset of menstrual bleeding and that, if the expected time of bleeding was socially inconvenient, then menstruation could be withheld entirely by continuing the pill (Baird, 1976). Since then, many women, in particular those who exercise, have continued to exploit OCs for additional non-contraceptive benefits. In a review of the literature, Bennell, White, and Crossley (1999) suggested that cycle manipulation was a secondary advantage to OC use in exercising females, after contraception. Similarly, Schaumberg and colleagues (2018) showed that 29 per cent of OC users manipulated menstruation at least 4 times a year and 74 per cent manipulated menstruation at least once per year. Interestingly, however, the prevalence of manipulation was not significantly different between recreationally active women, sub-elite, and elite athletes (72 per cent, 74 per cent, and 77 per cent, respectively) (Schaumberg et al., 2018). Sports competition, convenience, and special events or holidays were provided as reasons for menstrual tampering. These data further support the notion that hormonal contraceptives are being used by exercising females to alter and control bleeding which may have consequences on sports participation, performance, and health.

The effects of hormonal contraceptives on athletic performance

Although eliminating any potential negative effects of the menstrual cycle through hormonal contraceptive use is appealing to females, the consequences of hormonal contraceptives on performance remain unclear. Although there are many forms of hormonal contraceptives, OCs are the most prevalent form used by elite female athletes (Brynhildsen et al., 1997; Martin et al., 2017; Torstveit & Sundgot-Borgen, 2005) and the most widely studied hormonal contraceptive in previous literature, and, as such, is the focus of the remainder of this section.

The metabolic- and performance-based effects of OCs are poorly understood. Previous data and interpretation are not consistent on either the directional or the quantitative effects of OCs on athletic performance. These inconsistencies may be due, in part, to a lack of standardisation of the OC used (e.g., using high- and low-dose OCs in the same group). Failing to control for the type of OC used results in large inter- and intra-individual variation in endogenous hormone concentration, and an increase in the occurrence of type II errors (Elliott-Sale et al., 2013). In addition, in some studies endogenous hormone concentrations have not measured, and, as such, the degree of downregulation during pill-taking days and possible upregulation during pill-free days has been estimated. Authors need to be clear in their discussion of the concentration of exogenous synthetic hormones versus the resultant changes in endogenous reproductive hormone concentrations, as these cannot be described interchangeably. Due to the difference in preparations, and hence chemical constitution, the concomitant effects of all types and delivery methods of hormonal contraceptives on performance need to be considered. As athletic performance is a complex, multifaceted process, only the three main components of performance, namely strength, short-term, high-intensity ability and endurance capability, are covered in this section, as well as sport-specific performance tests.

Strength

In 1987, the International Olympic Committee banned the use of OCs containing norethindrone, a synthetic progestin with some anabolic, oestrogenic, and androgenic properties. At that time, some laboratories were unable to distinguish between the metabolites of norethindrone and nandrolone, the latter being a common anabolic-androgenic steroid (Duda, 1988). Although the ban was overturned within five months, the effects of OCs on strength are still inconclusive. Wirth and Lohman (1982) showed significantly greater handgrip endurance times and force output measurements made at 50 per cent maximum voluntary contraction, in eumenorrhoeic females compared to measures in OC users (eight non-specified OCs), despite observing no change in maximum voluntary contraction between the two groups. In 1996, Sarwar, Niclos, and Rutherford (1996) investigated the effects of OC use and non-use on maximal voluntary isometric force of the quadriceps and handgrip strength across two menstrual/pill cycles. Contrary to the non-OC users, for whom strength significantly increased prior to ovulation, strength did not fluctuate across the OC (monophasic combined; 0.02–0.035 mg ethinyl oestradiol and progestins in different doses) cycle. Similarly, Phillips, Sanderson, Birch, Bruce, and Woledge (1996) showed that maximum force production of the adductor pollicis muscle did not change throughout the OC cycle (non-specified OCs), compared to a significant 10 per cent increase in maximum voluntary force during the follicular phase of the menstrual cycle in eumenorrhoeic women. Elliott, Cable, and Reilly (2005) also showed that maximum force production of the first dorsal interosseous muscle did not fluctuate throughout the OC cycle (monophasic combined; 0.03–0.035 mg ethinyl oestradiol and 0.15–0.5 mg progestin), but nor did the strength of OC users differ when compared to the strength of eumenorrhoeic females measured during various phases of the menstrual cycle with significantly different oestrogen concentrations.

In order to examine the effect of different progestins on muscle strength, Peters and Burrows (2006) standardised the dose of ethinyl oestradiol (0.03 mg), but manipulated the potency and androgenicity of progestin (0.15 mg levonorgestrel, having a potency of 0.8 mg and an androgenicity of 1.25 mg, and 0.25 mg norgestimate, with a potency of 0.33 mg and androgenicity of 0.45 mg). They showed no significant differences in strength across the OC cycle, despite the androgenicity of levonorgestrel being higher than that of norgestimate. Most studies have not shown a change in strength between pill-taking and pill-free days (Ekenros, Hirschberg, Heijne, & Fridén, 2013; Elliott et al., 2005; Peters & Burrows, 2006; Sarwar et al., 1996). Rechichi and Dawson (2009), however, showed that reactive strength was affected by the withdrawal phase (pill-free days) in monophasic OC users using a variety of formulations. These researchers showed that reactive strength from a 30-cm drop was significantly lower in the late-withdrawal phase, compared with the early-withdrawal and pill-consumption phases, whereas reactive strength from a 45-cm drop was significantly lower in the early and late pill-withdrawal phase compared with the pill-consumption phase (Rechichi & Dawson, 2009). To date, no study has used one brand and type of OC, which is required to reduce the variability in exogenous hormone content and resultant endogenous hormone concentration (Elliott-Sale et al., 2013). Therefore, although the majority of evidence suggests that OCs do not affect strength, for an axiom conclusion to be drawn, further research is required to rigorously control for the different oestrogen and progestin dosages and preparations. Furthermore, several studies have used non-active participants (Elliott et al., 2005; Peters & Burrows, 2006; Sarwar et al., 1996). Future research should, therefore, be performed on exercising populations in order to assess the impact of OCs on performance.

With regards to strength training and OC use, Nichols, Hetzler, Villanueva, Stickley, and Kimura (2008) showed that OC users had similar gains in strength following a 12-week, preseason, strength training programme in collegiate softball and water polo players. They concluded that, within the limits of their study, combined OC use did not provide any additional androgenic stimulus beyond that provided by the training protocol. Ružić, Matković, and Leko (2003) showed that women taking an anti-androgenic OC (0.2 mg of cyproterone acetate) responded less well to a 16-week (3 days/week) training study than did combined OC (0.15 mg levonorgestrel) users, the latter showing a significant increase in fat-free mass and muscle strength. These findings indicate that the type of OC (anti-androgenic versus combined) can determine the effects of strength training in women.

Short-term, high-intensity exercise

Bushman, Masterson, and Nelsen (2006) showed that short-term, high-intensity performance, as represented by the Wingate test and Margaria-Kalamen staircase test, did not change across an OC cycle in moderately active women ($n = 17$). These findings are in agreement with those of Sunderland, Tunaley, Horner, Harmer, and Stokes (2011), who showed that all-out, 30-s sprint performance on a non-motorised treadmill was not affected by OC consumption or withdrawal in nine monophasic OC users. The OC users had similar peak and mean power outputs to their eumenorrhoeic counterparts. Lynch, De Vito, and Nimmo (2001) also showed that low-dosage, monophasic OCs did not influence intermittent high-intensity exercise performance in untrained females. In their study, nine women completed six intermittent, high-intensity, 20-s runs, and a final run to exhaustion, following 5–8 days and 19–21 days of pill consumption. Energy metabolism was also unchanged as determined by: peak blood lactate concentration; peak blood glycerol concentration; resting free-fatty acid concentration; peak blood glucose concentration; and peak capillary blood ammonia concentration. Similarly, Giacomoni, Bernard, Gavarry, Altare, and Falgairette (2000) showed no difference in the performance of three anaerobic tests – force-velocity, multi-jump, and squatting jump tests – in 10 monophasic OC users across three phases (days 1–4, 7–9 and 19–21) of an OC cycle. The collective evidence suggests that OCs do not affect short-term, high-intensity exercise performance.

Endurance performance

Endurance performance (cycling to voluntary exhaustion) was tested before and after four months of triphasic pill consumption in six moderately active women (Casazza, Suh, Miller, Navazio, & Brooks, 2002). There were no significant differences in endurance performance between the follicular and luteal phase of the menstrual cycle (i.e., prior to OC use). Similarly, there was no significant difference in peak oxygen consumption between days 22 and 28 (i.e., the withdrawal phase) and days 8–14 (i.e., pill-consumption phase) of the OC cycle. Oral contraceptive use did, however, result in a significant 11 per cent decrease in peak exercise capacity between the menstrual and OC cycle, suggesting that exogenous, ovarian hormones reduce endurance performance in moderately active women. Bryner, Toffle, Ullrich, and Yeater (1996) also tested endurance performance before and after 21 days of OC supplementation in ten women. They showed no effect of OC consumption (day 8 and day 21) on maximal oxygen consumption, attained during a modified Balke treadmill protocol, or run time to exhaustion. Unlike Casazza and colleagues (2002), Bryner and colleagues (1996) did not show any difference between the data obtained during the menstrual (follicular and luteal) and OC cycles. Rechichi, Dawson, and Goodman (2008) showed no significant difference in mean power output during a 1-hr cycle test when comparing the early- (days 2–3) and late- (days 6–7) withdrawal phases with the pill-consumption phase (days 13–17) in monophasic OC users. This evidence (Rechichi et al., 2008) and the work of Casazza and colleagues (2002) suggest that there are no differences in endurance performance between OC consumption and withdrawal, although, whether OC use versus non-use affects endurance performance remains unclear, due to the conflicting evidence of Casazza and colleagues (2002) and Bryner and colleagues (1996). Clearly, more studies are required before a conclusion can be reached.

Performance tests

While it appears that some individual components of performance might be influenced by OC use, their collective effect on performance is poorly understood. Few researchers have investigated the relationship between OC use and sport-specific performance tests in well-trained athletes. Rechichi and Dawson (2012) showed that 200-m swim time, mean stroke rate, peak heart rate and blood glucose were not affected by OC consumption or withdrawal in six competitive swimmers and water polo players. Interestingly, however, blood lactate was reduced, and pH increased during the withdrawal (pill-free) phase, which the authors attributed to a possible increase in fluid retention, plasma volume, and cellular alkalosis. Vaiksaar and colleagues (2011) showed no difference in sport-specific endurance performance (power output on an incremental test to voluntary exhaustion on a rowing ergometer) between two time points of the OC cycle, in recreationally trained rowers ($n = 9$). Similarly, Rechichi and Dawson (2009) showed no significant differences in countermovement jump performance and repeated sprint ability (total work and peak power), representing common team sport performance variables, in ten female team sport athletes at three phases of the OC cycle (early-withdrawal, late-withdrawal, and pill-consumption). In contrast, Lebrun, Petit, McKenzie, Taunton, and Prior (2003) showed a decrease in maximal oxygen consumption following the ingestion of one full cycle of a tricyclic OC in previously eumenorrhoeic, highly-trained female athletes participating in running, cycling, triathlon, rowing, and cross-country skiing. These authors also showed, however, that anaerobic capacity (anaerobic speed test), aerobic endurance (time to fatigue at 90 per cent maximal oxygen consumption), and isokinetic strength were unchanged as a result of OC use. Redman and Weatherby (2004) investigated whether anaerobic rowing power (10-s, all-out row) or capacity (1000-m rowing time trial) varied between two time points of a triphasic pill cycle in five elite and sub-elite rowers. Participants were tested on days 16–18 (i.e., pill-consumption phase) and days 26–28 (i.e., withdrawal phase), over three OC cycles. Although there were no significant differences in endogenous oestradiol and progesterone concentrations between the two phases, peak power output was significantly higher, and 1000-m rowing ergometer time was significantly shorter during the withdrawal phase, when exogenous hormones were absent. These findings suggest that anaerobic performance is hindered by the exogenous hormone supplementation experienced during pill consumption. The available evidence suggests that some, but not all, types of sport-specific tests are affected by OC use in trained athletes, but given the dearth of literature in this area, additional studies are warranted, and these studies should focus on testing larger numbers of athletes over more than one OC cycle, across a variety of sport-specific performance tests.

The effects of OCs on performance, and many of the components of performance, in exercising females are unclear. Indeed, there is surprisingly little high-quality research available on this topic, despite the high prevalence of OC use in athletic populations. It is difficult to make direct comparisons between previous studies due to variations in the type of OC pill used (combined or progesterone-only), phase of OC cycle investigated (consumption or withdrawal in monophasic and multiphasic pills), and the type of performance test used. Future research should compare homogenous groups of OC users with their eumenorrhoeic counterparts, investigate performance before and after OC consumption in the same individuals, and examine the potential changes in performance across different phases of an OC cycle. Upcoming work should also include other types of hormonal contraceptives, especially progesterone-only contraceptives, in line with their prevalence of use in sportswomen.

Practical recommendations based on research

It is difficult to make universal practical recommendations on the use of hormonal contraceptives for exercising females for two main reasons. First, there are numerous types and delivery methods of hormonal contraceptives, which result in large inter- and intra-individual variation in endogenous reproduc-tive hormone concentration, making homogenous comparisons almost impossible. Second, there is still insufficient, robust data on the effects of each type and delivery method of hormonal contraceptives on performance. These two issues preclude global recommendations on hormonal contracep-tives for an exercising population. Exercising females should take a more individual approach to hormonal contraceptive use, considering the positive and negative effects of their specific hormonal contraceptives on their per-formance and long-term health. They should freely discuss the effects of their hormonal contraceptives on their performance with their coach and should actively seek medical advice on the most appropriate type of hormo-nal contraceptive to use for their own health-related needs. It should be noted that the effects of hormonal contraceptives on health (e.g., bone health, and fertility) have not been discussed in this chapter, but that these effects are pertinent to the exercising female.

Real-world example

Martin and colleagues (2017) quoted one elite athlete as saying, 'Literally struggle to get out of bed so training is out of the question' during one phase of the menstrual cycle. Similar quotes were not reported by hormonal con-traceptive users, who reported less negative side effects than their eumenor-rhoeic counterparts did. In the short-term, hormonal contraceptive users appear to perceive less adverse health reactions than non-users; however, objective long-term health-related outcomes were not assessed.

Summary

The term 'hormonal contraceptives' defines a wide range of brands, prepara-tions/types (e.g., combined, progesterone-only, mono-/bi-/tri-phasic,), and delivery methods (e.g., oral pills, injections, implants, and patches). The primary role of hormonal contraceptives is to prevent pregnancy and to treat certain medical conditions, such as dysmenorrhoea, menorrhagia, and acne. Some athletes choose to use hormonal contraceptives so that they can manipulate their cycle and control the timing and frequency of bleeding. The effects of hormonal contraceptives on performance, and components of performance, remain unclear, which may be due to methodological differ-ences and non-homogenous populations, making direct comparisons between studies difficult. Exercising females should be encouraged to seek medical advice when deciding on whether or not to use hormonal contraceptives and should closely monitor the effects of the contraceptive on performance and on physical and emotional health and well-being.

References

Baird, D. (1976). Manipulation of the menstrual cycle. *Proceedings of the Royal Society of London. Series B, Biological Sciences, 195*(1118), 137–148.

Bennell, K., White, S., & Crossley, K. (1999). The oral contraceptive pill: A revolution for sportswomen? *British Journal of Sports Medicine, 33*(4), 231–238. https://doi.org/10.1136/bjsm.33.4.231.

Bryner, R. W., Toffle, R. C., Ullrich, I. H., & Yeater, R. (1996). Effect of low dose oral contraceptives on exercise performance. *British Journal of Sports Medicine, 30*(1), 36–40. https://doi.org/10.1136/bjsm.30.1.36.

Brynhildsen, J., Lennartsson, H., Klemetz, M., Dahlquist, P., Hedin, B., & Hammar, M. (1997). Oral contraceptive use among female elite athletes and age-matched controls and its relation to low back pain. *Acta Obstetricia et Gynecologica Scandinavica, 76*(9), 873–878.

Bushman, B., Masterson, G., & Nelsen, J. (2006). Anaerobic power performance and the menstrual cycle: Eumenorrheic and oral contraceptive users. *The Journal of Sports Medicine and Physical Fitness, 46*(1), 132–137.

Casazza, G. A., Suh, S.-H., Miller, B. F., Navazio, F. M., & Brooks, G. A. (2002). Effects of oral contraceptives on peak exercise capacity. *Journal of Applied Physiology (1985), 93*(5), 1698–1702. https://doi.org/10.1152/japplphysiol.00622.2002.

Cea-Soriano, L., García Rodríguez, L., Machlitt, A., & Wallander, M. A. (2014). Use of prescription contraceptive methods in the UK general population: A primary care study. *BJOG: An International Journal of Obstetrics & Gynaecology, 121*(1), 53–61. https://doi.org/10.1111/1471-0528.12465.

Davis, A. R., Westhoff, C., O'Connell, K., & Gallagher, N. (2005). Oral contraceptives for dysmenorrhea in adolescent girls: A randomized trial. *Obstetrics and Gynecology, 106*(1), 97–104.

Duda, M. (1988). IOC rescinds ban on birth control drug. *The Physician and Sportsmedicine, 16*(2), 175–179. https://doi.org/10.1080/00913847.1988.11709439.

Ekenros, L., Hirschberg, A. L., Heijne, A., & Fridén, C. (2013). Oral contraceptives do not affect muscle strength and hop performance in active women. *Clinical Journal of Sport Medicine, 23*(3), 202–207. https://doi.org/10.1097/JSM.0b013e3182625a51.

Elliott, K. J., Cable, N. T., & Reilly, T. (2005). Does oral contraceptive use affect maximum force production in women? *British Journal of Sports Medicine, 39*(1), 15–19. https://doi.org/10.1136/bjsm.2003.009886.

Elliott-Sale, K. J., Smith, S., Bacon, J., Clayton, D., McPhilimey, M., Goutianos, G., ... Sale, C. (2013). Examining the role of oral contraceptive users as an experimental and/or control group in athletic performance studies. *Contraception, 88*(3), 408–412. https://doi.org/10.1016/j.contraception.2012.11.023.

Giacomoni, M., Bernard, T., Gavarry, O., Altare, S., & Falgairette, G. (2000). Influence of the menstrual cycle phase and menstrual symptoms on maximal anaerobic performance. *Medicine and Science in Sports and Exercise, 32*(2), 486–492. https://doi.org/10.1097/00005768-200002000-00034.

Lebrun, C. M., Petit, M. A., McKenzie, D. C., Taunton, J. E., & Prior, J. C. (2003). Decreased maximal aerobic capacity with use of a triphasic oral contraceptive in highly active women: A randomised controlled trial. *British Journal of Sports Medicine, 37*(6), 315–320. https://doi.org/10.1136/bjsm.37.4.315.

Lynch, N. J., De Vito, G., & Nimmo, M. A. (2001). Low dosage monophasic oral contraceptive use and intermittent exercise performance and metabolism in humans. *European Journal of Applied Physiology, 84*(4), 296–301. https://doi.org/10.1007/s004210000380.

Martin, D., Sale, C., Cooper, S. B., & Elliott-Sale, K. J. (2017). Period prevalence and perceived side effects of hormonal contraceptive use and the menstrual cycle in elite athletes. *International Journal of Sports Physiology and Performance*, 1–22. https://doi.org/10.1123/ijspp. 2017–0330.

Milsom, I., & Andersch, B. (1984). Effect of various oral contraceptive combinations on dysmenorrhea. *Gynecologic and Obstetric Investigation, 17*(6), 284–292.

Nichols, A. W., Hetzler, R. K., Villanueva, R. J., Stickley, C. D., & Kimura, I. F. (2008). Effects of combination oral contraceptives on strength development in women athletes. *The Journal of Strength and Conditioning Research, 22*(5), 1625–1632. https://doi.org/10.1519/JSC.0b013e31817ae1f3.

Peters, C., & Burrows, M. (2006). Androgenicity of the progestin in oral contraceptives does not affect maximal leg strength. *Contraception, 74*(6), 487–491. https://doi.org/10.1016/j.contraception.2006.08.005.

Phillips, S. K., Sanderson, A. G., Birch, K., Bruce, S. A., & Woledge, R. C. (1996). Changes in maximal voluntary force of human adductor pollicis muscle during the menstrual cycle. *The Journal of Physiology, 496*(2), 551–557. https://doi.org/10.1113/jphysiol.1996.sp021706.

Rechichi, C., & Dawson, B. (2009). Effect of oral contraceptive cycle phase on performance in team sport players. *Journal of Science and Medicine in Sport, 12*(1), 190–195. https://doi.org/10.1016/j.jsams.2007.10.005.

Rechichi, C., & Dawson, B. (2012). Oral contraceptive cycle phase does not affect 200-m swim time trial performance. *The Journal of Strength and Conditioning Research, 26*(4), 961–967. https://doi.org/10.1519/JSC.0b013e31822dfb8b.

Rechichi, C., Dawson, B., & Goodman, C. (2008). Oral contraceptive phase has no effect on endurance test. *International Journal of Sports Medicine, 29*(4), 277–281.

Redman, L. M., & Weatherby, R. P. (2004). Measuring performance during the menstrual cycle: A model using oral contraceptives. *Medicine and Science in Sports and Exercise, 36*(1), 130–136. https://doi.org/10.1249/01.MSS.0000106181.52102.99.

Ružić, L., Matković, B. R., & Leko, G. (2003). Antiandrogens in hormonal contraception limit muscle strength gain in strength training: Comparison study. *Croatian Medical Journal, 44*(1), 65–68.

Sarwar, R., Niclos, B. B., & Rutherford, O. M. (1996). Changes in muscle strength, relaxation rate and fatiguability during the human menstrual cycle. *The Journal of Physiology, 493*(1), 267–272. https://doi.org/10.1113/jphysiol.1996.sp021381.

Schaumberg, M. A., Emmerton, L. M., Jenkins, D. G., Burton, N., W, Janse De Jonge, X. A. K., & Skinner, T. L. (2018). Use of oral contraceptives to manipulate menstruation in young, physically active women. *International Journal of Sports Physiology and Performance, 13*(1), 82–87. https://doi.org/10.1123/ijspp.2016-0689.

Sunderland, C., Tunaley, V., Horner, F., Harmer, D., & Stokes, K. A. (2011). Menstrual cycle and oral contraceptives' effects on growth hormone response to sprinting. *Applied Physiology, Nutrition, and Metabolism, 36*(4), 495–502. https://doi.org/10.1139/h11-039.

Torstveit, M. K., & Sundgot-Borgen, J. (2005). Participation in leanness sports but not training volume is associated with menstrual dysfunction: A national survey of 1276 elite athletes and controls. *British Journal of Sports Medicine, 39*(3), 141–147. https://doi.org/10.1136/bjsm.2003.011338.

Vaiksaar, S., Jürimäe, J., Mäestu, J., Purge, P., Kalytka, S., Shakhlina, L., & Jürimäe, T. (2011). No effect of menstrual cycle phase and oral contraceptive use on endurance performance in rowers. *The Journal of Strength and Conditioning Research, 25*(6), 1571–1578. https://doi.org/10.1519/JSC.0b013e3181df7fd2.

Wirth, J. C., & Lohman, T. G. (1982). The relationship of static muscle function to use of oral contraceptives. *Medicine and Science in Sports and Exercise, 14*(1), 16–20.

Wong, C. L., Farquhar, C., Roberts, H., & Proctor, M. (2009). Oral contraceptive pill as treatment for primary dysmenorrhoea. *Cochrane Database Systematic Reviews, 15(2):* CD002120.

5 Energy and the nutritional needs of the exercising female

Joan M. Eckerson

Introduction

Compared to males, females have unique metabolic and physiological differences that should be considered when developing nutritional strategies for optimal training, performance, and health. As with every athlete, specific energy and nutritional needs vary and depend upon several factors including the demands of the sport, environmental factors, and the current phase of training and competition. In this chapter, general guidelines to help meet the nutritional needs of the exercising female are provided, including: the importance of energy intake (EI) and energy availability; recommendations for carbohydrate, protein, and fat intake; the practice of dietary manipulation and nutrient timing for optimal performance and recovery; fluid needs; and requirements for micronutrients of primary health concern.

Aims of the chapter

The aims of the chapter are as follows:

1 To understand the importance of adequate EI as the foundation for determining nutritional requirements.
2 To identify the components that determine total daily energy expenditure including resting metabolic rate, the thermic effect of activity, and the thermic effect of food.
3 To calculate needs for adequate carbohydrate, protein, and fat intake based upon total energy needs for current state of training.
4 To understand the advantages and potential disadvantages of dietary strategies to enhance exercise performance including carbohydrate timing, protein timing, carbohydrate loading, and training with high and low carbohydrate availability.
5 To understand the importance of obtaining adequate intakes of several shortfall nutrients that are critical for optimal health and performance including calcium, iron, zinc, and magnesium.

6   To understand the effect of the menstrual cycle on nutritional requirements and substrate utilisation during exercise.

Energy requirements

Adequate EI is the foundation upon which the nutritional needs of the exercising female are built, since EI is crucial not only for peak performance, but
also for optimal physiological and metabolic function. Energy requirements
vary and depend upon several factors including the energy demands of the
sport, environmental issues (i.e., altitude, temperature), and the current
phase of training and competition. Failure to meet energy requirements not
only impairs performance and delays the recovery process, but may also
result in loss of fat-free mass (FFM) and bone density, and increases the risk
of menstrual dysfunction, injury, and illness (Thomas, Erdman, & Burke,
2016). It has traditionally been recognised that energy balance occurs when
EI is equal to total daily energy expenditure (TDEE). EI from food, beverages, and dietary supplements is commonly derived from 3–7-day food
records, multiple-pass 24-hr recall, food-frequency questionnaires, and
dietary history interviews. Under-reporting EI is very common and the error
increases as energy requirements increase (Heydenreich, Kayser, Schutz, &
Melzer, 2017). Therefore, because exercising females exhibit a high TDEE,
it is very likely that they under-report their EI.

Components that make up the TDEE include the basal metabolic rate
(BMR), the thermic effect of food (TEF), and the thermic effect of activity
(TEA). Because BMR measurements are difficult to obtain (no exercise for
12–18 hr and after an overnight sleep), it is usually more practical to measure
resting metabolic rate (RMR), which can be ~10 per cent higher. While the
RMR typically represents 60–80 per cent of TDEE for sedentary individuals,
it may only represent ~38–47 per cent of TDEE for elite athletes. The TEF
represents the energy expenditure associated with food consumption including
digestion, absorption, metabolism, and energy storage and accounts for ~10
per cent of TDEE for a mixed diet (Hedrick-Fink & Mikesky, 2018). The TEA
represents the energy demands associated with any physical activity and
includes energy expenditure from structured exercise (EEX), excess post-
exercise oxygen consumption (EPOC, commonly referred to as 'after burn' and
estimated to account for ~15 per cent of TDEE), and non-exercise activity
thermogenesis (NEAT, i.e., activities of daily living plus spontaneous physical
activity such as fidgeting) (Thomas et al., 2016). Therefore, it is important for
the exercising female to understand that TDEE is not simply equal to EEX,
since TDEE = RMR + TEF + NEAT + EEX + EPOC. The phase of the menstrual cycle may also influence TDEE, since it has been reported that RMR is
slightly increased during the luteal phase compared to the follicular phase
(Volek, Forsythe, & Kraemer, 2006). It may be advised, therefore, that exercising females consume more energy during the luteal phase of their menstrual
cycle to maintain energy requirements.

Laboratory methods to measure actual TDEE include direct and indirect calorimetry, and doubly labelled water that measures isotope excretion rates, such as deuterium. However, these methods are expensive, time consuming, and thus, are not practical in most professional or field settings. Several prediction equations are available to estimate RMR including the Harris–Benedict (Harris & Benedict, 1918) and Cunningham equations (Cunningham, 1980), as well as more recent calculations based upon the original Harris–Benedict equation (Mifflin et al., 1990; Roza & Shizgal, 1984). The RMR value is then multiplied by an appropriate activity factor to estimate TDEE (see Table 5.1).

Another model regarding the energy needs of the exercising female that is receiving increased research attention is the concept of 'energy availability' (EA). The term EA emerged from studies of the Female Athlete Triad and represents the energy available for normal body processes *after* taking into account energy expended from exercise (i.e., EEX) standardised to kg FFM: EA = EI − EEX/FFM. The concept of EA was first introduced by Loucks and colleagues following a series of investigations using females who found that an EA of 45 kcal/kg FFM per day was associated with energy balance and optimal health; whereas, a chronic reduction in EA of ≤30 kcal/kg FFM per day was associated with increased risks for impairments in the endocrine system affecting energy and bone metabolism, and the cardiovascular and reproductive systems (Loucks, Verdun, & Heath, 1998; Loucks & Thuma, 2003; Loucks, 2007; Loucks, Kiens, & Wright, 2011).

Example calculation for EA:

70 kg BM (body mass), 20% body fat, FFM = 56.0 kg, EI = 2600 kcal/day, EEX = 600 kcal/day
EA = (2600–600 kcal/day) ÷ 56 kg FFM = 35.7 kcal/kg FFM per day

Volek and colleagues (2006) have also reported that exercising females are at risk for menstrual dysfunction when EI is less than 1800–2000 kcal/day or <30 kcal/kg BM per day. In their review of the nutritional needs of female strength athletes, it was recommended that women who resistance train consume 39–44 kcal/kg BM per day and cautioned that women who consumed <30 kcal/kg BM per day, or the equivalent of <1800–2000 kcal per day, were at risk for energy imbalance disorders and menstrual cycle disturbances. Therefore, chronic low EA may compromise both short- and long-term exercise performance and impair endocrine function in exercising females. Factors that contribute to a low EA include disordered eating, intentional efforts to lose BM for a sport, or the unintentional failure to meet energy requirements during high volume training or competition (Loucks et al., 2011).

It is important to recognise that low EA is not the same as negative energy balance or weight loss, since a low EA may result in a decrease in RMR and a re-adjustment in energy balance to maintain BM at a lower EI

Table 5.1 Calculations to estimate energy requirements for females

---

Original Harris–Benedict equation (Harris & Benedict, 1918)
Resting metabolic rate (RMR) = 655.096 + (9.563 × weight in kg) + (1.850 × height in cm) − (4.676 × age)

Revised Harris–Benedict equation (Roza & Shizgal, 1984)
RMR = 447.593 + (9.247 × weight in kg) + (3.098 × height in cm) − (4.330 × age in years)

Revised Harris–Benedict equation (Mifflin et al., 1990)
RMR = (10 × weight in kg) + (6.25 × height in cm) − (5 × age in years) − 161

Cunningham equation (Cunningham, 1980)
Males and females
RMR = 500 + (22 × fat-free mass [FFM] in kg)

Dietary Reference Intake (DRI) method: estimated energy requirements for adult females (Institute of Medicine, 2005)
Females
354 − 6.91 (age) + physical activity level (PAL) × (9.36 × (weight in kg) + 726 × (height in metres)
PAL
   Sedentary: 1.0
   Low active: 1.12
   Active: 1.27
   Very active: 1.45

RMR calculations and activity factors for females (WHO, 1985)

Age	Equation (body weight [BW] in kg)	Activity factor
Females, 10 to 18 years old	RMR = (12.2 × BW) + 749	1.6–2.4
Females, 19 to 30 years old	RMR = (14.7 × BW) + 496	1.6–2.4
Females, 31 to 60 years old	RMR = (8.7 × BW) + 829	1.6–2.4

Example calculations for determining Total Daily Energy Expenditure(TDEE)[1]
Jill: 30 years old; height = 167.6 cm; weight stable = 54.5 kg; per cent body fat = 17.0%; FFM = 45.2 kg; a marathoner, running 96–130 km/week.
Her estimated range of energy requirements, considering an activity level of 1.6 (lower volume training) and 2.4 (higher volume training) using the various equations presented above is:

Harris–Benedict equation:
RMR = 655.096 + (1.850 × 167.6 cm) + (9.563 × 54.5 kg) − (4.676 × 30 years) = 1346 kcal
1346 kcal × 1.6 = 2153 kcal; 1346 kcal × 2.4 = 3230 kcal
TDEE range = 2153–3230 kcal

Cunningham equation:
RMR = 500 + 22 (45.2 kg) = 1494 kcal
1494 kcal × 1.6 = 2390 kcal; 1494 kcal × 2.4 = 3585 kcal
TDEE range = 2390–3585 kcal

World Health Organization equation:
RMR = (14.7 × 54.5 kg) + 496 = 1296 kcal
1296 kcal × 1.6 = 2074 kcal; 1296 kcal × 2.4 = 3110 kcal
TDEE range = 2074 − 3110 kcal

Note
1 This example shows that there are differences (~ ±300 kcal) between prediction equations, and that the range of Calories is quite large depending upon the activity factor selected. Therefore, it is recommended to calculate energy needs using different equations and activity factors depending upon training status (i.e., light training day, heavy training day, and rest day) to help determine an appropriate range of Calories. In practice, it may be recommended that Jill requires between 2100 and 3500 kcal/day depending upon her daily volume and intensity of training.

that is inadequate to maintain optimal health (Thomas et al., 2016). Although the EA threshold associated with impaired health and performance appears to occur across a continuum, research has shown that interventions to increase EA help restore endocrine function in exercising females; for example, Guebels, Kam, Maddalozzo, and Manore (2014) reported that increasing EA to 40 kcal/kg FFM per day restored menses in exercising females with previously reported menstrual dysfunction in less than 3 months. More on EA, as it relates to the Female Athlete Triad, is given in Chapter 6.

To summarise, estimating TDEE is not a clear science and requires calculating a range of Calories depending upon several factors discussed above. What is apparent, however, is that exercising females consuming <2000 kcal or <30 kcal/kg BM per day are at risk for menstrual dysfunction, and suboptimal health and performance.

Macronutrient intake

Carbohydrates

Carbohydrates are often referred to as the 'master fuel' because they provide energy for both aerobic and anaerobic exercise, and are exclusively used for energy by the central nervous system. Although body fat represents the largest capacity of stored energy and is a primary energy source during aerobic exercise, carbohydrates are necessary to metabolise fats and are the only macronutrient that can provide energy during maximal and supramaximal exercise. An adequate intake of carbohydrate is also essential to preserve FFM, since the body will break down muscle to convert to glucose when carbohydrate stores are low.

Carbohydrate is stored in the form of glycogen in the liver and skeletal muscle and can be manipulated by both exercise and dietary intake. The recommended range for carbohydrates expressed as a percentage of daily EI is 45–65 per cent of Calories, but can range as high as 70–75 per cent as training volume increases, or when 'carbohydrate loading' prior to competition while tapering training (Hedrick-Fink & Mikesky, 2018). Because daily carbohydrate needs vary depending upon factors such as the type and quantity of daily physical activity, demands of the sport, environmental conditions, and stage of training and competition, it is recommended that carbohydrate needs be calculated relative to BM versus a percentage of total EI. Guidelines for carbohydrate intake are presented in Table 5.2 and generally range from 5–8 g/kg for moderate-to-high intensity exercise for 1–3 hr, and up to 10 g/kg for extreme intensity and/or prolonged exercise. However, for most exercising females engaged in regular training, a range of 5–7 g/kg is likely adequate.

Unfortunately, the results of several studies indicate that many exercising females do not meet their individual carbohydrate needs. For example,

Table 5.2 Guidelines for carbohydrate, protein, and fat intake for exercising females

Daily carbohydrate needs for energy and recovery[1]

Low	Low-intensity exercise (<1 hr/day)	3–5 g/kg BM; 55–65% of total Calories
Moderate	Moderate-intensity exercise (~1–2 hr/day)	5–7 g/kg BM; 55–65% of total Calories
High	Moderate-to-high intensity exercise (~2–3 hr/day)	6–8 g/kg BM; 55–65% of total Calories
Very high	Moderate-to-high intensity exercise (>4–5 hr/day)	8–10+ g/kg BM; 65–70% of total Calories

Guidelines to promote carbohydrate availability during training and competition

General fuelling	Events <90 min	5–8 g/kg BM/24 hr consistent with daily energy needs	
Carbohydrate loading	Events >90 min of continuous/intermittent moderate-to-high intensity exercise	8+ g/kg BM/24 hr for 3–4 days	Requires 30–35% increase in total energy intake; taper training 1–2 days prior to event
Pre-event fuelling	Prior to exercise of >60 min	1–4 g/kg BM consumed 1–4 hr prior to exercise	The timing, amount, and type of carbohydrate are chosen to meet the needs of the event and preferences/experiences of the individual
During short duration exercise	<45 min	Generally not needed	
During high-intensity continuous exercise	45–75 min	Small amounts and/or mouth rinse	High glycaemic sport drinks and gels
During prolonged moderate-to-high intensity continuous or intermittent exercise	1.0–2.5 hr	30–60 g/hr	Moderate-to-high glycaemic foods and drinks depending upon the nature of the activity, hydration needs, and gut comfort
During ultra-endurance exercise	>2.5–3.0 hr	Up to 90 g/hr	Same recommendation as above; products containing multiple transportable carbohydrates result in higher rates of carbohydrate oxidation
Recovery between repeated bouts of moderate-to-high intensity exercise	<8 hr recovery between two exercise bouts	1–2 g/kg BM/hr for 4–6 hr	Moderate-to-high glycaemic carbohydrate-rich foods and drinks

continued

Table 5.2 Continued

General recovery	Within 2–4 hr post-exercise	1.0–1.5 g/kg BM every 2 hr for 6 hr	100 g consumed within the first 30 min post-exercise if possible, to optimise glycogen repletion; carbohydrate meal consumed with protein in a 2:1 to 3:1 ratio
Daily protein needs for the exercising female[2]			
Endurance athletes		1.2–1.6 g/kg BM	Distributed in a meal plan that provides 25–40 g at least 3 times per day of high quality animal- and/ or plant-based protein. During periods of energy restriction, injury, or intense training, amounts >2.0 g/kg BM may be warranted
Strength athletes		1.4–2.0 g/kg BM	
Team sport athletes		1.4–1.7 g/kg BM	
Pre-event fuelling	4 hr prior to exercise	57–113 g	Lean protein sources; avoid full-fat dairy, high-fat cuts of meat, and nuts
During exercise	Generally not needed, but may confer some benefit during prolonged endurance events	0.1–0.2 g/kg BM	Branched chain amino acids (leucine, isoleucine, and valine) as part of a carbohydrate drink
Recovery from exercise	0–2 hr post-exercise	0.25–0.30 g/kg BM (~10 g)	Essential amino acids preferred
Recommendation for daily fat intake			
All exercising females		≥1.0 g/kg BM; at least 20% of total Calories	Balance of lean cuts of animal protein with natural sources of saturated fat, and polyunsaturated and monounsaturated fat from fish, seeds, avocados, nuts, oils, etc.

Notes

1 The following represents general guidelines that need to be individualised depending upon total energy needs, phase of training/competition, and training response. Adapted from Burke, Hawley, Wong, and Jeukendrup, 2011.

2 The recommended range to support metabolism, tissue repair and modelling, and protein turnover is 1.2–2.0 g/kg BM per day. Recommendations for general protein needs are adapted from Jager et al., 2017.

Gibson, Stuart-Hill, Martin, and Gaul (2011) reported that 51.5 per cent of female football (soccer) players consumed <5 g/kg per day, and Burke, Cox, Culmmings, and Desbrow (2001) found that female athletes consumed 30 per cent less carbohydrate relative to BM than did males who participated in the same sport, and did not meet energy requirements. Because depleted glycogen stores are associated with fatigue and a greater perception of effort, it is critical that the exercising female consume adequate amounts of carbohydrates prior to exercise, during exercise, and in recovery, to maintain carbohydrate availability.

Carbohydrates consumed in meals and snacks 1–4 hr prior to exercise will augment liver and muscle glycogen stores, especially following an overnight fast, and may provide a source of glucose during exercise (Thomas et al., 2016). A common recommendation is to consume 1 g/kg BM for each hour leading up to exercise. For example, as much as 4 g/kg of carbohydrate could be consumed as part of a pre-game meal, 4 hr before competition or training, whereas 1 hr prior to competition, a much lower amount (~1 g/kg) is recommended as a snack or in beverage form.

Recommendations for the amount and types of carbohydrate intake during exercise depend upon the duration of the activity, and carbohydrates are typically ingested in the form of a drink or sports-gel as a matter of convenience and easy digestibility (Table 5.2). It has also been suggested that performance may be enhanced by consuming multiple transportable carbohydrates, which are a combination of saccharides that use different glucose transporters, and may increase the rate of carbohydrate oxidation and reduce gastrointestinal symptoms associated with carbohydrate ingestion during exercise (Rossi, 2017). Mouth rinsing with carbohydrates to stimulate the central nervous system to detect their presence is another tactic used for short-term exercise, and has been reported to improve performance by 2–3 per cent through improved pacing and a decreased perception of effort (Burke & Dziedzic, 2013).

Glycogen repletion is a primary goal of recovery post-exercise, especially between two bouts of moderate-to-high intensity exercise performed on the same day. The rate of glycogen resynthesis is only ~5 per cent per hour. Therefore, early consumption of moderate-to-high glycaemic carbohydrates at a rate of 1.0–1.2 kg BM/h during the first 4–6 hr is recommended for refuelling (Thomas et al., 2016). When recovery time is >24 hr, there is greater flexibility with regard to timing and the types of carbohydrates that can be consumed; however, it is recommended that carbohydrates be consumed with a rich source of protein in a 2:1 ratio within 2–4 hr to promote higher glycogen repletion (Hedrick-Fink & Mikesky, 2018).

Carbohydrate loading

Carbohydrate loading, also known as glycogen supercompensation, practised for several days prior to endurance competition, has been shown to delay the onset of fatigue by ~20 per cent for exercise lasting longer than 90 min and, therefore, is a common strategy used by endurance athletes to optimise performance. The carbohydrate loading 'threshold' to experience an ergogenic effect has been reported to range between 8 and 10 g/kg (Wismann & Willoughby, 2006). Compared to males, exercising females oxidise proportionately more lipid and less carbohydrate during endurance exercise that is explained, in part, by higher oestrogen concentrations in females. The ability to spare muscle glycogen via increased lipid oxidation also supports the finding that females perform as well as, or better than, men during ultra-endurance events >66 km (Bam, Noakes, Juritz, & Dennis, 1997). Although there are sex differences in carbohydrate oxidation, Tarnopolsky (2000) reported that when females consumed >8 g/kg BM per day, they demonstrated similar increases in muscle glycogen compared to men; however, it required that they increase their total EI by 34 per cent during the loading period for four days. This increase in EI also makes sense from a practical standpoint, since a carbohydrate intake of >8 g/kg BM for many exercising females using their usual EI would represent 80–90 per cent or more of the daily allowance of Calories and would result in suboptimal intakes of protein and fat. As an example, for a 55 kg distance runner, an intake of 8 g/kg BM translates to 440 g or 1762 kcal. If she normally consumes 2100 kcal, her carbohydrate intake at 8 g/kg BM represents 84 per cent of her total daily EI. However, by consuming an additional 630 kcal (2100 × 0.30) per day during those four days of carbohydrate loading, or 2730 kcal/d, the carbohydrate intake represents 64 per cent of her daily EI (1762/2730 kcal), which falls within recommended ranges.

Effects of the menstrual cycle on carbohydrate availability

As previously mentioned, oestrogen affects carbohydrate oxidation and, therefore, will fluctuate with the menstrual cycle. Higher glycogen storage and lower carbohydrate oxidation have been observed during the luteal phase, when oestrogen and progesterone circulation are increased compared to the follicular phase, particularly in the early phase when both progesterone and oestrogen are depressed. Therefore, it may be warranted to increase carbohydrate intake during the follicular phase to maintain or increase glycogen stores (Rossi, 2017), which coincides with the recommendation to increase daily EI during this phase, since RMR has been reported to be lower during the same phase of the menstrual cycle.

Training with high and low carbohydrate availability

Strategies that restrict carbohydrate availability during training, such as training in a fasted state or limiting carbohydrate intake during an exercise session to increase glycogen storage later and compete 'high', have received considerable research attention. In fact, several variations of both 'training low' and 'training high' have been proposed and are currently being used by athletes as part of their periodised training programme (Jeukendrup, 2017). Training with low carbohydrate availability appears to be most prevalent and is intended to increase lipid oxidation and mitochondrial enzyme activity to spare glycogen and enhance exercise capacity. Although several training low studies have shown beneficial effects in terms of cell signalling and gene expression to increase lipid oxidation, few have shown any meaningful effects on performance (Bartlett, Hawley, & Morton, 2015; Jeukendrup, 2017; Psilander, Frank, Flockhart, & Sahlin, 2013; Stellingwerff, 2013), and there is concern that the practice could potentially be misused by exercising females and, consequently, impair training by affecting their ability to sustain high training intensities and volume (Thomas et al., 2016). In addition, low glycogen availability during intense training may result in immunosuppression and increase the risk of infection and illness (Gleeson, Nieman, & Pedersen, 2004), and result in muscle protein breakdown (Taylor et al., 2013). Because there is no clear evidence that training low (or training high) enhances exercise performance, it is recommended that the exercising female maintain a diet that achieves their nutrition goals and provides adequate glycogen availability that complements their periodised training programme.

Protein

Protein is a major component of the body structure and has a role in virtually all body processes including immune and endocrine function, and in tissue growth, maintenance, and repair. Like recommendations for carbohydrate, protein requirements are not static and vary depending upon many factors including training status (i.e., a new training stimulus requires higher intakes), stage of training, carbohydrate availability, and, most importantly, EI and EA. The recommended range for dietary protein intake to support metabolism, repair, remodelling, and protein turnover is 1.2–2.0 g/kg BM per day for exercising females (15–35 per cent of Calories); and higher intakes may be warranted (~2.3 g/kg BM per day) during periods of intense training, injury, or when EI is low, to spare FFM (Jäger et al., 2017; Mettler, Mitchell, & Tipton, 2010).

The position stand of the International Society of Sport Nutrition for protein and exercise (Jäger et al., 2017) recommends that active individuals consume between 1.4 and 2.0 g/kg BM per day of protein, and that endurance athletes consume levels at the lower end of the range, and strength/power athletes ingest levels at the higher end. Individuals involved in team sports or who engage in high-intensity intermittent activities should ingest levels in the middle of the range. Exercising females who consume an adequate EI, particularly in the form of carbohydrate, typically consume adequate amounts of protein for both training and competition. However, it is important to note that exercising females involved in sports that require a low BM, may be at risk for low protein intake due to low EA.

It is recommended that daily protein intake be reached with a meal plan that provides a regular distribution of moderate amounts of high-quality protein foods throughout the day and following strenuous bouts of exercise, since an unequal distribution is less effective for maintaining muscle mass and function (Arentson-Lantz, Clairmont, Paddon-Jones, Tremblay, & Elango, 2015; Thomas et al., 2016). In addition, because the body has a limited ability to store protein, there is no advantage in consuming excessive amounts of protein in one meal (Paddon-Jones & Rasmussen, 2009). A meal plan that provides between 25 and 40 g (or 0.25–0.30 g/kg BM per meal) of high-quality protein at least 3 times a day and includes animal protein or combinations of plant-based proteins, may be an effective strategy for optimising muscle protein synthesis (MPS) and preserving muscle mass and function (Arentson-Lantz et al., 2015; Jäger et al., 2017; Phillips, 2014).

Protein intake before, during, and after exercise

Exercising females require more dietary protein than their sedentary peers due to increased protein oxidation and breakdown during training, and the need to resynthesise protein and diminish proteolytic cellular activity during recovery (Jäger et al., 2017). Therefore, strategically planned protein intake timed around training is essential for maintaining (or increasing) muscle mass, ensuring adequate recovery, and promoting optimal health, including immune function. Classic investigations by Lemon, Berardi, and Noreen (2002), Wolfe and Miller (1999), and Tipton et al. (2001) have shown that when essential amino acids (EAA) are consumed prior to exercise they may provide energy for cells, decrease protein breakdown (catabolism) during exercise, and increase MPS during recovery.

Although the focus should be on carbohydrate prior to training or competition, small amounts of lean protein (57–113 g) can be consumed within 4 hr prior to exercise. Protein sources higher in fat (full-fat dairy, high-fat cuts of meat, and nuts) are not recommended in the time leading up to exercise, since they take longer to digest and increase the risk of intestinal distress during performance. Protein is not a major source of energy during exercise, since the process of converting amino acids to glucose (gluconeogenesis) in the liver is slow. However, the branched chain amino acids (BCAA), leucine, isoleucine, and valine are different in that they represent a readily available energy source for the muscle. Although BCAA ingestion during exercise does not appear to enhance performance, it has been shown to decrease the rate of protein degradation and delay glycogen depletion, particularly in individuals with reduced glycogen stores, and may help with mental fatigue (Jäger et al., 2017).

There are sex differences in protein metabolism. Compared to males, females oxidise less protein both at rest and during exercise. In a study by Tarnopolsky, MacDougall, Atkinson, Tarnopolsky, and Sutton (1990), it was found that 24-hr urinary nitrogen excretion (a marker of protein utilisation) was significantly higher in males following a bout of endurance exercise, while no significant difference was observed in females. The findings were confirmed in follow-up studies by the same laboratory, in which it was shown that males oxidised more leucine during rest and exercise, which may be explained by the effects of oestrogen and/or by sex differences in hepatic regulation of the rate-limiting enzyme branched chain-2-oxodehydrogenase (McKenzie et al., 2000; Phillips, Atkinson, Tarnopolsky, & MacDougall, 1993). Although protein catabolism during exercise has been reported to increase throughout the luteal phase of the menstrual cycle due to higher circulating levels of progesterone or a lower oestrogen to progesterone ratio (Kriengsinyos, Wykes, Goonewardene, Ball, & Pencharz, 2004), it appears to be attenuated with carbohydrate supplementation (Bailey, Zacher, & Mittleman, 2000). Therefore, the influence of ovarian hormones on metabolism during exercise may be secondary to substrate availability, energy status, and exercise intensity.

Protein intake is critical for post-exercise recovery in muscle, since proteolysis (protein breakdown) is diminished and MPS is increased resulting in an 'anabolic window' and an enhanced opportunity to achieve positive protein balance (i.e., nitrogen balance) in the muscle. During recovery, MPS appears to be similar in males and females; however, it has been reported that the increase in muscle protein fractional synthetic rate (fraction of the protein pool synthesised per unit time) is attenuated in females indicating that they may need to consume more protein post-exercise to elicit the same anabolic response (Volek et al., 2006). Most research suggests that MPS is optimised when ~10 g of EAA are consumed immediately post-exercise for up to 2 hr, which translates to 0.25–0.30 g/kg BM, and that the increase in MPS following EAA ingestion continues for 24 hr (Rossi, 2017; Thomas et al., 2016). It has also been reported that ingesting proteins high in EAA post-exercise, such as whey protein, which is easily digested and is rich in BCAA, results in improved immune function and reduced muscle soreness (Jäger et al., 2017).

In summary, an adequate intake of protein is essential for the exercising female to optimise MPS, minimise proteolysis, and preserve FFM. Therefore, consuming a moderate amount of high-quality protein at each meal (~25–40 g) and ~10 g of EAA up to 2 hr post-exercise is recommended for optimal health and muscle function.

Fat

Fat is not only an important fuel source during exercise, but is also a major component of cell membranes, is necessary for the absorption of fat-soluble vitamins, maintains hormone balance, and provides a source of essential free-fatty acids (FFA); therefore, it has several structural and functional roles in the body. Despite the importance of obtaining enough fat in the diet, many exercising females restrict their intake because of a belief that it may increase body fat and compromise performance (Larson-Meyer, Newcomer, & Hunter, 2002). It is generally recommended that athletes consume *at least* 20 per cent of their EI as fat (≥1.0 g/kg BM) with a range to as much as 40 per cent; however, for many women, fat may only account for 10–15 per cent of daily calorific intake (Hausswirth & Le Meur, 2011; Thomas et al., 2016). Exercising females involved in sports that require a weigh-in (e.g., combat sports, rowing, and Olympic weightlifting) or a low body weight (e.g., gymnastics, figure skating, diving, dance, and cross-country running) are especially prone to limit their fat intake, which may lead to disordered eating and more serious conditions associated with the Female Athlete Triad.

The major fats that contribute to energy production include plasma FFA, intramuscular triglycerides (IMTG), and adipose tissue, which represents the major storage form of triglycerides. Both adipose and IMTG stores supply FA to the muscle and, depending upon the duration and intensity of exercise, may account for between 30 and 70 per cent of substrate utilisation (Hausswirth & Le Meur, 2011; Maher & Tarnopolsky, 2013). Therefore, low-fat diets not only compromise health, but they also decrease IMTG stores, which, in turn, may negatively impact performance and recovery from exercise. For example, Larson-Meyer and colleagues (2002) found that female endurance athletes, who were in energy balance, needed to consume at least 30 per cent of their EI from fat to replete IMTG stores, and Decombaz, Fleith, Hoppeler, Kreis, and Boesch (2000) found that when fat intake was suboptimal, IMTG depletion continued for up to two days after exercise, which could impair exercise performance on subsequent days of training.

It is generally well recognised that females oxidise more fat during endurance exercise than men, as indicated by a lower respiratory exchange ratio and glycerol tracer studies that show females have a higher lipolytic rate at intensities ranging from 45–65 per cent of their maximum oxygen consumption. Although the exact mechanism for the higher fat use is not entirely clear, factors including oestrogen, differences in enzyme concentrations involved in the mitochondrial breakdown of FA, higher IMTG stores, and a greater per cent area of type I muscle fibres in females, may all play a role (Maher & Tarnopolsky, 2013; Rossi, 2017).

Recently, there has been some renewed interest in high-fat, low carbohydrate diets to increase fat oxidation and spare glycogen. However, enhanced rates of fat oxidation can only maintain an exercise capacity achieved by diets that promote high carbohydrate availability at moderate intensities, whereas performance at higher intensities is impaired due to a downregulation of carbohydrate metabolism, even when glycogen is available (Thomas et al., 2016). Although there may be some situations in which a higher fat diet may be warranted, most exercising females train and compete at high intensities, and therefore, a higher fat intake at the expense of carbohydrate is generally not recommended.

Fat provides more than twice the energy per gram (9 kcal/g) compared to the other macronutrients (protein and carbohydrate: 4 kcal/g), which can help the exercising female achieve energy balance. Therefore, it is recommended that athletes consume at least 20 per cent ($\geq 1.0 \text{g/kg}$ BM) of their EI in the form of unprocessed fats, since intakes less than 15 per cent of total Calories increase the risk of deficiencies in essential FA and the fat-soluble vitamins D and E (Hausswirth & Le Meur, 2011). To obtain a healthy balance of FA in the diet, including the essential omega-3 and omega-6 FA, it is recommended to consume lean animal protein with natural sources of saturated fat (poultry, beef, pork), as well as monounsaturated and polyunsaturated FA found in nuts, seeds, fatty fish (salmon, trout), flaxseed oil, olive oil, canola oil, and avocados. In addition, there is strong evidence that omega-3 FA found in fatty fish, walnuts, flaxseed, soybeans, and canola oil are beneficial to the cardiovascular system by lowering triglyceride levels and blood pressure, and by decreasing atherosclerotic plaques and inflammation and, therefore, may have positive effects on blood flow and muscle pain during exercise (Hedrick-Fink & Mikesky, 2018).

Fluid and electrolytes

Water is the most essential of all the nutrients, second only to oxygen for maintaining life, and accounts for ~55–65 per cent of total BM. Body water is lost through the kidneys (urine), skin (sweat), lungs, and faeces, and it is imperative that daily water intake is equal to water loss to maintain hydration. The goals of hydration during exercise are to maintain electrolyte balance and plasma volume, since a water loss of only 2–3 per cent BM can lead to a decrease in muscle function and strength performance (Judelson et al., 2007). The general recommended intake for exercising females is 2.7 L per day, which represents intake from drinking water, watery foods, and other water-containing beverages. However, hydration needs will vary depending upon BM, environmental factors, and exercise intensity and duration. For most exercising females, ~100–200 ml every 10–20 min (0.4–0.8 L/hr) during exercise will help maintain BM and prevent dehydration. Plain water is typically adequate for training sessions lasting <1 hr; however, a sports drink containing electrolytes is recommended for longer exercise sessions.

Micronutrients

Micronutrients include vitamins and minerals and, although they do not provide energy directly, they play a critical role in the metabolism of fats, protein, and carbohydrate, and deficiencies can result in serious health problems. Exercising females who restrict EI, eliminate food groups, or have poor diets, likely have deficiencies in several micronutrients of concern, including calcium, vitamin D, iron, and magnesium, that can have a negative impact on health and performance.

Iron

Iron is an important component of haemoglobin and myoglobin in red blood cells and, therefore, is critical for aerobic exercise and endurance training, since these carry oxygen to body tissues and muscle. Iron also has a role in energy production as a co-factor for enzymes, and is involved in immune function and brain development. The two types of dietary iron include haem and non-haem. Haem iron has greater bioavailability and is found only in animal foods such as beef, fish, and poultry. Non-haem iron is found in plant foods including soya, dried fruit, legumes, fortified cereals, green-leafy vegetables, and wholegrains, and its bioavailability can be improved when ingested with vitamin C or haem sources (Hedrick-Fink & Mikesky, 2018).

Exercising females are at an increased risk of iron deficiency, with or without anaemia, as a result of several factors including limited iron intake from haem food sources and low EI (~6 mg iron is consumed per 1000 kcal), foot-strike haemolysis, menstrual blood loss, training at high altitude, injury, urinary and sweat loss, and overuse of nonsteroidal anti-inflammatory drugs (Rossi, 2017; Thomas et al., 2016). It has been estimated that as many as 56–60 per cent of exercising females have iron deficiency without anaemia, which is typically defined as ferritin levels (storage form of iron in cells) ≤25 ng/ml; and 20 per cent have iron-deficiency anaemia (IDA), defined as haemoglobin levels <12 g/dl and ferritin levels <20 ng/ml (Rossi, 2017). When an exercising female is diagnosed with IDA, oral iron supplementation under the care of a physician is usually warranted, as well as improvements in diet, and limiting activities that contribute to iron loss, such as blood donation and weight bearing activities. Reversing IDA can take up to 3–6 months; therefore, adopting eating strategies that encourage the intake of foods with haem iron and non-haem iron with vitamin C is recommended to maintain iron status and prevent IDA from developing.

Calcium and vitamin D

Calcium is important for building, repairing, and maintaining bone tissue, as well as muscle contraction, blood clotting, nerve impulse conduction, and fluid regulation. Vitamin D is necessary for the absorption of calcium and phosphorus, and plays a role in immunity, muscle function, and cardiovascular health (Hedrick-Fink & Mikesky, 2018). It has been suggested that most exercising females do not receive adequate intakes of calcium and vitamin D due to several factors including disordered eating, elimination of dairy/calcium-rich foods from their diet, low EI intake, and menstrual dysfunction, which increases their risk for stress fractures (Rossi, 2017; Thomas et al., 2016). The recommended intake for calcium for women between the ages of 19 and 50 years is 1000 mg/d. However, exercising females at risk of calcium deficiency for the above mentioned reasons may require as much as 1500–2000 mg/day with 800–2000 IU of vitamin D to optimise bone health and help prevent stress fractures (Lappe et al., 2008; Thomas et al., 2016). In a study by Lappe and colleagues (2008), female Naval recruits who received 2000 mg of calcium and 800 IU of vitamin D per day during 8 weeks of basic training experienced 20 per cent fewer stress fractures compared to recruits who received a placebo. Therefore, when calcium and vitamin D intake is adequate, there is a decreased risk for bone injury and stress fracture in exercising females.

Although increasing the intake of calcium-rich foods (dairy, green-leafy vegetables, tofu, sardines with bones, and fortified cereals) should be the primary focus for improving a deficiency, calcium supplements may be warranted, particularly for exercising females who are following Calorie-restricted diets. In this case, it is important to note that not all calcium supplements are created equally. Calcium citrate is the most bioavailable form and does not need to be consumed with food, but is more expensive than other forms. Calcium carbonate supplements are less expensive and have higher amounts of calcium per tablet, but are not as bioavailable as calcium citrate and need to be consumed with food for optimal absorption. Calcium supplements derived from oyster shells or bone meal may contain lead and should be avoided. In addition, it is best to consume calcium supplements alone at a dosage of <500 mg for optimal absorption, since it competes for absorption with iron and zinc (Hedrick-Fink & Mikesky, 2018).

There is some controversy among scientists regarding the definition of vitamin D deficiency; however, it is most commonly accepted that vitamin D levels >20 ng/ml are sufficient and that levels >40 ng/ml are optimal (Cannell, Hollis, Sorenson, Taft, & Anderson, 2009). Daily vitamin D requirements are difficult to obtain naturally through food; therefore, supplementation is typically warranted. Vitamin D is primarily synthesised in the skin from exposure to ultraviolet B (UVB) light rays. Therefore, in addition to the factors discussed above, exercising females at risk for vitamin D deficiency also include those who train and compete indoors or during non-peak UVB hours, and those living at latitudes above 37° North or South of the equator. It is important to note, however, that athletes living in temperate climates who train outdoors may be vitamin D deficient due the use of sunscreen. The clinical practice guidelines of the Endocrine Society (Holick et al., 2011) recommend a vitamin D intake of between 1500–2000 IU daily for adults >18 years, which is significantly higher than the recommendation from the Institute of Medicine (600 IU) (Ogan & Pritchett, 2013). Backx and colleagues (2016) recently reported that 2210 IU/day for 3 months restored serum vitamin D to optimal levels in exercising females who were either sufficient or deficient. Therefore, it is recommended that exercising females ingest between 1000–2000 IU of vitamin D daily through food and/or vitamin D_3 supplementation for optimal health and performance.

Magnesium and zinc

Magnesium plays a vital role in bioenergetics and is important for bone and cardiovascular health, protein synthesis, blood clotting, serves as a co-factor for hundreds of enzymatic reactions, and may also play a role in blood pressure regulation and the prevention of muscle cramps (Volpe, 2015). Magnesium is not normally considered when discussing nutritional considerations for exercising females who consume a balanced diet, but vegetarians, vegans, and athletes who participate in sports that require a lower BM, may have inadequate intakes, which could impair carbohydrate, fat, and protein metabolism, as well as, hormonal and cardiovascular function (Thomas et al., 2016). Exercising females who ingest rich sources of magnesium, including green-leafy vegetables, whole grains, legumes, nuts and seafood, are likely meeting recommended levels (310–320 mg/d) and will not likely benefit from supplementation; however, symptoms such as muscle weakness, cramping, and irritability could indicate a magnesium deficiency (<220 mg/d).

Like magnesium, zinc is also a component of several enzymes necessary for carbohydrate, protein, and fat metabolism, and is involved in protein synthesis. Zinc is also important for several body processes including wound healing and immunity, tissue growth and repair, and gene expression (Thomas et al., 2016). Therefore, adequate zinc intake is important for performance and recovery from exercise. The recommendation for zinc intake is 8 mg per day for women and supplementation is not usually necessary if exercising females are consuming zinc-rich foods in the diet such as beef and other dark meats, fish, eggs, whole grains, legumes, and dairy products. Because it has been suggested that zinc may help prevent upper respiratory infections and relieve cold symptoms, zinc supplementation is practised by some female athletes. The effectiveness of zinc for preventing colds remains unclear; however, it should be noted that high levels of zinc can interfere with the absorption of iron and copper (Hedrick-Fink & Mikesky, 2018).

Real-world example

Calculating the energy needs of a female cyclist

Sofia is a 24-year-old experienced cyclist who is currently riding 100–240 km/week. She weighs 61 kg and is 168 cm in height. Using the tables and recommendations throughout this chapter, we can calculate her recommended intakes for carbohydrate (CHO), protein (PRO), and fat (FAT) relative to her BM to meet her energy requirements and maintain her current weight.

Example 1: Since she is an endurance athlete and using Table 5.2, you may recommend that she consume 6.0 g/kg CHO; 1.4 g/kg PRO; and 1.5 g/kg FAT

6.0 g/kg × 61 kg = 366 g CHO × 4 kcal/g = 1464 kcal (56% kcal)
1.4 g/kg × 61 kg = 85 g PRO × 4 kcal/g = 340 kcal (13% kcal)
1.5 g/kg × 61 kg = 91 g FAT × 9 kcal/g = 819 kcal (31% kcal)
Total kcal   **2623 kcal**

Example 2: Using the World Health Organization calculator for RMR and activity factors in Table 5.1:

RMR = (14.7 × 61 kg) + 496 = 1393 kcal; RMR × 1.6 activity factor = 2223 kcal; RMR × 2.4 activity factor = 3343 kcal; average of the range = 2783 kcal (2223 + 3343 kcal ÷ 2)

Considering a recommended macronutrient distribution of 60 per cent CHO; 15 per cent PRO; and 25 per cent FAT:

2783 kcal × 0.60 = 1670 kcal ÷ 4 kcal/g = 417.5 g; 417.5 g ÷ 61 kg BM = 6.8 g/kg CHO
2783 kcal × 0.15 = 417 kcal ÷ 4 kcal/g = 104 g; 104 g ÷ 61 kg BM = 1.70 g/kg PRO
2783 kcal × 0.25 = 696 kcal ÷ 9 kcal/g = 77 g; 77 g ÷ 61 kg BM = 1.3 g/kg FAT

Note: When determining energy requirements, values expressed relative to BM are the most important to consider (i.e., g/kg BM value); therefore, when allocating a recommended percentage distribution for the macronutrients, the values relative to BM should *always* be calculated, to make sure they fall within recommended ranges.

Summary

To ensure optimal health, performance, and recovery, it is imperative for exercising females to consume energy that is adequate in amount and timing to meet their individual training needs, since low EA results in loss of FFM, menstrual dysfunction, suboptimal bone density, and increases their risk of illness and injury. Adequate EI is dependent upon several factors including meeting targets for carbohydrate, protein, and fat, as well as meeting needs for hydration. Exercising females who restrict EI or avoid individual foods or food groups are also at risk for inadequate intakes of several nutrients of concern including calcium, vitamin D, iron, magnesium, and zinc, in which case, supplementation may be warranted.

References

Arentson-Lantz, E., Clairmont, S., Paddon-Jones, D., Tremblay, A., & Elango, R. (2015). Protein: A nutrient in focus. *Applied Physiology, Nutrition, and Metabolism, 40*(8), 755–761. https://doi.org/10.1139/apnm-2014-0530.

Backx, E. M., Tieland, M., Maase, K., Kies, A. K., Mensink, M., van Loon, L. J., & de Groot, L. C. (2016). The impact of 1-year vitamin D supplementation on vitamin D status in athletes: A dose-response study. *European Journal of Clinical Nutrition, 70*(9), 1009–1014. https://doi.org/10.1038/ejcn.2016.133.

Bailey, S. P., Zacher, C. M., & Mittleman, K. D. (2000). Effect of menstrual cycle phase on carbohydrate supplementation during prolonged exercise to fatigue. *Journal of Applied Physiology, 88*(2), 690–697. https://doi.org/10.1152/jappl.2000.88.2.690.

Bam, J., Noakes, T. D., Juritz, J., & Dennis, S. C. (1997). Could women outrun men in ultramarathon races? *Medicine and Science in Sports and Exercise, 29*(2), 244–247.

Bartlett, J. D., Hawley, J. A., & Morton, J. P. (2015). Carbohydrate availability and exercise training adaptation: Too much of a good thing? *European Journal of Sport Science, 15*(1), 3–12. https://doi.org/10.1080/17461391.2014.920926.

Burke, L. M., Cox, G. R., Culmmings, N. K., & Desbrow, B. (2001). Guidelines for daily carbohydrate intake: Do athletes achieve them? *Sports Medicine, 31*(4), 267–299.

Burke, L. M. & Dziedzic. C. E. (2013). Carbohydrate requirements for the female athlete. In K. A. Beals (Ed.), *Nutrition and the female athlete: From research to practice* (pp. 25–50). Boca Raton, FL: CRC Press.

Burke, L. M., Hawley, J. A., Wong, S. H. S., & Jeukendrup, A. E. (2011). Carbohydrates for training and competition. *Journal of Sports Sciences, 29*(Suppl 1), S17–S27. https://doi.org/10.1080/02640414.2011.585473.

Cannell, J. J., Hollis, B. W., Sorenson, M. B., Taft, T. N., & Anderson, J. J. (2009). Athletic performance and vitamin D. *Medicine and Science in Sports and Exercise, 41*(5), 1102–1110. https://doi.org/10.1249/MSS.0b013e3181930c2b.

Cunningham, J. J. (1980). A reanalysis of the factors influencing basal metabolic rate in normal adults. *The American Journal of Clinical Nutrition, 33*(11), 2372–2374. https://doi.org/10.1093/ajcn/33.11.2372.

Decombaz, J., Fleith, M., Hoppeler, H., Kreis, R., & Boesch, C. (2000). Effect of diet on the replenishment of intramyocellular lipids after exercise. *European Journal of Nutrition, 39*(6), 244–247.

Gibson, J. C., Stuart-Hill, L., Martin, S., & Gaul, C. (2011). Nutrition status of junior elite Canadian female soccer athletes. *International Journal of Sport Nutrition and Exercise Metabolism, 21*(6), 507–514.

Gleeson, M., Nieman, D. C., & Pedersen, B. K. (2004). Exercise, nutrition and immune function. *Journal of Sports Sciences, 22*(1), 115–125. https://doi.org/10.1080/0264041031000140590.

Guebels, C. P., Kam, L. C., Maddalozzo, G. F., & Manore, M. M. (2014). Active women before/after an intervention designed to restore menstrual function: Resting metabolic rate and comparison of four methods to quantify energy expenditure and energy availability. *International Journal of Sport Nutrition and Exercise Metabolism, 24*(1), 37–46. https://doi.org/10.1123/ijsnem.2012-0165.

Harris, J. A., & Benedict, F. G. (1918). A biometric study of human basal metabolism. *Proceedings of the National Academy of Sciences of the United States of America, 4*(12), 370–373.

Hausswirth, C., & Le Meur, Y. (2011). Physiological and nutritional aspects of post-exercise recovery: Specific recommendations for female athletes. *Sports Medicine, 41*(10), 861–882. https://doi.org/10.2165/11593180-000000000-00000.

Hedrick-Fink, H., & Mikesky, A. (2018). *Practical applications in sports nutrition* (5th ed.). Burlington, MA: Jones & Bartlett Learning.

Heydenreich, J., Kayser, B., Schutz, Y., & Melzer, K. (2017). Total energy expenditure, energy intake, and body composition in endurance athletes across the training season: A systematic review. *Sports Medicine – Open, 3*(1), 8-017-0076-1. https://doi.org/10.1186/s40798-017-0076-1.

Holick, M. F., Binkley, N. C., Bischoff-Ferrari, H. A., Gordon, C. M., Hanley, D. A., Heaney, R. P., … Endocrine Society. (2011). Evaluation, treatment, and prevention of vitamin D deficiency: An endocrine society clinical practice guideline. *The Journal of Clinical Endocrinology and Metabolism, 96*(7), 1911–1930. https://doi.org/10.1210/jc.2011-0385.

Institute of Medicine. (2005). *Dietary reference intakes for energy, carbohydrate, fiber, fat, fatty acids, cholesterol, protein, and amino acids.* Washington, DC: The National Academies Press. https://doi.org/10.17226/10490.

Jäger, R., Kerksick, C. M., Campbell, B. I., Cribb, P. J., Wells, S. D., Skwiat, T. M., … Antonio, J. (2017). International society of sports nutrition position stand: Protein and exercise. *Journal of the International Society of Sports Nutrition, 14*, 20-017-0177-8. https://doi.org/10.1186/s12970-017-0177-8.

Jeukendrup, A. E. (2017). Periodized nutrition for athletes. *Sports Medicine, 47*(Suppl 1), 51–63. https://doi.org/10.1007/s40279-017-0694-2.

Judelson, D. A., Maresh, C. M., Farrell, M. J., Yamamoto, L. M., Armstrong, L. E., Kraemer, W. J., … Anderson, J. M. (2007). Effect of hydration state on strength, power, and resistance exercise performance. *Medicine and Science in Sports and Exercise, 39*(10), 1817–1824. https://doi.org/10.1249/mss.0b013e3180de5f22.

Kriengsinyos, W., Wykes, L. J., Goonewardene, L. A., Ball, R. O., & Pencharz, P. B. (2004). Phase of menstrual cycle affects lysine requirement in healthy women. *American Journal of Physiology, Endocrinology and Metabolism, 287*(3), E489–496. https://doi.org/10.1152/ajpendo.00262.2003.

Lappe, J., Cullen, D., Haynatzki, G., Recker, R., Ahlf, R., & Thompson, K. (2008). Calcium and vitamin D supplementation decreases incidence of stress fractures in female navy recruits. *Journal of Bone and Mineral Research: The Official Journal of the American Society for Bone and Mineral Research, 23*(5), 741–749. https://doi.org/10.1359/jbmr.080102.

Larson-Meyer, D. E., Newcomer, B. R., & Hunter, G. R. (2002). Influence of endurance running and recovery diet on intramyocellular lipid content in women: A 1H NMR study. *American Journal of Physiology. Endocrinology and Metabolism, 282*(1), E95–E106. https://doi.org/10.1152/ajpendo.2002.282.1.E95.

Lemon, P. W., Berardi, J. M., & Noreen, E. E. (2002). The role of protein and amino acid supplements in the athlete's diet: Does type or timing of ingestion matter? *Current Sports Medicine Reports, 1*(4), 214–221.

Loucks, A. B. (2007). Low energy availability in the marathon and other endurance sports. *Sports Medicine, 37*(4–5), 348–352. https://doi.org/37NaN19.

Loucks, A. B., Kiens, B., & Wright, H. H. (2011). Energy availability in athletes. *Journal of Sports Sciences, 29*(Suppl 1), S7–S15. https://doi.org/10.1080/02640414.2011.588958.

Loucks, A. B., & Thuma, J. R. (2003). Luteinizing hormone pulsatility is disrupted at a threshold of energy availability in regularly menstruating women. *The Journal of Clinical Endocrinology and Metabolism, 88*(1), 297–311. https://doi.org/10.1210/jc.2002-020369.

Loucks, A. B., Verdun, M., & Heath, E. M. (1998). Low energy availability, not stress of exercise, alters LH pulsatility in exercising women. *Journal of Applied Physiology, 84*(1), 37–46. https://doi.org/10.1152/jappl.1998.84.1.37.

Maher, A. C., & Tarnopolsky, M. A. (2013). Substrate utilization in female athletes. In K. A. Beals (Ed.), *Nutrition and the female athlete: From research to practice* (pp. 1–23). Boca Raton, FL: CRC Press.

McKenzie, S., Phillips, S. M., Carter, S. L., Lowther, S., Gibala, M. J., & Tarnopolsky, M. A. (2000). Endurance exercise training attenuates leucine oxidation and BCOAD activation during exercise in humans. *American Journal of Physiology, Endocrinology and Metabolism, 278*(4), E580–E587. https://doi.org/10.1152/ajpendo.2000.278.4.E580.

Mettler, S., Mitchell, N., & Tipton, K. D. (2010). Increased protein intake reduces lean body mass loss during weight loss in athletes. *Medicine and Science in Sports and Exercise, 42*(2), 326–337. https://doi.org/10.1249/MSS.0b013e3181b2ef8e.

Mifflin, M. D., St Jeor, S. T., Hill, L. A., Scott, B. J., Daugherty, S. A., & Koh, Y. O. (1990). A new predictive equation for resting energy expenditure in healthy individuals. *The American Journal of Clinical Nutrition, 51*(2), 241–247. https://doi.org/10.1093/ajcn/51.2.241.

Ogan, D., & Pritchett, K. (2013). Vitamin D and the athlete: Risks, recommendations, and benefits. *Nutrients, 5*(6), 1856–1868. https://doi.org/10.3390/nu5061856.

Paddon-Jones, D., & Rasmussen, B. B. (2009). Dietary protein recommendations and the prevention of sarcopenia. *Current Opinion in Clinical Nutrition and Metabolic Care, 12*(1), 86–90. https://doi.org/10.1097/MCO.0b013e32831cef8b.

Phillips, S. M. (2014). A brief review of critical processes in exercise-induced muscular hypertrophy. *Sports Med., 44* (Suppl 1), S71–S77. https://doi.org/10.1007/s40279-014-0152-3.

Phillips, S. M., Atkinson, S. A., Tarnopolsky, M. A., & MacDougall, J. D. (1993). Gender differences in leucine kinetics and nitrogen balance in endurance athletes. *Journal of Applied Physiology, 75*(5), 2134–2141. https://doi.org/10.1152/jappl.1993.75.5.2134.

Psilander, N., Frank, P., Flockhart, M., & Sahlin, K. (2013). Exercise with low glycogen increases PGC-1alpha gene expression in human skeletal muscle. *European Journal of Applied Physiology, 113*(4), 951–963. https://doi.org/10.1007/s00421-012-2504-8.

Rossi, K. A. (2017). Nutritional aspects of the female athlete. *Clinics in Sports Medicine, 36*(4), 627–653. https://doi.org/S0278-5919(17)30054-6.

Roza, A. M., & Shizgal, H. M. (1984). The Harris Benedict equation reevaluated: Resting energy requirements and the body cell mass. *The American Journal of Clinical Nutrition, 40*(1), 168–182. https://doi.org/10.1093/ajcn/40.1.168.

Stellingwerff, T. (2013). Contemporary nutrition approaches to optimize elite marathon performance. *International Journal of Sports Physiology and Performance, 8*(5), 573–578. https://doi.org/2013-0092.

Tarnopolsky, L. J., MacDougall, J. D., Atkinson, S. A., Tarnopolsky, M. A., & Sutton, J. R. (1990). Gender differences in substrate for endurance exercise. *Journal of Applied Physiology, 68*(1), 302–308. https://doi.org/10.1152/jappl.1990.68.1.302.

Tarnopolsky, M. A. (2000). Gender differences in metabolism; nutrition and supplements. *Journal of Science and Medicine in Sport, 3*(3), 287–298. https://doi.org/S1440-2440(00)80038-9.

Taylor, C., Bartlett, J. D., van de Graaf, C. S., Louhelainen, J., Coyne, V., Iqbal, Z., … Morton, J. P. (2013). Protein ingestion does not impair exercise-induced AMPK signalling when in a glycogen-depleted state: Implications for train-low compete-high. *European Journal of Applied Physiology, 113*(6), 1457–1468. https://doi.org/10.1007/s00421-012-2574-7.

Thomas, D. T., Erdman, K. A., & Burke, L. M. (2016). Position of the academy of nutrition and dietetics, dietitians of Canada, and the American College of Sports Medicine Nutrition and athletic performance. *Journal of the Academy of Nutrition and Dietetics, 116*(3), 501–528. https://doi.org/S2212-2672(15)01802-X.

Tipton, K. D., Rasmussen, B. B., Miller, S. L., Wolf, S. E., Owens-Stovall, S. K., Petrini, B. E., & Wolfe, R. R. (2001). Timing of amino acid-carbohydrate ingestion alters anabolic response of muscle to resistance exercise. *American Journal of Physiology, Endocrinology and Metabolism, 281*(2), E197–E206. https://doi.org/10.1152/ajpendo.2001.281.2.E197.

Volek, J. S., Forsythe, C. E., & Kraemer, W. J. (2006). Nutritional aspects of women strength athletes. *British Journal of Sports Medicine, 40*(9), 742–748. https://doi.org/bjsm.2004.016709.

Volpe, S. L. (2015). Magnesium and the athlete. *Current Sports Medicine Reports, 14*(4), 279–283. https://doi.org/10.1249/JSR.0000000000000178.

Wismann, J., & Willoughby, D. (2006). Gender differences in carbohydrate metabolism and carbohydrate loading. *Journal of the International Society of Sports Nutrition, 3*, 23–34. https://doi.org/10.1186/1550-2783-3-1-28.

Wolfe, R. R., & Miller, S. L. (1999). Amino acid availability controls muscle protein metabolism. *Diabetes, Nutrition & Metabolism, 12*(5), 322–328.

World Health Organization. (1985). Energy and protein requirements. Report of a joint FAO/WHO/UNU Expert Consultation. *World Health Organization Technical Report Series, 724*, 1–206. Retrieved from www.ncbi.nlm.nih.gov/pubmed/3937340.

6 The Female Athlete Triad

Mary Jane De Souza, Kristen J. Koltun,
Emily A. Southmayd, and Nicole C. Aurigemma

Introduction

In the early 1990s, researchers identified a medical syndrome that was impacting the health of female athletes (Nattiv, Agostini, Drinkwater, & Yeager, 1994). This medical syndrome, to be defined as the Female Athlete Triad (Triad), was named in 1994 (Nattiv et al., 1994) as a syndrome initiated by inadequate energy intake to meet the exercise energy expenditure needs of an athlete, and was associated with poor reproductive and bone health. In 1997, the American College of Sports Medicine published the first position stand on the Triad (Otis, Drinkwater, Johnson, Loucks, & Wilmore, 1997). As research advances informed the field of a better understanding of the interrelationships among eating behaviours, energy, reproduction, and bone health, the Triad was updated in 2007 and presented as a continuum of severity (Figure 6.1) (Nattiv et al., 2007). In 2014, the Female Athlete Triad Coalition published a set of guidelines for the prevention, detection, and treatment of the Triad that included an evidence-based risk assessment tool and scoring system to define athlete eligibility for sport participation and return to play following diagnosis and treatment for the Triad (De Souza et al., 2014a; De Souza et al., 2014b).

The updated Triad model (Nattiv et al., 2007) describes a continuum of severity, ranging from a 'healthy' starting point to an 'unhealthy' endpoint. At the 'healthy' ends of the continuum, energy status is adequate, menstrual cycles are ovulatory and occur at regular intervals of 26–32 days (i.e., eumenorrhoeic), and bone health is within a healthy range. At the extreme 'unhealthy' endpoints of the continuum, energy status is inadequate with or without disordered eating, and functional hypothalamic amenorrhoea (FHA: the absence of menses for at least three months that is hypothalamic in origin), and low bone mineral density (BMD) are present. The 2007 continuum model highlights intermediate, or 'subclinical', midpoints of the Triad components that may progress to more severe 'clinical' endpoints, such as disordered eating progressing to eating disorders, or luteal phase defects and anovulation in the menstrual cycle progressing to FHA (Nattiv et al., 2007). In the 2014 Treatment and Return to Play Guidelines published by the

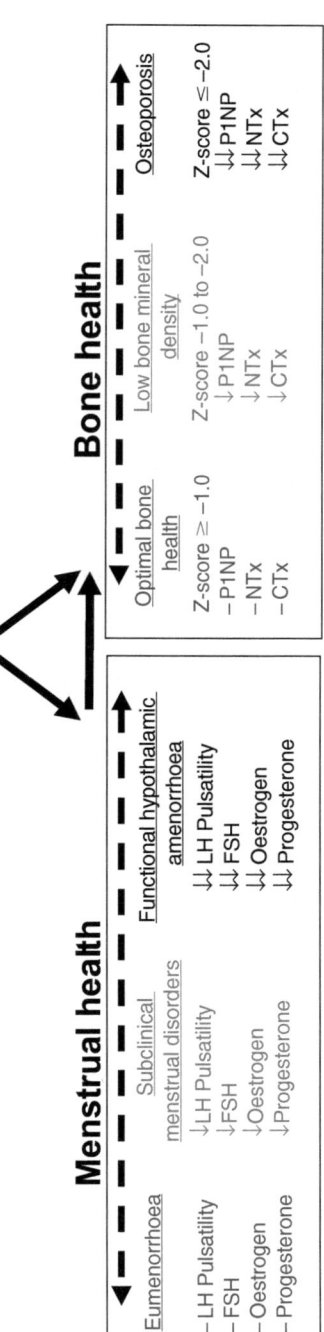

Energy availability

Optimal EA	Reduced EA with and without disordered eating	Low EA with and without disordered eating
– REE	↓ REE	↓↓REE
– TT₃	↓ TT₃	↓↓ TT₃
– Ghrelin	↔ Ghrelin	↑↑ Ghrelin
– PYY	↔ PYY	↑↑ PYY
– Leptin	↓ Leptin	↓↓ Leptin
– IGF-1	↓ IGF 1	↓↓ IGF-1
– Cortisol	↑ Cortisol	↑↑ Cortisol

Key: EA – energy availability; REE – resting energy expenditure; TT3 – total triiodothyronine; PYY – peptide YY; IGF – 1-insulin-like growth factor-1

Menstrual health

Eumenorrhoea	Subclinical menstrual disorders	Functional hypothalamic amenorrhoea
– LH Pulsatility	↓LH Pulsatility	↓↓ LH Pulsatility
– FSH	↓FSH	↓↓ FSH
– Oestrogen	↓Oestrogen	↓↓ Oestrogen
– Progesterone	↓Progesterone	↓↓ Progesterone

Key: LH – luteinising hormone; FSH – follicle-stimulating hormone

Bone health

Optimal bone health	Low bone mineral density	Osteoporosis
Z-score ≥ –1.0	Z-score –1.0 to –2.0	Z-score ≤ –2.0
– P1NP	↓P1NP	↓↓ P1NP
– NTx	↓NTx	↓↓ NTx
– CTx	↓CTx	↓↓ CTx

Key: P1NP – procollagen Type-1 propeptide; NTx – N-terminal telopeptide; CTx – C-terminal telopeptide

Figure 6.1 The Female Athlete Triad.

Note

The Triad represents a spectrum of energy availability, menstrual health, and bone health status. Within each health category, individuals may vary from optimal health (light grey), compromised health (lightest grey) to a pathological health status (black).

Female Athlete Triad Coalition (De Souza et al., 2014a; De Souza et al., 2014b), Triad researchers emphasised the importance of prevention and early intervention to prevent Triad problems from advancing to serious health outcomes, including clinical eating disorders, such as anorexia nervosa, FHA, and osteoporosis (De Souza et al., 2014a; De Souza et al., 2014b; Nattiv et al., 2007).

Aims of the chapter

The aims of the chapter are as follows:

1   To describe the physiology of all three components of the Triad (i.e., low energy availability, and disordered eating behaviours, menstrual disturbances, and bone health).
2   To detail the prevalence of the Triad in female athletes and exercising women.
3   To discuss prevention and treatment strategies for the Triad and describe the expected timeline of recovery for each Triad component.

Overview of the Female Athlete Triad

The athletes most often impacted by the Triad include those participating in sports that emphasise leanness, such as cross-country running, gymnastics, and figure skating (Beals & Manore, 2002; De Souza et al., 2014a; Nattiv et al., 2007); however, athletes participating in any sport can experience the syndrome, including women who are participating in sport and exercise for health and fitness reasons, who are not competitive athletes (De Souza et al., 1998; De Souza et al., 2010). Additionally, although this chapter focuses on the female athlete, a similar syndrome is experienced by male athletes, and current research is underway to improve our understanding of Triad physiology in exercising men (Tenforde, Barrack, Nattiv, & Fredericson, 2016).

Triad researchers emphasise that a diagnosis of the Triad does not require the simultaneous presence of all three Triad components (low energy availability with or without disordered eating, menstrual disturbances, and low bone density); the presence of one or more of the Triad components warrants a diagnosis of the Triad (De Souza et al., 2014a; De Souza et al., 2014b; Nattiv et al., 2007). Among female athletes, the prevalence of any one component of the Triad ranges from 16 to 60 per cent, the prevalence of any two Triad components ranges from 3 to 27 per cent, and the prevalence of all three Triad conditions presenting concurrently ranges from 0 to 16 per cent (Gibbs, Williams, & De Souza, 2013a). The prevalence of all Triad components is increased in sports that emphasise leanness.

Energy availability and disordered eating behaviours

Low energy availability, defined below, is considered to be the root cause of the Triad (Nattiv et al., 2007). In the context of the Triad, energy availability is calculated as energy intake (kcal) minus exercise energy expenditure (kcal) divided by fat-free mass (FFM) or lean body mass (kg) (Loucks, 2007). Low energy availability, defined as a value below 30 kcal/kg FFM/day, is associated with detrimental physiological changes in reproductive, metabolic, and bone health (Ihle & Loucks, 2004; Loucks & Thuma, 2003), and although its prevalence is not well documented, the only study to date ($n = 80$) reports that this condition affects 6 per cent of female high school athletes (Hoch et al., 2009). Low energy availability can develop secondary to a variety of pathways, including clinical eating disorders, disordered eating behaviours, intentional weight loss without disordered eating, and inadvertent undereating (De Souza et al., 2014b). In the majority of Triad cases, energy intake is not sufficient to meet the demands of exercise-related energy expenditure resulting in a prolonged energy deficit and low energy availability (Gibbs et al., 2013a).

Disordered eating behaviours can include dietary cognitive restraint, drive for thinness (DT), laxative or diuretic use, and self-induced vomiting (Joy, Kussman, & Nattiv, 2016) and are more common in athletes than non-athletes (Sundgot-Borgen & Torstveit, 2004), especially in athletes who participate in sports that emphasise leanness (Sundgot-Borgen, 1993). Dietary cognitive restraint, which is the conscious restriction of food intake relating to disordered eating and/or clinical eating disorders, is often associated with low energy availability and has been observed in 13–42 per cent (Sundgot-Borgen & Torstveit, 2004) of exercising females. Similarly, a high DT has been described as one of the principal features of disordered eating (Garner, 1991), and may be a key component preceding the development of the Triad. DT is associated with attitudes and behaviours revolving around the desire to be thinner, as well as a preoccupation with weight, dieting, and fear of weight gain (Garner, 1991). Because higher DT may be related to behavioural changes reflective of dietary energy restriction, it follows that a high DT is often associated with suppressed resting energy expenditure in exercising women (Gibbs, Williams, Scheid, Toombs, & De Souza, 2011). Additionally, in exercising women with high DT, there is a greater prevalence of severe menstrual disturbances (Gibbs et al., 2011), highlighting the relationship between behaviour-induced energy restriction and menstrual dysfunction.

In response to a prolonged energy deficit and low energy availability, physiological adaptations occur to conserve energy for the processes most essential for immediate survival. Specifically, energy is shunted away from processes such as growth and reproduction in favour of the more pressing needs of thermoregulation, cellular maintenance, and locomotion (Wade & Schneider, 1992). Metabolic shifts are evidenced through endocrinological changes that may include reductions in the concentration of total triiodothyronine (TT_3) (Harber, Petersen, & Chilibeck, 1998), leptin (Thong, McLean, & Graham, 2000), and insulin-like growth factor-1 (IGF-1), and elevations in concentrations of growth hormone (Waters, Qualls, Dorin, Veldhuis, & Baumgartner, 2001) and cortisol (Laughlin & Yen, 1996).

A series of well-designed, short-term laboratory experiments demonstrated the association of energy availability with alterations in markers of reproductive (Loucks, Verdun, & Heath, 1998), metabolic (Loucks & Thuma, 2003), and bone (Ihle & Loucks, 2004) health. These experiments provided evidence for the existence of a threshold of energy availability, determined to be 30 kcal/kg FFM/day (Loucks & Thuma, 2003), below which negative physiological adaptations occur and severe clinical sequelae associated with impaired metabolic, reproductive, and bone health may develop. However, this concept has recently been challenged, as Lieberman, De Souza, Wagstaff, and Williams (2017) reported that no specific value of energy availability emerged as a threshold below which menstrual disturbances were induced in sedentary women undergoing an exercise and diet intervention designed to test the relationships between energy availability and menstrual function. However, an inverse linear relationship between energy availability and the development of menstrual disturbances was reported, such that energy availability below 30 kg/kcal FFM/day increased the probability of menstrual disturbances by greater than 50 per cent (Lieberman et al., 2017). Notably, these data support the use of energy availability as a predictor of menstrual disturbances, and the Female Athlete Triad Coalition endorses a recommendation to maintain energy availability goals of at least 45 kcal/kg FFM/day to avoid clinical sequelae associated with the Triad (De Souza et al., 2014b).

Consistent with the hypometabolic state resulting from a chronic energy deficit, markers of low energy availability in exercising women include suppressed concentrations in serum TT_3 and a concomitant decrease in resting energy expenditure (REE) (De Souza et al., 2007; Dominguez, Laughlin, Nelson, & Yen, 1997). Specifically, compared to women with eumenorrhoeic, ovulatory menstrual cycles, exercising women with menstrual disturbances often present with significantly lower REE and TT_3 concentrations and these alterations occur in a dose-dependent manner, such that women with the most severe menstrual disturbances have the lowest REE and TT_3 concentrations (De Souza et al., 2007). Laboratory assessments of energy status and reproductive and bone health have used the ratio of measured/predicted REE to identify low energy availability, operationally defining energy deficiency as a ratio of measured/predicted REE ≤ 0.90 (De Souza, Hontscharuk, Olmsted, Kerr, & Williams, 2007; Gibbs et al., 2011; Scheid, Williams, West, VanHeest, & De Souza, 2009); however, further work is required to confirm the diagnostic credibility of this value.

Conceptually, energy availability is a simplistic calculation, as it requires measurements of energy intake, exercise energy expenditure, and body composition only. This is in contrast to the concept of energy balance (also discussed in Chapter 5), which requires quantification of non-exercise energy expenditure, REE, and the thermic effect of food (Donahoo, Levine, & Melanson, 2004). Thus, energy availability is a more tangible and attainable measure. However, there are limitations to the use of energy availability since it relies on self-report measures of dietary intake and exercise, which are susceptible to modifications during the reporting period and inaccurate reporting (Heaney, O'Connor, Gifford, & Naughton, 2010). The limitations associated with measuring energy availability will translate to difficulties in reliably diagnosing low energy availability, so additional variables should be taken into consideration, including weight stability and body mass index (BMI). While the aforementioned compensatory metabolic mechanisms often result in weight loss, weight stability should not be used for diagnosis, as it has been reported in women with amenorrhoea (Myerson et al., 1991). Additionally, a BMI of $<18.5\,\text{kg/m}^2$ or <85 per cent of expected body weight, as proposed by the Female Athlete Triad Coalition (De Souza et al., 2014b), may be helpful in screening for low energy availability; however, this should be corroborated by diet and exercise logs.

Traditionally, energy availability has been assessed over 24-hr periods, but recent findings (Fahrenholtz et al., 2017; Vescovi & VanHeest, 2016) have brought attention to the importance of within-day fluctuations as well. Athletes often cannot meet their energy needs for complex reasons, including having to plan meals around intensive training and travel schedules in addition to work or school schedules, and while they may meet their 24-hr energy availability goals, there may be periods of acute energy deficiency throughout the day. One case study reported that a high-level triathlete experienced an energy deficit of $>300\,\text{kcal}$ for 6 hr of the day, with the largest single hour deficit in excess of $1000\,\text{kcal}$ (Vescovi & VanHeest, 2016). Other recent findings conclude that there were no differences in 24-hr energy availability between athletes with menstrual disturbances compared to eumenorrhoeic athletes; however, those with menstrual disturbances spent more time in an energy deficient state, although within-day energy availability values were not reported (Fahrenholtz et al., 2017). Although continual assessment of energy availability (rather than measuring 24-hr average energy availability) is time consuming and requires additional burden on the athletes and investigators, it may be an important consideration for practitioners.

Of the three Triad components, recovery from a state of low energy availability can be realised relatively quickly and is essential for the recovery of the other two components. In cases of unintentional low energy availability, assessing energy needs and providing nutritional education should be a first step (De Souza et al., 2014b). Often, athletes may need to eat based on scheduling rather than rely on feelings of hunger. Ghrelin and peptide YY are appetite-regulating hormones that are both elevated in amenorrhoeic athletes and may play an aetiological role in the development of an energy deficiency and low energy availability by sending competing hunger messages resulting in an overall suppression of appetite (De Souza, Leidy, O'Donnell, Lasley, & Williams, 2004; Scheid et al., 2009). In cases where disordered eating or frank eating disorders, such as anorexia nervosa or bulimia nervosa, are present, a multidisciplinary team consisting of a physician, mental health professional, and dietician should be organised to develop personalised care for the athlete and target the behaviours (Joy et al., 2016).

Menstrual disturbances associated with the Triad

Alterations in the production and secretion of reproductive hormones occur at each level of the reproductive axis, including the hypothalamus, pituitary gland, and ovaries (the menstrual cycle is discussed in more detail in Chapter 3). The spectrum of menstrual disturbances associated with the Triad ranges from subclinical menstrual disturbances, including luteal phase defects and anovulation, to the most severe menstrual disturbances, including oligomenorrhoea and FHA (Figure 6.2) (De Souza et al., 1998; De Souza et al., 2010). Optimal menstrual function is characteristically dependent on the availability of metabolic fuel (Wade & Schneider, 1992), and the reliance of reproductive function on food availability and energy balance is well established. In exercising females and athletes, several studies have demonstrated the causal role of low energy availability on suppression of menstrual function (Bullen et al., 1985; Loucks & Thuma, 2003; Williams, Helmreich, Parfitt, Caston-Balderrama, & Cameron, 2001). In fact, Williams and colleagues (2001) demonstrated a dose-response relationship between the magnitude of energy deficiency and the frequency of exercise-related menstrual disturbances in untrained eumenorrhoeic women who underwent prescribed exercising energy deficit. However, these menstrual changes related to energy deficit are not permanent. Increasing energy by way of increased food intake reversed menstrual disturbances related to energy restriction, without reducing exercise volume in non-human primates (Williams et al., 2001; Williams, Helmreich et al., 2001).

Subclinical menstrual disturbances are the least severe menstrual disturbances observed in athletes and are often difficult to detect because both luteal phase defects and anovulation present without any change in menstrual cycle length, and present with hormonal patterns that are difficult to detect without detailed hormonal analyses (De Souza et al., 2010). Indeed, in order to identify luteal phase defects and anovulation, daily hormonal assessments of oestrogen, progesterone, and luteinising hormone are necessary (De Souza et al., 2010). Luteal phase defects are characterised by a short luteal phase of < 10 days in length, an inadequate luteal phase that is characterised by suppressed progesterone production, or both (De Souza, 2003; McNeely & Soules, 1988). Anovulatory cycles are characterised by an inadequate oestrogen priming peak, and the subsequent absence of a significant luteinising hormone peak and the failure to ovulate and to subsequently

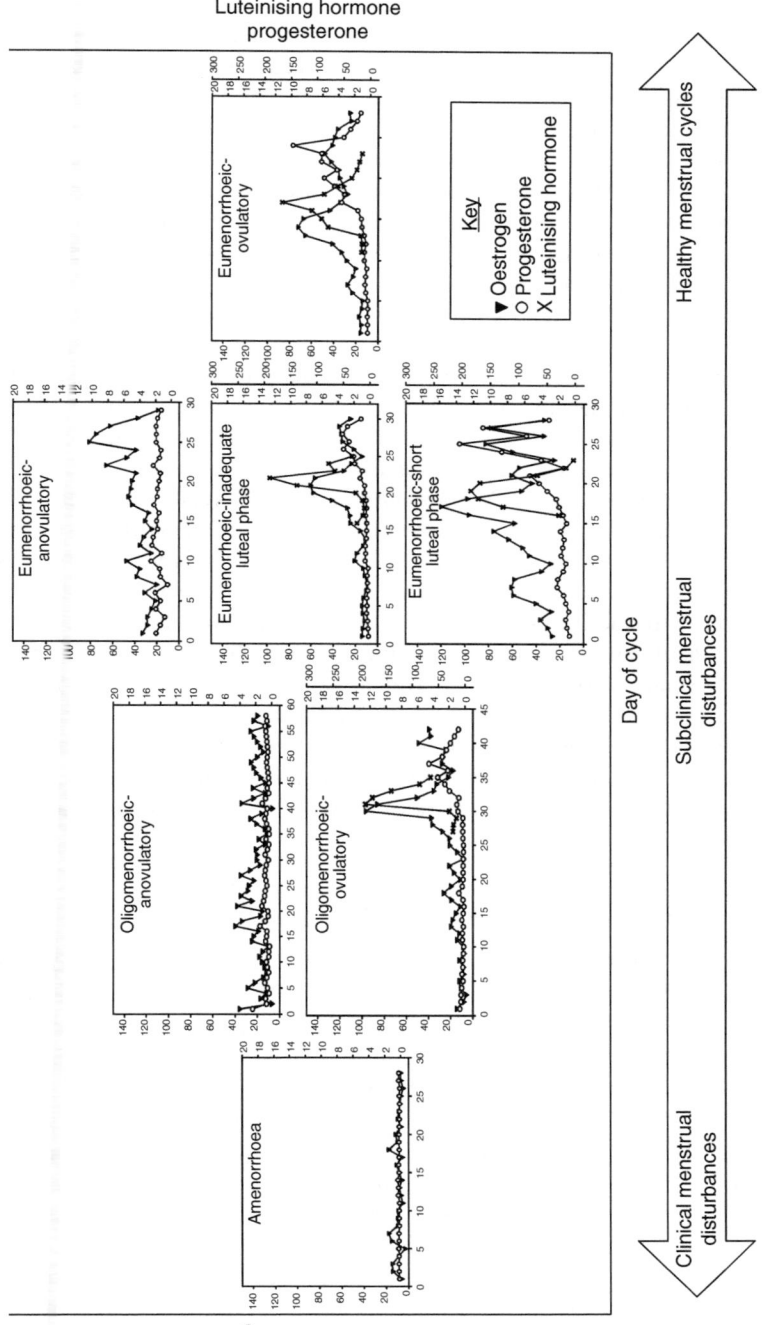

Figure 6.2 Reproductive hormone profiles across the spectrum of menstrual cycle types.

produce a corpus luteum and, as such, substantial amounts of progesterone (De Souza et al., 2010; Soules et al., 1989). Reductions in follicle-stimulating hormone during the luteal-follicular transition in association with luteal phase defects and anovulation may cause delayed follicular maturation, and thus, a decrease in oestrogen production from the developing follicles (De Souza et al., 1998).

FHA associated with the Triad is characterised by decreased luteinising hormone pulse frequency and increased luteinising hormone pulse amplitude at the level of the pituitary gland, leading to chronic hypo-oestrogenism. Amenorrhoea is easy to detect since menses is absent for several months. FHA is typically defined as the absence of menses for at least three months or less than five menses in 12 months in a woman who has previously menstruated (Gordon et al., 2017). Amenorrhoea can also present as primary amenorrhoea, which is the failure to menstruate by age 15 in the presence of normal secondary sex characteristic development (American Society for Reproductive Medicine, 2008; Gordon et al., 2017). Oligomenorrhoea associated with the Triad is specifically defined as the presence of irregular and inconsistent menstrual cycle intervals of 36–90 days (De Souza et al., 2010). Oligomenorrhoeic cycles can present with or without an ovulatory event, and attention must be given to rule out irregular and inconsistent cycles that are secondary to hyperandrogenism (De Souza et al., 2010). Although the impact of severe menstrual disturbances on reproductive potential and fertility is unfavourable, consequences appear to be acute and do not cause permanent infertility (Beitins, McArthur, Turnbull, Skrinar, & Bullen, 1991; Bullen et al., 1985). Upon recovery of optimal energy status, exercising women with menstrual disturbances can recover normal menstrual function, allowing proper follicular growth and development and conception without complication (Beitins et al., 1991; Bullen et al., 1985; Dueck, Matt, Manore, & Skinner, 1996; Kopp-Woodroffe, Manore, Dueck, Skinner, & Matt, 1999).

Bone health in the Female Athlete Triad

Low energy availability and energy deficiency have both direct and indirect effects on bone health (discussed also in Chapter 7). The described metabolic perturbations that occur in response to inadequate energy intake, including decreased concentrations of leptin and IGF-1, have direct implications for bone formation (Combs, Nicholls, Duncan Bassett, & Williams, 2011; Guntur & Rosen, 2013; Turner et al., 2013). Specifically, leptin is an adipokine that upregulates osteoblast proliferation and bone formation, such that in mouse models, knock-out of leptin genes results in decreases in BMD and bone formation that are rescued with leptin administration (Turner et al., 2013). IGF-1, the majority of which is produced hepatically, is directly involved in osteoblast differentiation, and thus bone formation, and osteoblast-specific knock-out of IGF-1 results in decreased bone formation and bone mass (Govoni et al., 2007; Guntur & Rosen, 2013). While changes in metabolic hormones, as a direct result of energy deficiency, impair bone formation, energy deficiency indirectly impairs bone health through its impacts on the reproductive axis. As described on p. 74, suppression of reproduction at the level of the hypothalamus, pituitary, and ovaries results in downregulation of oestrogen and progesterone concentrations. One important role of oestrogen is to inhibit osteoblast apoptosis and promote osteoclast apoptosis resulting in a net effect of downregulation of bone resorption relative to bone formation (Weitzmann & Pacifici, 2006). If women are oestrogen deficient, as occurs in clinical and subclinical menstrual disturbances associated with the Triad, bone osteoclast activity is likely upregulated, promoting excess bone resorption.

With prolonged energy and oestrogen deficiency associated with the Triad, changes in bone metabolism result in measurable structural changes to bone that extend beyond changes in BMD, which can be assessed by both two- and three-dimensional bone imaging. Clinically, areal (two-dimensional) BMD can be assessed at the total body, hip, and/or spine to diagnose low BMD. In premenopausal women, Z-scores are used to assess the number of standard deviations an individual's BMD measurement is from an average measurement in a healthy reference population of her same age and ethnicity. In female athletes, a Z-score ≤ -1.0 is a red-flag for further investigation, especially considering the typical osteogenic benefit of sport participation (Nattiv et al., 2007). When low BMD is defined as a Z-score between -1.0 and -2.0 at the lumbar spine or hip, the prevalence of low BMD in athletes has been reported to be 0–40 per cent; more conservative approaches that define low BMD as a Z-score ≤ -2.0 result in a prevalence of 0–16 per cent in female athletes (Gibbs, Williams, & De Souza, 2013b). Dual energy X-ray absorptiometry measurements of hip geometry demonstrate compromised bone structure in addition to low BMD at the hip (Ackerman et al., 2013; Mallinson et al., 2016) and three-dimensional imaging techniques, such as peripheral quantitative computed tomography (pQCT) and high resolution pQCT reveal compromised volumetric BMD, bone geometry, bone microarchitecture, and estimated bone strength of the radius and tibia as a result of energy and/or oestrogen deficiency in female athletes (Ackerman et al., 2012; Southmayd, Mallinson, Williams, Mallinson, & De Souza, 2016).

The age at which an athlete experiences the Triad can have a profound impact on the severity of clinical outcomes. Specifically, if an athlete is energy- and oestrogen-suppressed during adolescence and young adulthood, she may be especially at risk for poor bone outcomes, as this is the window of time during which peak bone mass is achieved. Lifetime maximal BMD occurs by the end of the third decade of life and the time from puberty to the early 20s represents a crucial time period in which intrinsic and extrinsic factors have a potent ability to alter the course of bone modelling and remodelling. Failure to achieve an optimal peak bone mass during adolescence and young adulthood can predispose women to osteoporosis and related fragility fractures later in life, especially when the woman reaches menopause and experiences inevitable and dramatic declines in BMD (Weaver et al., 2016). More imminently, low BMD in athletes increases the risk of bone stress injury (e.g., stress fractures), which preclude participation in sport for weeks to months (Barrack et al., 2014). Up to 20 per cent of sports injuries are stress fractures (Fredericson, Jennings, Beaulieu, & Matheson, 2006), an estimated 80 per cent of which occur in the lower extremities (Kahanov, Eberman, Games, & Wasik, 2015). Compared to males, active females demonstrate a substantially greater proportion of all stress fracture cases as well. For instance, in a study of female military recruits, stress fracture incidence was 4 per cent in females while only 2 per cent in males (Sheehan et al., 2003). As the occurrence of one stress fracture increases the risk of future fractures (Rauh, Macera, Trone, Shaffer, & Brodine, 2006; Tenforde et al., 2017), it is important to address the underlying aetiology of bone stress injury, which is often due to energy and oestrogen deficiency associated with the Triad, before bone health is irreversibly compromised.

Unfortunately, depending on the severity of bone loss and the age at which suboptimal bone health occurs, it is not certain that bone can be fully recovered. Drinkwater and colleagues (Drinkwater et al., 1984) first demonstrated significantly lower BMD at the lumbar spine in amenorrhoeic compared to eumenorrhoeic distance runners, later reporting that in those that gained weight and resumed menstrual function, though BMD was improved compared to those that remained amenorrhoeic, BMD was still 12 per cent lower than the runners that had always been eumenorrhoeic (Drinkwater, Nilson, Ott, & Chesnut, 1986). Warren and colleagues (2002) replicated this finding in young ballerinas, reporting that amenorrhoeic dancers who resumed menses, while improving BMD by an average of 17 per cent, still had significantly lower BMD than dancers who were always eumenorrhoeic. Thus, the best strategy is to maintain bone health, as complete recovery of bone loss or a 'catch up' to healthy BMD is not guaranteed. For further information on bone health, see Chapter 7.

Treatment strategies for bone health in athletes with the Triad should address energy deficiency as the aetiological basis of Triad sequelae. Mallinson and colleagues (2013) published case studies detailing the benefits of increasing calorific intake over the course of 12 months in amenorrhoeic exercising women, reporting resumption of menses in concert with significant alterations in bone metabolism to favour bone formation and downregulate bone resorption. Despite the positive outcomes demonstrated with nutritional therapy, clinicians will often prescribe combined oral contraceptive (OC) therapy to 'regulate' menstrual function in those with menstrual disturbances; however, this strategy will result in withdrawal bleeding that masks menstrual dysfunction and does not address the energy deficiency component. Multiple studies demonstrate that OC therapy only results in modest, if any, increases in BMD in athletes and does not normalise BMD (Grinspoon et al., 2003; Rickenlund et al., 2004; Warren, Miller, Olson,

Grinspoon, & Friedman, 2005). The Female Athlete Triad Coalition promotes that athlete with the Triad should be treated with non-pharmacological treatment strategies, namely addressing energy deficiency with nutritional interventions, before pharmacological treatment strategies are considered (De Souza et al., 2014a, 2014b). If nutritional therapy for 1 year fails to improve health outcomes or if new fractures occur during non-pharmacological management, pharmacological strategies may be considered (De Souza et al., 2014a, 2014b). Due to the potential harmful effects of OC therapy on bone health due to hepatic first-pass effects suppressing IGF-1 concentrations and bone formation (Karlsson, Edén, & von Schoultz, 1990), transdermal oestrogen therapy with oral progestin is a potential alternative. Preliminary data in adolescent girls with anorexia nervosa suggest that just 6 months of transdermal oestrogen therapy with cyclic oral progestin can significantly increase lumbar spine BMD (Misra et al., 2011). Future research on such therapy in athletes with less severe energy deficiency associated with the Triad is warranted before this strategy becomes mainstream treatment.

Practical recommendations based on research

The Female Athlete Triad Coalition endorses the following recommendations for athletes with the Female Athlete Triad (De Souza et al., 2014a, 2014b):

- Screening for the Triad should take place as part of the preparticipation physical exam prior to sport participation. Screening questions should address risk factors including: (1) history of menstrual irregularities and amenorrhoea; (2) history of stress fractures; (3) history of critical comments about eating or weight from parent, coach, or teammate; (4) history of depression; (5) history of dieting; (6) personality factors like perfectionism and obsessiveness; (7) pressure to lose weight and/or frequent weight cycling; (8) early start of sport-specific training; (9) over-training; (10) recurrent and non-healing injuries; and (11) inappropriate coaching behaviour.
- When an athlete or exercising woman is diagnosed with the Triad, non-pharmacological nutritional therapy should be the first line of treatment. Nutrition therapy should aim to increase energy intake by ~20–30 per cent above baseline energy needs to result in a weight gain of 0.5 kg every 7–10 days. Weight monitoring may be used to track progress and compliance.
- If inadvertent undereating is the cause of low energy availability, nutritional education should be implemented by a sports dietitian.
- If eating disorders/disordered eating are present, proper psychological and/or nutritional counselling should be prescribed.
- A multidisciplinary team should be enlisted to best treat the athlete, including a sports medicine physician, athletic trainer, sports dietitian,

mental health practitioner, coaches, and parents, as appropriate and available for the athlete's level of training.

Real-world examples

Collegiate distance runner

Sarah was a 20-year-old runner on her university's varsity cross-country team. Her training consisted of running 50 miles (80 km) per week and weight training three days per week for 45 min per session. When Sarah started running at the collegiate level at age 18, her periods became irregular and by age 19 had stopped altogether. During this time, Sarah's bodyweight declined by ~2 kg, but her body fat percentage significantly decreased from 25 to 15 per cent. When Sarah suffered from a stress fracture in her tibia, she consulted a sports medicine physician, who diagnosed Sarah with the Female Athlete Triad. Sarah was advised to increase her food intake to support her exercise training, which she attempted by adding a protein bar before her workouts and switching from drinking skimmed milk to drinking low-fat milk for added calories. After six months of nutritional therapy, Sarah had gained 1 kg, resumed menses, and has not had a recurrent fracture.

Recreationally active woman

Megan is a 24-year-old woman who, between the ages of 21 and 23, lost about 13.5 kg by dieting and increasing her physical activity substantially. Megan is in 'the best shape of her life' and now partakes in recreational fitness, to include group fitness classes three times per week, running about five miles (8 km) twice a week, and occasional weight lifting at the gym. Megan's periods have been irregular for about a year, with cycle lengths ranging from 45–70 days. Megan's physician did a full workup to rule out hyperandrogenism and any other organic cause of menstrual disturbances, eventually prescribing combined OCs in order to 'regulate' Megan's cycles. After 6 months of OC use, Megan decided that she wanted to stop the pill due to side effects and her menstrual cycles returned to being irregular. Megan also began suffering from a nagging injury in her ankle that was slow to heal. Consequently, Megan had to take time off from exercising to rest her ankle and, in the span of one month, Megan gained 2 kg. When Megan's ankle healed and she returned to her exercise routine, she was surprised to see that her menstrual cycles became more normal, which she attributed to the small amount of weight gain and improved energy balance.

Summary

The Female Athlete Triad model represents over 30 years of research investigating the complex interrelationships between energy, reproduction, and bone, with the goal of maintaining the overall health and well-being of female athletes. Based on the evidence described, ensuring adequate nutritional intake is foundational for preserving optimal reproductive and bone function, and, although recovery from some aspects of the Triad are possible, it remains unclear whether complete recovery can be achieved. Based on this, efforts focused on the prevention, screening, and early identification of athletes at risk for development of the Triad is essential.

References

Ackerman, K. E., Pierce, L., Guereca, G., Slattery, M., Lee, H., Goldstein, M., & Misra, M. (2013). Hip structural analysis in adolescent and young adult oligo-amenorrheic and eumenorrheic athletes and nonathletes. *The Journal of Clinical Endocrinology and Metabolism, 98*(4), 1742–1749. https://doi.org/10.1210/jc.2013-1006.

Ackerman. K. E., Putman, M., Guereca, G., Taylor, A. P., Pierce, L., Herzog, D. B., ... Misra, M. (2012). Cortical microstructure and estimated bone strength in young amenorrheic athletes, eumenorrheic athletes and non-athletes. *Bone, 51*(4), 680–687. https://doi.org/10.1016/j.bone.2012.07.019.

American Society for Reproductive Medicine. (2008). Current evaluation of amenorrhea. *Fertility and Sterility, 90*(5 Suppl), S219–S225. https://doi.org/10.1016/j.fertnstert.2008.08.038.

Barrack, M. T., Gibbs, J. C., De Souza, M. J., Williams, N. I., Nichols, J. F., Rauh, M. J., & Nattiv, A. (2014). Higher incidence of bone stress injuries with increasing female athlete triad-related risk factors: A prospective multisite study of exercising girls and women. *The American Journal of Sports Medicine, 42*(4), 949–958. https://doi.org/10.1177/0363546513520295.

Beals, K. A., & Manore, M. M. (2002). Disorders of the female athlete triad among collegiate athletes. *International Journal of Sport Nutrition and Exercise Metabolism, 12*(3), 281–293.

Beitins, I. Z., McArthur, J. W., Turnbull, B. A., Skrinar, G. S., & Bullen, B. A. (1991). Exercise induces two types of human luteal dysfunction: Confirmation by urinary free progesterone. *The Journal of Clinical Endocrinology and Metabolsim, 72*(6), 1350–1358. https://doi.org/10.1210/jcem-72-6-1350.

Bullen, B. A., Skrinar, G. S., Beitins, I. Z., Vonmering, G., Turnbull, B. A., & Mcarthur, J. W. (1985). Induction of menstrual disorders by strenuous exercise in untrained women. *The New England Journal of Medicine, 312*(21), 1349–1353. https://doi.org/10.1056/Nejm198505233122103.

Combs, C. E., Nicholls, J. J., Duncan Bassett, J. H., & Williams, G. R. (2011). Thyroid hormones and bone development. *Minerva Endocrinologica, 36*(1), 71–85.

De Souza, M. J. (2003). Menstrual disturbances in athletes: A focus on luteal phase defects *Medicine & Science in Sports & Exercise, 35*(9), 1553–1563. https://doi.org/10.1249/01.MSS.0000084530.31478.DF.

De Souza, M. J., Hontscharuk, R., Olmsted, M., Kerr, G., & Williams, N. I. (2007). Drive for thinness score is a proxy indicator of energy deficiency in exercising women. *Appetite, 48*(3), 359–367. https://doi.org/10.1016/j.appet.2006.10.009.

De Souza, M. J., Lee, D. K., VanHeest, J. L., Scheid, J. L., West, S. L., & Williams, N. I. (2007). Severity of energy-related menstrual disturbances increases in proportion to indices of energy conservation in exercising women. *Fertility and Sterility, 88*(4), 971–975. https://doi.org/10.1016/j.fertnstert.2006.11.171.

De Souza, M. J., Leidy, H. J., O'Donnell, E., Lasley, B., & Williams, N. I. (2004). Fasting ghrelin levels in physically active women: Relationship with menstrual disturbances and metabolic hormones. *The Journal of Clinical Endocrinology & Metabolism, 89*(7), 3536–3542. https://doi.org/10.1210/jc.2003-032007.

De Souza, M. J., Miller, B. E., Loucks, A. B., Luciano, A. A., Pescatello, L. S., Campbell, C. G., & Lasley, B. L. (1998). High frequency of luteal phase deficiency and anovulation in recreational women runners: blunted elevation in follicle-stimulating hormone observed during luteal-follicular transition. *The Journal of Clinical Endocrinology & Metabolism, 83*(12), 4220–4232. https://doi.org/10.1210/jcem.83.12.5334.

De Souza, M. J., Nattiv, A., Joy, E., Misra, M., Williams, N. I., Mallinson, R. J., ... Matheson, G. (2014a). 2014 Female Athlete Triad Coalition consensus statement on treatment and return to play of the female athlete triad: 1st International Conference held in San Francisco, CA, May 2012, and 2nd International Conference held in Indianapolis, Indiana, May 2013. *Clinical Journal of Sport Medicine, 24*(2), 96–119. https://doi.org/10.1097/JSM.0000000000000085.

De Souza, M. J., Nattiv, A., Joy, E., Misra, M., Williams, N. I., Mallinson, R. J., ... Expert Panel. (2014b). 2014 Female Athlete Triad coalition consensus statement on treatment and return to play of the female athlete triad: 1st International Conference held in San Francisco, California, May 2012 and 2nd International Conference held in Indianapolis, Indiana, May 2013. *British Journal of Sports Medicine, 48*(4), 289. https://doi.org/10.1136/bjsports-2013-093218.

De Souza, M. J., Toombs, R. J., Scheid, J. L., O'Donnell, E., West, S. L., & Williams, N. I. (2010). High prevalence of subtle and severe menstrual disturbances in exercising women: Confirmation using daily hormone measures. *Human Reproduction, 25*(2), 491–503. https://doi.org/10.1093/humrep/dep411.

Dominguez, C. E., Laughlin, G. A., Nelson, J. C., & Yen, S. S. (1997). Altered binding of serum thyroid hormone to thyroxine-binding globulin in women with functional hypothalamic amenorrhea. *Fertility and Sterility, 68*(6), 992–996.

Donahoo, W. T., Levine, J. A., & Melanson, E. L. (2004). Variability in energy expenditure and its components. *Current Opinion in Clinical Nutrition & Metabolic Care, 7*(6), 599–605.

Drinkwater, B. L., Nilson, K., Chesnut, C. H., 3rd, Bremner, W. J., Shainholtz, S., & Southworth, M. B. (1984). Bone mineral content of amenorrheic and eumenorrheic athletes. *The New England Journal of Medicine, 311*(5), 277–281. https://doi.org/10.1056/NEJM198408023110501.

Drinkwater, B. L., Nilson, K., Ott, S., & Chesnut, C. H., 3rd. (1986). Bone mineral density after resumption of menses in amenorrheic athletes. *Journal of the American Medical Association, 256*(3), 380–382.

Dueck, C. A., Matt, K. S., Manore, M. M., & Skinner, J. S. (1996). Treatment of athletic amenorrhea with a diet and training intervention program. *International Journal of Sport Nutrition, 6*(1), 24–40.

Fahrenholtz, I. L., Sjödin, A., Benardot, D., Tornberg, A. B., Skouby, S., Faber, J., ... Melin, A. K. (2017). Within-day energy deficiency and reproductive function in female endurance athletes. *Scandinavian Journal of Medicine & Science in Sports.* https://doi.org/10.1111/sms.13030.

Fredericson, M., Jennings, F., Beaulieu, C., & Matheson, G. O. (2006). Stress fractures in athletes. *Topics in Magnetic Resonance Imaging, 17*(5), 309–325. https://doi.org/10.1097/RMR.0b013e3180421c8c.

Garner, D. M. (1991). *Eating disorder inventory-2. Professional manual.* Odessa, FL: Psychological Assessment Research.

Gibbs, J. C., Williams, N. I., & De Souza, M. J. (2013a). Prevalence of individual and combined components of the female athlete triad. *Medicine & Science in Sports & Exercise, 45*(5), 985–996. https://doi.org/10.1249/MSS.0b013e31827e1bdc.

Gibbs, J. C., Williams, N. I., & De Souza, M. J. (2013b). Prevalence of individual and combined components of the female athlete triad. *Medicine & Science in Sports & Exercise, 45*(5), 985–996. https://doi.org/10.1249/MSS.0b013e31827e1bdc.

Gibbs, J. C., Williams, N. I., Scheid, J. L., Toombs, R. J., & De Souza, M. J. (2011). The association of a high drive for thinness with energy deficiency and severe menstrual disturbances: confirmation in a large population of exercising women. *International Journal of Sport Nutrition and Exercise Metabolism, 21*(4), 280–290.

Gordon, C. M., Ackerman, K. E., Berga, S. L., Kaplan, J. R., Mastorakos, G., Misra, M., ... Warren, M. P. (2017). Functional hypothalamic amenorrhea: An Endocrine Society Clinical Practice Guideline. *The Journal of Clinical Endocrinology and Metabolism.* https://doi.org/10.1210/jc.2017-00131.

Govoni, K. E., Wergedal, J. E., Florin, L., Angel, P., Baylink, D. J., & Mohan, S. (2007). Conditional deletion of insulin-like growth factor-I in collagen type 1alpha2-expressing cells results in postnatal lethality and a dramatic reduction in bone accretion. *Endocrinology, 148*(12), 5706–5715. https://doi.org/10.1210/en.2007-0608.

Grinspoon, S. K., Friedman, A. J., Miller, K. K., Lippman, J., Olson, W. H., & Warren, M. P. (2003). Effects of a triphasic combination oral contraceptive containing norgestimate/ethinyl estradiol on biochemical markers of bone metabolism in young women with osteopenia secondary to hypothalamic amenorrhea. *The Journal of Clinical Endocrinology & Metabolism, 88*(8), 3651–3656. https://doi.org/10.1210/jc.2003-030033.

Guntur, A. R., & Rosen, C. J. (2013). IGF-1 regulation of key signaling pathways in bone. *BoneKEy Reports, 2,* 437. https://doi.org/10.1038/bonekey.2013.171.

Harber, V. J., Petersen, S. R., & Chilibeck, P. D. (1998). Thyroid hormone concentrations and muscle metabolism in amenorrheic and eumenorrheic athletes. *Canadian Journal of Applied Physiology, 23*(3), 293–306.

Heaney, S., O'Connor, H., Gifford, J., & Naughton, G. (2010). Comparison of strategies for assessing nutritional adequacy in elite female athletes' dietary intake. *International Journal of Sport Nutrition and Exercise Metabolism, 20*(3), 245–256.

Hoch, A. Z., Pajewski, N. M., Moraski, L., Carrera, G. F., Wilson, C. R., Hoffmann, R. G., ... Gutterman, D. D. (2009). Prevalence of the female athlete triad in high school athletes and sedentary students. *Clinical Journal of Sport Medicine, 19*(5) 421–428. https://doi.org/10.1097/JSM.0b013e3181b8c136.

Ihle, R. & Loucks, A. B. (2004). Dose-response relationships between energy availability and bone turnover in young exercising women. *Journal of Bone Mineral Research, 19*(8), 1231–1240. https://doi.org/10.1359/JBMR.040410.

Joy, E., Kussman, A., & Nattiv, A. (2016). 2016 update on eating disorders in athletes: A comprehensive narrative review with a focus on clinical assessment and management. *British Journal of Sports Medicine, 50*(3), 154–162. https://doi.org/10.1136/bjsports-2015-095735.

Kahanov, L., Eberman, L. E., Games, K. E., & Wasik, M. (2015). Diagnosis, treatment, and rehabilitation of stress fractures in the lower extremity in runners. *Open Access Journal of Sports Medicine, 6,* 87–95. https://doi.org/10.2147/OAJSM.S39512.

Karlsson, R., Edén, S., & von Schoultz, B. (1990). Altered growth hormone secretion during oral contraception. *Gynecologic and Obstetric Investigation, 30*(4), 234–238. https://doi.org/10.1159/000293276.

Kopp-Woodroffe, S. A., Manore, M. M., Dueck, C. A., Skinner, J. S., & Matt, K. S. (1999). Energy and nutrient status of amenorrheic athletes participating in a diet and exercise training intervention program. *International Journal of Sport Nutrition, 9*(1), 70–88.

Laughlin, G. A., & Yen, S. S. (1996). Nutritional and endocrine-metabolic aberrations in amenorrheic athletes. *Journal of Clinical Endocrinology & Metabolism, 81*(12), 4301–4309.

Lieberman, J. L., De Souza, M. J., Wagstaff, D. A., & Williams, N. I. (2017). Menstrual disruption with exercise is not linked to an energy availability threshold. *Medicine & Science in Sports & Exercise, 50*(3), 551–561. https://doi.org/10.1249/MSS.0000000000001451.

Loucks, A. B. (2007). Low energy availability in the marathon and other endurance sports. *Sports Medicine, 37*(4–5), 348–352. https://doi.org/10.2165/00007256-200737040-00019.

Loucks, A. B., & Thuma, J. R. (2003). Luteinizing hormone pulsatility is disrupted at a threshold of energy availability in regularly menstruating women. *Journal of Clinical Endocrinology & Metabolism, 88*(1), 297–311. https://doi.org/10.1210/jc.2002-020369.

Loucks, A. B., Verdun, M., & Heath, E. M. (1998). Low energy availability, not stress of exercise, alters LH pulsatility in exercising women. *Journal of Applied Physiology (1985), 84*(1), 37–46.

Mallinson, R. J., Williams, N. I., Gibbs, J. C., Koehler, K., Allaway, H. C., Southmayd, E., & De Souza, M. J. (2016). Current and past menstrual status is an important determinant of femoral neck geometry in exercising women. *Bone, 88,* 101–112. https://doi.org/10.1016/j.bone.2016.01.030.

Mallinson, R. J., Williams, N. I., Olmsted, M. P., Scheid, J. L., Riddle, E. S., & De Souza, M. J. (2013). A case report of recovery of menstrual function following a nutritional intervention in two exercising women with amenorrhea of varying duration. *Journal of the International Society of Sports Nutrition, 10,* 34. https://doi.org/10.1186/1550-2783-10-34.

McNeely, M. J., & Soules, M. R. (1988). The diagnosis of luteal phase deficiency: A critical review. *Fertility and Sterility, 50*(1), 1–15.

Misra, M., Katzman, D., Miller, K. K., Mendes, N., Snelgrove, D., Russell, M., … Klibanski, A. (2011). Physiologic estrogen replacement increases bone density in adolescent girls with anorexia nervosa. *Journal of Bone and Mineral Research, 26*(10), 2430–2438. https://doi.org/10.1002/jbmr.447.

Myerson, M., Gutin, B., Warren, M. P., May, M. T., Contento, I., Lee, M., … Brooks-Gunn, J. (1991). Resting metabolic rate and energy balance in amenorrheic and eumenorrheic runners. *Medicine & Science in Sports & Exercise, 23*(1), 15–22.

Nattiv, A., Agostini, R., Drinkwater, B., & Yeager, K. K. (1994). The female athlete triad. The inter-relatedness of disordered eating, amenorrhea, and osteoporosis. *Clinics in Sports Medicine, 13*(2), 405–418.

Nattiv, A , Loucks, A. B., Manore, M. M., Sanborn, C. F., Sundgot-Borgen, J., & Warren M. P. (2007). American College of Sports Medicine position stand. The female athlete triad. *Medicine & Science in Sports & Exercise, 39*(10), 1867–1882. https://doi.org/10.1249/mss.0b013e318149f111.

Otis, C. L , Drinkwater, B., Johnson, M., Loucks, A., & Wilmore, J. (1997). American College of Sports Medicine position stand. The Female Athlete Triad. *Medicine & Science in Sports & Exercise, 29*(5), i–ix.

Rauh, M. J., Macera, C. A., Trone, D. W., Shaffer, R. A., & Brodine, S. K. (2006). Epidemiology of stress fracture and lower-extremity overuse injury in female recruits *Medicine & Science in Sports & Exercise, 38*(9), 1571–1577. https://doi.org/10.1249/01.mss.0000227543.51293.9d.

Rickenlurd, A., Carlström, K., Ekblom, B., Brismar, T. B., Von Schoultz, B., & Hirschberg, A. L. (2004). Effects of oral contraceptives on body composition and physical performance in female athletes. *The Journal of Clinical Endocrinology & Metabolism, 89*(9), 4364–4370. https://doi.org/10.1210/jc.2003-031334.

Scheid, J. L., Williams, N. I., West, S. L., VanHeest, J. L., & De Souza, M. J. (2009). Elevated PYY is associated with energy deficiency and indices of subclinical disordered eating in exercising women with hypothalamic amenorrhea. *Appetite 52*(1), 184–192. https://doi.org/10.1016/j.appet.2008.09.016.

Sheehan, K. M., Murphy, M. M., Reynolds, K., Creedon, J. F., White, J., & Kazel, M. (2003). The response of a bone resorption marker to marine recruit training. *Military Medicine, 168*(10), 797–801.

Soules, M. R., McLachlan, R. I., Ek, M., Dahl, K. D., Cohen, N. L., & Bremner, W. J. (1989). Luteal phase deficiency: Characterization of reproductive hormones over the menstrual cycle. *The Journal of Clinical Endocrinology & Metabolism, 69*(4), 804–812. https://doi.org/10.1210/jcem-69-4-804.

Southmayd, E. A., Mallinson, R. J., Williams, N. I., Mallinson, D. J., & De Souza, M. J. (2016). Unique effects of energy versus estrogen deficiency on multiple components of bone strength in exercising women. *Osteoporosis International, 28*(4), 1365–1376. https://doi.org/10.1007/s00198-016-3887-x.

Sundgot-Borgen, J. (1993). Prevalence of eating disorders in elite female athletes. *International Journal of Sport Nutrition, 3*(1), 29–40.

Sundgot-Borgen, J., & Torstveit, M. K. (2004). Prevalence of eating disorders in elite athletes is higher than in the general population. *Clinical Journal of Sport Medicine, 14*(1), 25–32.

Tenforde A. S., Barrack, M. T., Nattiv, A., & Fredericson, M. (2016). Parallels with the female athlete triad in male athletes. *Sports Medicine, 46*(2), 171–182. https://doi.org/10.1007/s40279-015-0411-y.

Tenforde A. S., Carlson, J. L., Chang, A., Sainani, K. L., Shultz, R., Kim, J. H., … Fredericson, M. (2017). Association of the female athlete triad risk assessment stratification to the development of bone stress injuries in collegiate athletes. *The American Journal of Sports Medicine, 45*(2), 302–310. https://doi.org/10.1177/0363546516676262.

Thong, F. S., McLean, C., & Graham, T. E. (2000). Plasma leptin in female athletes: relationship with body fat, reproductive, nutritional, and endocrine factors. *Journal of Applied Physiology, 88*(6), 2037–2044.

Turner, R. T., Kalra, S. P., Wong, C. P., Philbrick, K. A., Lindenmaier, L. B., Boghossian, S., & Iwaniec, U. T. (2013). Peripheral leptin regulates bone formation. *Journal of Bone and Mineral Research, 28*(1), 22–34. https://doi.org/10.1002/jbmr.1734.

Vescovi, J. D., & VanHeest, J. L. (2016). Case Study: Impact of Inter- and Intra-Day Energy parameters on bone health, menstrual function, and hormones in an elite junior female triathlete. *International Journal of Sport Nutrition and Exercise Metabolsim, 26*(4), 363–369. https://doi.org/10.1123/ijsnem.2015-0282.

Wade, G. N., & Schneider, J. E. (1992). Metabolic fuels and reproduction in female mammals. *Neuroscience Biobehavioral Review, 16*(2), 235–272.

Warren, M. P., Brooks-Gunn, J., Fox, R. P., Holderness, C. C., Hyle, E. P., & Hamilton, W. G. (2002). Osteopenia in exercise-associated amenorrhea using ballet dancers as a model: A longitudinal study. *The Journal of Clinical Endocrinology & Metabolism, 87*(7), 3162–3168. https://doi.org/10.1210/jcem.87.7.8637.

Warren, M. P., Miller, K. K., Olson, W. H., Grinspoon, S. K., & Friedman, A. J. (2005). Effects of an oral contraceptive (norgestimate/ethinyl estradiol) on bone mineral density in women with hypothalamic amenorrhea and osteopenia: An open-label extension of a double-blind, placebo-controlled study. *Contraception, 72*(3), 206–211. https://doi.org/10.1016/j.contraception.2005.03.007.

Waters, D. L., Qualls, C. R., Dorin, R., Veldhuis, J. D., & Baumgartner, R. N. (2001). Increased pulsatility, process irregularity, and nocturnal trough concentrations of growth hormone in amenorrheic compared to eumenorrheic athletes. *The Journal of Clinical Endocrinology & Metabolism, 86*(3), 1013–1019. https://doi.org/10.1210/jcem.86.3.7361.

Weaver, C. M., Gordon, C. M., Janz, K. F., Kalkwarf, H. J., Lappe, J. M., Lewis, R., ... Zemel, B. S. (2016). The National Osteoporosis Foundation's position statement on peak bone mass development and lifestyle factors: A systematic review and implementation recommendations. *Osteoporosis International, 27*(4), 1281–1386. https://doi.org/10.1007/s00198-015-3440-3.

Weitzmann, M. N., & Pacifici, R. (2006). Estrogen deficiency and bone loss: An inflammatory tale. *The Journal of Clinical Investigation, 116*(5), 1186–1194. https://doi.org/10.1172/JCI28550.

Williams, N. I., Caston-Balderrama, A. L., Helmreich, D. L., Parfitt, D. B., Nosbisch, C., & Cameron, J. L. (2001). Longitudinal changes in reproductive hormones and menstrual cyclicity in cynomolgus monkeys during strenuous exercise training: Abrupt transition to exercise-induced amenorrhea. *Endocrinology, 142*(6), 2381–2389. https://doi.org/10.1210/endo.142.6.8113.

Williams, N. I., Helmreich, D. L., Parfitt, D. B., Caston-Balderrama, A., & Cameron, J. L. (2001). Evidence for a causal role of low energy availability in the induction of menstrual cycle disturbances during strenuous exercise training. *The Journal of Clinical Endocrinology & Metabolism, 86*(11), 5184–5193. https://doi.org/10.1210/jcem.86.11.8024.

7 Bone health and the exercising female

Jacky Forsyth and Karen Hind

Introduction

The benefits of regular exercise throughout the lifespan are well recognised, with certain types of exercise more beneficial to bone than others. In contrast, high levels of endurance exercise, and participation in sports that emphasise leanness, have been associated with low bone strength, bone loss, and elevated stress fracture risk. In females, these skeletal problems are mainly reported in athletes displaying Female Athlete Triad conditions, arising from relative energy deficit and/or functional hypothalamic amenorrhoea.

In this chapter, the following will be addressed: the issues that the exercising female may encounter due to low bone density as a result of relative energy deficit (purposeful or inadvertent), menstrual dysfunction, and endogenous and exogenous changes in oestrogen that occur across the lifespan; and how to optimise bone health for the exercising female, to ensure athletic success, and longevity of an athletic career.

Aims of the chapter

The aims of the chapter are as follows:

1   To examine the physiological processes involved in bone remodelling, and the effect of oestrogen and energy deficiency on bone turnover.
2   To evaluate the research on the interplay between endocrinology, exercise, and bone health.
3   To examine strategies to support bone health for the exercising female and how to effectively maximise bone strength.

Osteoporosis

Osteoporosis is characterised by low bone mineral density (BMD) and architectural deterioration of bone. For women, bone loss and osteoporosis are of particularly concern, since around 50 per cent of females suffer an osteoporotic fracture in their lifetime (Randell et al., 1995). Common sites of fragility fracture are the femoral neck, distal radius, and vertebrae. Fractures can lead to a loss of independence, a reduction in quality of life, and an increase in premature mortality. Osteoporosis is known as a 'silent disease' in that bone loss is not realised until fracture. Thereafter, secondary prevention is key. Nonetheless, the most tangible approach to reducing fracture risk is through primary prevention. The maximisation of bone mass during adolescence, maintaining optimal bone mass during the premenopausal years, and reducing the rate of postmenopausal bone loss are critical for avoiding osteoporotic bone fracture.

The measurement of bone

The most widely used and universally recognised method for bone health assessment is dual energy X-ray absorptiometry (DXA). This method provides a highly precise measurement of BMD (Carey & Delaney, 2017; Hind, Oldroyd, & Truscott, 2010), and uses low iodising radiation with bone density evaluations typically equivalent, or less, than 2 days of natural background radiation. A bone density assessment by DXA usually includes scans of both the lumbar spine and total hip, with each scan only taking several minutes. Areal BMD (g/cm^2) measured by DXA is a robust predictor of fracture risk (Cummings et al., 1993). The Z- and T-score scales measure the deviation from age- and sex-matched and young normal mean values, respectively, and are calibrated in SD (standard deviation) units. A 1-SD decline in BMD results in around a doubling of fracture risk (Marshall, Johnell, & Wedel, 1996).

In postmenopausal females, osteoporosis is defined as a BMD T-score that is −2.5 or less, and osteopaenia as a BMD T-score that is between −1.0 and −2.4 (Kanis & Kanis, 1994). In people aged under 50 years, low BMD is identified as a Z-score that is equal to or less than −2.0, although −1.0 also indicates suboptimum BMD, particularly for exercising females who require stronger bones for repetitive or higher impact activities. The definitions of osteoporosis and low BMD for age, are further described in the official Positions of the International Society for Clinical Densitometry (Schousboe, Shepherd, Bilezikian, & Baim, 2013).

Volumetric BMD is assessed using medical imaging such as peripheral quantitative computed tomography (pQCT). This method can clearly distinguish between the different types of bone tissue, and high resolution pQCT systems provide advanced information on the bone microarchitecture, which is an independent risk factor for fracture. Over the last decade, studies of bone architecture in female athletes from various sports demonstrate the osteogenic effects of loading (e.g., Kontulainen, Sievänen, Kannus, Pasanen, & Vuori, 2003; Nikander, Sievänen, Uusi-Rasi, Heinonen, & Kannus, 2006). Athletes with amenorrhoea demonstrate lower cortical volumetric BMD (Ackerman et al., 2011), which suggests an increased risk of fracture as a result of menstrual disturbances.

Bone structure and bone turnover

There are two types of bone tissue – cortical and trabecular, which differ according to structure, function, and location. In cortical bone, the structural unit is the Haversian system or osteon, which runs the length of the bone, and consists of concentric layers or lamellae. Cortical bone has a high resistance to torque, and has a slow bone turnover rate. It is found on the outer surfaces of most bones and in the shafts of long bones.

Trabecular bone consists of a matrix, called trabeculae. This mesh-like design enables trabecular bone to withstand sudden stresses that occur through the joints during loading. Bone remodelling takes place predominantly within trabecular bone, and it is where haematopoiesis and mineral (calcium and phosphate) metabolism take place. Trabecular bone is more associated with osteoporosis, and more sensitive to oestrogen deficiency (Beerthuizen et al., 2000). It is found mainly at the ends of long bones, and in the internal portions of other bones, such as the spine and pelvis. Approximately 80 per cent of the skeleton consists of cortical bone, and 20 per cent of trabecular bone (Eriksen, Axelrod, & Melsen, 1994).

There are five main types of bone cell: bone-lining cells, osteoprogenitor cells, osteoblasts, osteocytes, and osteoclasts. Bone-lining cells remain on the bone surface when there is no active bone growth. Osteoprogenitor cells are derived from mesenchymal stem cells, and differentiate into osteoblasts, the bone-forming cells, found at the bone surface. Osteocytes are the mature bone cells, found deep within the bone matrix in small lacunae (spaces), and are also central to mechanotransduction (sensing and responding to mechanical loading). Osteoclasts, derived from osteoclastic precursors, develop and differentiate to become mature, bone-resorbing cells.

Throughout life, bone is in a constant state of remodelling through bone resorption (removal) and bone formation. Bone remodelling occurs in response to the need for calcium in the extracellular fluid, to mechanical stress on the bone (e.g., through exercise), and to changes in hormones. Following bone resorption, osteoblasts migrate to the resorption pit, and secrete collagen and various proteins, creating osteoid, which is uncalcified bone tissue. Osteoblasts assist with the calcification of the osteoid, involving the secretion of alkaline phosphatase, osteocalcin, and osteonectin (Florencio-Silva et al., 2015). The whole remodelling cycle takes approximately three months.

Endocrine and hormone effects

Bone turnover is modulated by a wide variety of hormones/endocrine activity. Of primary importance for women's bone health is the hormone oestrogen, which comprises a group of steroid hormones (oestradiol, oestriol, and oestrone), produced by the ovaries in women and in small amounts by the male testes and adrenal cortex. Oestrogen has a necessary role in the development and maintenance of BMD. Deficiencies, such as that arising from the menopause, can bring rapid bone loss. Oestrogen deficiency can also occur in young women, who exercise excessively and/or eat too little; secondary hypothalamic amenorrhoea (present when a female, with previously normal menstrual cycles, has fewer than three menstrual cycles per year) is an acquired gonadal-releasing hormone deficiency, leading to ovarian suppression, and a deficiency of the sex steroids.

The interaction of oestrogen within the bone remodelling process involves tumour necrosis factor (TNF) cells: RANKL (the name is derived from Receptor Activator of Nuclear factor Kappa-B Ligand), RANK (Receptor Activator of Nuclear factor Kappa-B), and osteoprotegerin (OPG) (Rosen, 2013; Scheurer, 2013). RANKL is expressed by osteoblasts, and plays a key role in bone resorption, through its binding with its receptor, RANK, which is expressed on the surface of osteoclast precursors. This binding activates signalling pathways that promote fusion, differentiation, and maturation of osteoclasts. Osteoblasts also express OPG, which works as a decoy receptor for RANKL, by preventing the binding of RANKL to RANK.

With optimal oestrogen levels, RANKL expression by osteoblasts is inhibited, and OPG blocks the binding of RANKL to RANK; osteoclastic activity is reduced. Suboptimal levels of oestrogen (leading to an increase in pro-inflammatory cytokines, such as interleukin-1 [IL-1]) result in an increased expression of RANKL (Schett, 2011). Osteoprotegerin, which also decreases, is unable to block the binding of RANKL to RANK, being overwhelmed by the excessive expression of RANKL. Increased osteoclastic activity results and outstrips the pace of osteoblastic activity, leading to net bone loss (Marques et al., 2013; Xiong & O'Brien, 2012). Oestrogen also exerts its influence on bone formation through an increase in pro-inflammatory cytokines (Manolagas, 2013).

There are several other hormones, relevant to women that can influence bone metabolism. Increases in follicle-stimulating hormone (FSH) (for example during the perimenopause, prior to a notable reduction in oestrogen, or in subclinical menstrual dysfunction) can impact bone metabolism through osteoclast FSH receptors and FSH-increased expression of RANKL (Colaianni, Cuscito, & Colucci, 2013). Reductions in testosterone promote osteoclastogenesis and decrease bone formation and calcium absorption (Chen, Kaji, Kanatani, Sugimoto, & Chihara, 2004). In women, as in men, androgens also have independent effects on bone development (Manolagas, O'Brien, & Almeida, 2013).

Exercise and bone health

Bone adapts to its habitual loading environment and responds to a wide range of biochemical and physical stimuli. In particular, the musculoskeletal loading sustained during exercise is a major osteogenic stimulus. Exercise has an undisputed role for the attainment of peak bone mass, and the subsequent maintenance of bone as a prophylaxis against osteoporosis. The mechanism by which bone adapts to loading is well described in the mechanostat theory (Frost, 1987), which proposes that survival of the skeleton depends or the functional coordination of bone modelling and remodelling, and that when all else is equal, individuals who are physically active will possess stronger bones than their less active peers. Evidencing the mechanostat, superior bone strength is frequently reported in female athletes from sports such as gymnastics, running, and alpine skiing compared to non-athletic peers or athletes from non-weightbearing sports (Hind, Gannon, Whatley, Cooke, & Truscott, 2012; Sievänen et al., 2015), as well as positive skeletal effects from impact- or resistance-exercise (Tucker, Strong, LeCheminant, & Bailey, 2015; Watson et al., 2018).

Cellular responses to loading

At the molecular level, osteocytes sense bone loading through impacts (gravitational) or directly from muscle forces upon bone. Osteocyte mechanosensation is facilitated through plasma membrane disruption (Yu et al., 2017). When bone is loaded, movement of interstitial fluid creates shear stress on the cell membrane of the osteocytes instigating mechanotransduction processes (Robling & Turner, 2009). Osteocytes respond through calcium signalling to osteoblasts and osteoclasts (Marques et al., 2013), which leads to a decrease in RANKL/OPG ratio (Robling & Turner, 2009). Loading of bone also downregulates sclerostin expression via osteocytes (Xiong & O'Brien, 2012), which increases bone formation via relieving inhibition of canonical Wnt signalling in osteoblasts and through regulating OPG, which suppresses the resorptive activity of osteoclasts (Galea, Lanyon, & Price, 2017).

Optimal exercise for bone health

Animal studies have provided important insights for our understanding of the key components of an optimal exercise programme. It has been clearly demonstrated that dynamic rather than static loads, high strain magnitudes, high strain rates, rapid strain reversal, and unusual frequency distributions provide optimal osteogenic stimuli (Ehrlich & Lanyon, 2002; Rubin, Sommerfeldt, Judex, & Qin, 2001). The duration of load and the number of loading cycles appear to be of minor importance, whereas rest periods between bouts of loading have a positive role (Robling, Burr, & Turner, 2000).

In humans, exercise that mimics the loading patterns identified in animal studies, have been successful in increasing bone health. For instance, jumping interventions are particularly efficacious for improving femoral BMD, and especially if undertaken as short-discrete bouts (Babatunde & Forsyth, 2013; Babatunde, Forsyth, & Gidlow, 2012; Martyn-St James & Carroll, 2010; Zhao, Zhao, & Zhang, 2014). In contrast, walking and jogging bring about relatively modest improvements in bone health (Martyn-St James & Carroll, 2008; Palombaro, 2005), likely reflecting the habituation and desensitisation to the continuous loading and repetitive nature of these activities. Athletes involved in non-weightbearing sports, such as cyclists, can have lower BMD than athletes participating in weightbearing sports, to a level that is similar to, or less than, their non-active peers (Campion et al., 2010; Hind et al., 2012). It is also important to consider that the skeletal response to loading is localised to the focus of strain, which means that any changes in bone mass and structure are site specific. This localisation is clearly demonstrated through greater bone strength in the dominant versus non-dominant forearms of racquet sports' players (Ducher, Tournaire, Meddahi-Pellé, Berhamou, & Courteix, 2006; Kontulainen et al., 2003), in the upper body of gymnasts (Burt, Greene, Ducher, & Naughton, 2013), and in the greater BMD of the lower limbs compared to the spine in long-distance runners (Hind, Truscott, & Evans, 2006).

As well as gravitational loading, skeletal muscles provide an osteogenic driving force. Resistance training programmes can be designed to develop muscle and bone strength throughout the whole body and resistance can be adjusted to suit the level of the individual. Regular strength training is associated with higher BMD in female distance runners regardless of amenorrhoea (Hind et al., 2006), and in intervention studies improved BMD in premenopausal women and prematurely menopausal women have been reported following resistance training (Watson et al., 2018; Winters-Stone et al., 2013). From the evidence to date, exercise programmes should include not only gravitational, impact loading to the skeleton, but also exercises that develop muscle strength.

The Female Athlete Triad and bone health

The Female Athlete Triad is characterised by the three inter-related components of low energy availability, altered menstrual function, and low BMD. Reduced energy availability or relative energy deficit is the key driver of the Triad and occurs when there is a failure to match calorific energy intake with exercise energy expenditure. Over time, energy deficit can negatively affect bone health in female athletes through: (a) effects on the hypothalamic-pituitary-ovarian axis; and (b) effects on metabolic hormones and substrates. The Triad is covered in more detail in Chapter 6.

Athletes with longstanding functional hypothalamic amenorrhoea have been shown to benefit less from the osteogenic effects of exercise (Ackerman et al., 2012; Bonis, Loftin, Speaker, & Kontos, 2009). Even subtle alterations in the oestrogen/progesterone imbalance (e.g., regular menstruation but alterations in luteinising hormone), as seen in subclinical ovulatory disturbances, may adversely impact bone, particularly at trabecular-bone-dominant sites, such as the spine (Li, Hitchcock, Barr, Yu, & Prior, 2014). With optimal levels of oestrogen, exercise brings a greater osteogenic response than either exercise alone or oestrogen alone (Balasch, 2003).

Other endocrine disturbances from energy deficit include hypercortisolaemia, growth hormone resistance, reductions in insulin-like growth factor-1 (IGF-1) and suppressed 3,5,3 triiodothyronine ('low T3 syndrome') (Zanker & Cooke, 2004). Each have been shown to influence bone turnover; for example, hypercortisolaemia limits osteoblastic function and increases osteoclastic activity (Bressot et al., 1979), while reductions in IGF-1 retard the activity of osteoblasts and bone collagen synthesis (Yakar et al., 2002). In studies where an energy deficit has been experimentally induced in exercising females, significant reductions in IGF-1 and total triiodothyronine (TT_3), with corresponding reductions in bone formation, have been demonstrated, indicating that low energy availability directly affects bone metabolism (Ihle & Loucks, 2004). Prolonged relative energy deficit also brings disruptions in the body's nitrogen balance (Zanker & Cooke, 2004), which can lead to further negative effects on skeletal integrity through a loss of muscle mass and muscle strength (Kortebein, Ferrando, Lombeida, Wolfe, & Evans, 2007).

In the short-term, amenorrhoea and energy deficit in female athletes are associated with an increased risk for skeletal injury such as stress fracture and stress reaction (Barrack et al., 2014). There have been case reports of displaced femoral-neck fractures in amenorrhoeic female long-distance runners after continuing to run on untreated femoral-neck stress fractures (Goolsby, Barrack, & Nattiv, 2012; Okamoto, Arai, Hara, Tsuzihara, & Kubo, 2010). These athletes also had a history of disordered eating and low body mass. The long-term effects on bone strength are unclear but researchers indicate that, in some cases, bone density is recoverable through weight gains and resumption of menses, at least by the age of 30 years (Hind, 2008; Hind, Zanker, & Truscott, 2011).

Contraceptives and bone health

The effects of contraceptives on bone health and performance in female athletes has been a topic of much interest over the last few decades. Hormone-based contraceptives are used, by some, for the purposes of regulating or manipulating menses and associated symptoms, as well for its intended purpose (see Chapter 4 for a full review). The BMD of combined oral contraceptive (OC) users has been found to be lower than that of non-users (Hartard et al., 2007; Prior et al., 2001), although many researchers have found no change in BMD with OC use (e.g., Hind, Truscott, & Carroll, 2008; Nappi, Bifulco, Tommaselli, Gargano, & Di Carlo, 2012). The mixed findings concerned with OC use might be explained by the ratio of progesterone to oestradiol found in the different OC preparations (Nappi et al., 2012), and the type of concomitant exercise undertaken. The use of OCs might also lower the set point for mechanical adaptation as a result of exercise (Hartard, Bottermann, Bartenstein, Jeschke, & Schwaiger, 1997; Weaver et al., 2001).

Using progesterone-only contraception, in particular Depot Medroxyprogesterone Acetate (DMPA), also known as Depo-Provera®, can decrease BMD, especially with sustained use, among adolescents and with advancing age (Curtis & Martins, 2006; Shaarawy, El-Mallah, Seoudi, Hassan, & Mohsen, 2006). The use of DMPA and concurrent engagement in high levels of exercise may not be as beneficial to bone health as exercise undertaken without DMPA use (Babatunde & Forsyth, 2014). In the hypo-oestrogenic state, mechanical strain, brought about through exercise, could downregulate oestrogen receptor-alpha (ERα) expression (Zaman, Cheng, Jessop, White, & Lanyon, 2000) and hence impair the osteocytes' signalling capability. It is, therefore, important, to self-regulate hormone-based contraceptive use, and to check bone health and oestrogen status regularly.

The menopause, exercise, and bone health

The menopause (which is reviewed in Chapter 20) can negatively impact bone metabolism and lead to net bone loss. In response, there have been numerous studies to explore the effectiveness of exercise for protecting bone health in postmenopausal women. The results have been mixed and are likely to reflect differences in exercise modalities and exercise compliance (Howe et al., 2011; Kelley & Kelley, 2006). In interventions that have included high-impact activity, such as impact loading and jumping, BMD improvements have been modest (Bolton et al., 2012), although others have reported more beneficial osteogenic effects (Borer, Fogleman, Gross, La New, & Dengel, 2007). Positive effects have also been reported from interventions where high-magnitude joint loading has been achieved through resistance training (Marques, Mota, & Carvalho, 2012; Watson, Weeks, Weis, Horan, & Beck, 2015). Exercise for this population may counteract the negative effects of hypo-oestrogenism, but it needs to be targeted.

Practical recommendations based on research

- Exercising females should ensure that energy needs are well balanced with sufficient energy intake to support normal menstruation and bone health and reduce the risk of injuries including stress fracture.
- The Female Athlete Triad includes negative consequences for bone strength and, therefore, exercising females, their coaches, and support teams, should recognise signs, and seek positive interventions.
- Training programmes for the exercising female, regardless of age or menstrual status, should consist of bone-targeted, multicomponent exercise, such as muscle-strengthening exercise, and exercise that is dynamic, of high impact, discrete (with rest bouts), and unusual, with all areas of the body targeted.

Real-world example

A 21-year-old, international-level, female, long-distance runner displayed all three components of the Female Athlete Triad, with significant, and prolonged energy deficit. At first presentation, she was running around 88 km/ week, her body mass was 44.3 kg and her lumbar spine, total hip, and total body BMD Z-scores were –2.2, –0.5, and –0.3, respectively. She suffered a stress fracture of the left sacrum at first presentation and of the third metatarsal two years later. Six years later, following a recovery plan of 20 weeks consisting of cognitive behavioural therapy, weight gain (10 kg), improved dietary intake, and reduced training load (88 to 22 km/week), she regained menstrual function, and BMD. Her lumbar spine, hip, and total body BMD Z-scores improved to –0.6, 0.1, and –0.1, respectively. Restoration of fertility was indicated by pregnancy, following only four months of regular menstruation. This real-world example suggests that bone density and fertility may be recovered in formerly amenorrhoeic and osteopaenic athletes, through diet, weight gain, and return of menstruation.

Summary

Energy balance and adequate levels of oestrogen are important for the exercising female, since both are key mediators of bone remodelling. Decrements to bone health can also occur through the use of certain contraceptives, such as progesterone-only contraceptives, and through changes in hormones as a result of menopause. Exercise that specifically targets the bone, such as dynamic, high-impact, muscle-strengthening, and discrete bouts of exercise are important for the exercising female, especially when oestrogen is suboptimal, or when the usual exercise undertaken is non-weightbearing.

References

Ackerman, K. E., Nazem, T., Chapko, D., Russell, M., Mendes, N., Taylor, A. P., … Misra, M. (2011). Bone microarchitecture is impaired in adolescent amenorrheic athletes compared with eumenorrheic athletes and nonathletic controls. *The Journal of Clinical Endocrinology & Metabolism, 96*(10), 3123–3133. https://doi. org/10.1210/jc.2011-1614.

Ackerman, K. E., Putman, M., Guereca, G., Taylor, A. P., Pierce, L., Herzog, D. B., … Misra, M. (2012). Cortical microstructure and estimated bone strength in young amenorrheic athletes, eumenorrheic athletes and non-athletes. *Bone, 51*(4), 680–687. https://doi.org/10.1016/j.bone.2012.07.019.

Babatunde, O., & Forsyth, J. (2013). Effects of lifestyle exercise on premenopausal bone health: A randomised controlled trial. *Journal of Bone and Mineral Metabolism, 32*(5), 563–572. https://doi.org/10.1007/s00774-013-0527-9.

Babatunde, O., & Forsyth, J. (2014). Association between depot medroxyprogesterone acetate (DMPA), physical activity and bone health. *Journal of Bone and Mineral Metabolism, 32*(3). https://doi.org/10.1007/s00774-013-0497-y.

Babatunde, O. O., Forsyth, J. J., & Gidlow, C. J. (2012). A meta-analysis of brief high-impact exercises for enhancing bone health in premenopausal women. *Osteoporosis International, 23*(1), 109–119. https://doi.org/10.1007/s00198-011-1801-0.

Balasch, J. (2003). Sex steroids and bone: Current perspectives. *Human Reproduction Update, 9*(3), 207–222. https://doi.org/10.1093/humupd/dmg017.

Barrack, M. T., Gibbs, J. C., De Souza, M. J., Williams, N. I., Nichols, J. F., Rauh, M. J., & Nattiv, A. (2014). Higher incidence of bone stress injuries with increasing female athlete triad-related risk factors. *The American Journal of Sports Medicine, 42*(4), 949–958. https://doi.org/10.1177/0363546513520295.

Beerthuizen, R., van Beek, A., Massai, R., Mäkäräinen, L., Hout, J. in't, & Bennink, H. C. (2000). Bone mineral density during long-term use of the progestagen contraceptive implant Implanon® compared to a non-hormonal method of contraception. *Human Reproduction, 15*(1), 118–122. https://doi.org/10.1093/humrep/15.1.118.

Bolton, K. L., Egerton, T., Wark, J., Wee, E., Matthews, B., Kelly, A., ... Bennell, K. L. (2012). Effects of exercise on bone density and falls risk factors in postmenopausal women with osteopenia: A randomised controlled trial. *Journal of Science and Medicine in Sport, 15*(2), 102–109. https://doi.org/10.1016/j.jsams.2011.08.007.

Bonis, M., Loftin, M., Speaker, R., & Kontos, A. (2009). Body composition of elite, eumenorrheic and amenorrheic, adolescent cross-country runners. *Pediatric Exercise Science, 21*(3), 318–328.

Borer, K. T., Fogleman, K., Gross, M., La New, J. M., & Dengel, D. (2007). Walking intensity for postmenopausal bone mineral preservation and accrual. *Bone, 41*(4), 713–721. https://doi.org/10.1016/j.bone.2007.06.009.

Bressot, C., Meunier, P., Chapuy, M., Lejeune, E., Edouard, C., & Darby, A. (1979). Histomorphometric profile, pathophysiology and reversibility of corticosteroid-induced osteoporosis. *Metabolic Bone Disease and Related Research, 1*(4), 303–311. https://doi.org/10.1016/0221-8747(79)90024-9.

Burt, L. A., Greene, D. A., Ducher, G., & Naughton, G. A. (2013). Skeletal adaptations associated with pre-pubertal gymnastics participation as determined by DXA and pQCT: A systematic review and meta-analysis. *Journal of Science and Medicine in Sport, 16*(3), 231–239. https://doi.org/10.1016/j.jsams.2012.07.006.

Campion, F., Nevill, A. M., Karlsson, M. K., Lounana, J., Shabani, M., Fardellone, P., & Medelli, J. (2010). Bone status in professional cyclists. *International Journal of Sports Medicine, 31*(7), 511–515. http://doi.org/10.1055/s-0029-1243616.

Carey, J. J., & Delaney, M. F. (2017). Utility of DXA for monitoring, technical aspects of DXA BMD measurement and precision testing. *Bone, 104*, 44–53. https://doi.org/10.1016/j.bone.2017.05.021.

Chen, Q., Kaji, H., Kanatani, M., Sugimoto, T., & Chihara, K. (2004). Testosterone Increases Osteoprotegerin mRNA Expression in Mouse Osteoblast Cells. *Hormone and Metabolic Research, 36*(10), 674–678. https://doi.org/10.1055/s-2004-826013.

Colaianni, G., Cuscito, C., & Colucci, S. (2013). Review article FSH and TSH in the regulation of bone mass: The pituitary/immune/bone axis. *Clinical and Developmental Immunology, 2013*. https://doi.org/0.1155/2013/382698.

Cummings, S. R., Browner, W., Cummings, S. R., Black, D. M., Nevitt, M. C., Browner, W., ... Vogt, T. M. (1993). Bone density at various sites for prediction of hip fractures. *The Lancet, 341*(8837), 72–75. https://doi.org/10.1016/0140-6736(93)92555-8.

Curtis, K. M., & Martins, S. L. (2006). Progestogene-only contraception and bone mineral density: a systematic review. *Contraception, 73*, 470–487. https://doi.org/10.1016/j.contraception.2005.12.010.

Ducher, G., Tournaire, N., Meddahi-Pellé, A., Benhamou, C. L., & Courteix, D. (2006). Short-term and long-term site-specific effects of tennis playing on trabecular and cortical bone at the distal radius. *Journal of Bone and Mineral Metabolism, 24*(6), 484–490. https://doi.org/10.1007/s00774-006-0710-3.

Ehrlich, P. J., & Lanyon, L. E. (2002). Mechanical strain and bone cell function: A review. *Osteoporosis International, 13*(9), 688–700. https://doi.org/10.1007/s001980 200095.

Eriksen, E. F., Axelrod, D. W., & Melsen, F. (1994). *Bone histomorphometry. An official publication of the American Society for Bone and Mineral Research*. Philadelphia, PA: Lippincott, Williams and Wilkins.

Florencio-Silva, R., Rodrigues, G., Sasso-Cerri, E., Simões, M. J., & Cerri, P. S. (2015). Biology of bone tissue: structure, function, and factors that influence bone cells. *BioMed Research International, 2015*, 1–17. https://doi.org/10.1155/2015/421746.

Frost, H. M. (1987). Bone 'mass' and the 'mechanostat': A proposal. *The Anatomical Record, 219*(1), 1–9. https://doi.org/10.1002/ar.1092190104.

Galea, G. L., Lanyon, L. E., & Price, J. S. (2017). Sclerostin's role in bone's adaptive response to mechanical loading. *Bone, 96*, 38–44. https://doi.org/10.1016/j.bone.2016.10.008.

Goolsby, M. A., Barrack, M. T., & Nattiv, A. (2012). A displaced femoral neck stress fracture in an amenorrheic adolescent female runner. *Sports Health: A Multidisciplinary Approach, 4*(4), 352–356. https://doi.org/10.1177/1941738 111429929.

Hartard, M., Bottermann, P., Bartenstein, P., Jeschke, D., & Schwaiger, M. (1997). Effects on bone mineral density of low-dose oral contraceptives compared to and combined with physical activity. *Contraception, 55*, 87–90.

Hartard, M., Kleinmond, C., Wiseman, M., Weissenbacher, E. R., Felsenberg, D., & Erben, R. G. (2007). Detrimental effect of oral contraceptives on parameters of bone mass and geometry in a cohort of 248 young women. *Bone, 40*(2), 444–450. https://doi.org/10.1016/j.bone.2006.08.001.

Hind, K. (2008). Recovery of bone mineral density and fertility in a former amenorrheic athlete. *Journal of Sports Science & Medicine, 7*(3), 415–418. Retrieved from www.ncbi.nlm.nih.gov/pubmed/24149911.

Hind, K., Gannon, L., Whatley, E., Cooke, C., & Truscott, J. (2012). Bone cross-sectional geometry in male runners, gymnasts, swimmers and non-athletic controls: A hip-structural analysis study. *European Journal of Applied Physiology, 112*(2), 535–541. https://doi.org/10.1007/s00421-011-2008-y.

Hind, K., Oldroyd, B., & Truscott, J. G. (2010). In vivo precision of the GE Lunar iDXA densitometer for the measurement of total-body, lumbar spine, and femoral bone mineral density in adults. *Journal of Clinical Densitometry, 13*(4), 413–417. https://doi.org/10.1016/j.jocd.2010.06.002.

Hind, K., Truscott, J., & Carroll, S. (2008). Case report: Female athlete triad in monozygotic twins. *The Physician and Sportsmedicine, 36*(1), 119–124. https://doi.org/10.3810/psm.2008.12.20.

Hind, K., Truscott, J. G., & Evans, J. A. (2006). Low lumbar spine bone mineral density in both male and female endurance runners. *Bone, 39*(4), 880–885. https://doi.org/10.1016/j.bone.2006.03.012.

Hind, K., Zanker, C., & Truscott, J. (2011). Five-year follow-up investigation of bone mineral density by age in premenopausal elite-level long-distance runners. *Clinical Journal of Sport Medicine, 21*(6), 521–529. https://doi.org/10.1097/JSM.0b013e3182377257.

Howe, T. E., Shea, B., Dawson, L. J., Downie, F., Murray, A., Ross, C., … Creed, G. (2011). Exercise for preventing and treating osteoporosis in postmenopausal women. *Cochrane Database of Systematic Reviews,* (7). https://doi.org/10.1002/14651858.CD000333.pub2.

Ihle, R., & Loucks, A. B. (2004). Dose-response relationships between energy availability and bone turnover in young exercising women. *Journal of Bone and Mineral Research, 19*(8), 1231–1240. https://doi.org/10.1359/JBMR.040410.

Kanis, J. A., & Kanis, J. A. (1994). Assessment of fracture risk and its application to screening for postmenopausal osteoporosis: Synopsis of a WHO report. *Osteoporosis International, 4*(6), 368–381. https://doi.org/10.1007/BF01622200.

Kelley, G. A., & Kelley, K. S. (2006). Exercise and bone mineral density at the femoral neck in postmenopausal women: A meta-analysis of controlled clinical trials with individual patient data. *American Journal of Obstetrics and Gynecology, 194*(3), 760–767. https://doi.org/10.1016/j.ajog.2005.09.006.

Kontulainen, S., Sievänen, H., Kannus, P., Pasanen, M., & Vuori, I. (2003). Effect of long-term impact-loading on mass, size, and estimated strength of humerus and radius of female racquet-sports players: A peripheral quantitative computed tomography study between young and old starters and controls. *Journal of Bone and Mineral Research, 18*(2), 352–359. https://doi.org/10.1359/jbmr.2003.18.2.352.

Kortebein, P., Ferrando, A., Lombeida, J., Wolfe, R., & Evans, W. J. (2007). Effect of 10 days of bed rest on skeletal muscle in healthy older adults. *The Journal of the American Medical Association, 297*(16), 1769. https://doi.org/10.1001/jama.297.16.1772-b.

Li, D., Hitchcock, C. L., Barr, S. I., Yu, T., & Prior, J. C. (2014). Negative spinal bone mineral density changes and subclinical ovulatory disturbances – prospective data in healthy premenopausal women with regular menstrual cycles. *Epidemiologic Reviews, 36*(1), 137–147. https://doi.org/10.1093/epirev/mxt012.

Manolagas, S. C. (2013). Steroids and osteoporosis: The quest for mechanisms. *Journal of Clinical Investigation, 123*(5), 1919–1921. https://doi.org/10.1172/JCI68062.

Manolagas, S. C., O'Brien, C. A., & Almeida, M. (2013). The role of estrogen and androgen receptors in bone health and disease. *Nature Reviews Endocrinology, 9*(12), 699–712. https://doi.org/10.1038/nrendo.2013.179.

Marques, E. A., Mota, J., & Carvalho, J. (2012). Exercise effects on bone mineral density in older adults: A meta-analysis of randomized controlled trials. *Age, 34*(6), 1493–1515. https://doi.org/10.1007/s11357-011-9311-8.

Marques, E. A., Mota, J., Machado, L., Sousa, F., Coelho, M., Moreira, P., & Carvalho, J. (2011). Multicomponent training program with weight-bearing exercises elicits favorable bone density, muscle strength, and balance adaptations in older women. *Calcified Tissue International, 88*(2), 117–129. https://doi.org/10.1007/s00223-010-9437-1.

Marques, E. A., Mota, J., Viana, J. L., Tuna, D., Figueiredo, P., Guimarães, J. T., & Carvalho, J. (2013). Response of bone mineral density, inflammatory cytokines, and biochemical bone markers to a 32-week combined loading exercise programme in older men and women. *Archives of Gerontology and Geriatrics*, 57(2), 226–233. https://doi.org/10.1016/j.archger.2013.03.014.

Marshall, D., Johnell, O., & Wedel, H. (1996). Meta-analysis of how well measures of bone mineral density predict occurrence of osteoporotic fractures. *British Medical Journal*, 312(7041), 1254–1259. https://doi.org/10.1136/bmj.312. 7041.1254.

Martyn-St James, M., & Carroll, S. (2008). Meta-analysis of walking for preservation of bone mineral density in postmenopausal women. *Bone*, 43(3), 521–531. https:// doi.org.10.1016/j.bone.2008.05.012.

Martyn-St James, M., & Carroll, S. (2010). Effects of different impact exercise modalities on bone mineral density in premenopausal women: A meta-analysis. *Journal of Bone and Mineral Metabolism*, 28(3), 251–267. https://doi.org/10.1007/ s00774-009-0139-6.

Nappi, C., Bifulco, G., Tommaselli, G. A., Gargano, V., & Di Carlo, C. (2012). Hormonal contraception and bone metabolism: A systematic review. *Contraception*, 86(6), 606–621. https://doi.org/10.1016/j.contraception.2012.04.009.

Nikander, R., Sievänen, H., Uusi-Rasi, K., Heinonen, A., & Kannus, P. (2006). Loading modalities and bone structures at nonweight-bearing upper extremity and weight-bearing lower extremity: A pQCT study of adult female athletes. *Bone*, 39(4), 886–894. https://doi.org/10.1016/j.bone.2006.04.005.

Okamoto, S., Arai, Y., Hara, K., Tsuzihara, T., & Kubo, T. (2010). A displaced stress fracture of the femoral neck in an adolescent female distance runner with female athlete triad: A case report. *BMC Sports Science, Medicine and Rehabilitation*, 2(1), 6. https://doi.org/10.1186/1758-2555-2-6.

Palombaro, K. M. (2005). Effects of walking-only interventions on bone mineral density at various skeletal sites: a meta-analysis. *Journal of Geriatric Physical Therapy*, 28(3), 102–107.

Prior, J. C., Kirkland, S. A., Joseph, L., Kreiger, N., Murray, T. M., Hanley, D. A., … Tenenhouse, A. (2001). Oral contraceptive use and bone mineral density in premenopausal women: cross-sectional, population-based data from the Canadian Multicentre Osteoporosis Study. *Canadian Medical Association Journal*, 165(8), 1023–1029.

Randell, A., Sambrook, P. N., Nguyen, T. V., Lapsley, H., Jones, G., Kelly, P. J., & Eisman, J. (1995). Direct clinical and welfare costs of osteoporotic fractures in elderly men and women. *Osteoporosis International*, 5(6), 427–432.

Robling, A. G., Burr, D. B., & Turner, C. H. (2000). Partitioning a daily mechanical stimulus into discrete loading bouts improves the osteogenic response to loading. *Journal of Bone and Mineral Research*, 15(8), 1596–1602. https://doi. org/10.1359/jbmr.2000.15.8.1596.

Robling, A. G., & Turner, C. H. (2009). Mechanical signaling for bone modeling and remodeling. *Critical Reviews in Eukaryotic Gene Expression*, 19(4), 319–338.

Rosen, C. J. (Ed.). (2013). *Primer on the metabolic bone diseases and disorders of mineral metabolism*. Ames, USA: John Wiley & Sons, Inc. https://doi.org/10.1002/9781118453926.

Rubin, C. T., Sommerfeldt, D. W., Judex, S., & Qin, Y. X. (2001). Inhibition of osteopenia by low magnitude, high-frequency mechanical stimuli. *Drug Discovery Today*, 6(16), 848–858. https://doi.org/10.1016/S1359-6446(01)01872-4.

Schett, G. (2011). Effects of inflammatory and anti-inflammatory cytokines on the bone *European Journal of Clinical Investigation*, 41(12), 1361–1366. https://doi. org/10.1111/j.1365-2362.2011.02545.x.

Scheurer, H. (2013). *Osteoblasts: Morphology, functions and clinical implications: Morphology, functions and clinical implications.* Hauppauge: Nova.

Schousboe, J. T., Shepherd, J. A., Bilezikian, J. P., & Baim, S. (2013). Executive summary of the 2013 International Society for Clinical Densitometry Position Development Conference on Bone Densitometry. *Journal of Clinical Densitometry, 16*(4), 455–466. https://doi.org/10.1016/j.jocd.2013.08.004.

Shaarawy, M., El-Mallah, S. Y., Seoudi, S., Hassan, M., & Mohsen, I. A. (2006). Effects of the long-term use of depot medroxyprogesterone acetate as hormonal contraceptive on bone mineral density and biochemical markers of bone remodeling. *Contraception, 74*(4), 297–302. https://doi.org/10.1016/j.contraception.2006.04.003.

Sievänen, H., Zagorski, P., Drozdzowska, B., Vähä-Ypyä, H., Boron, D., Adamczyk, P., & Pluskiewicz, W. (2015). Alpine skiing is associated with higher femoral neck bone mineral density. *Journal of Musculoskeletal & Neuronal Interactions, 15*(3), 264–269.

Tucker, L. A., Strong, J. E., LeCheminant, J. D., & Bailey, B. W. (2015). Effect of two jumping programs on hip bone mineral density in premenopausal women: a randomized controlled trial. *American Journal of Health Promotion, 29*(3), 158–164. https://doi.org/10.4278/ajhp. 130430-QUAN-200.

Watson, S. L., Weeks, B. K., Weis, L. J., Harding, A. T., Horan, S. A. & Beck, B. R. (2018). High-intensity resistance and impact training improves bone mineral density and physical function in postmenopausal women with osteopenia and osteoporosis: The LIFTMOR randomized controlled trial. *Journal of Bone and Mineral Research, 33*(2), 211–220. https://doi.org/10.1002/jbmr.3284.

Watson, S. L., Weeks, B. K., Weis, L. J., Horan, S. A., & Beck, B. R. (2015). Heavy resistance training is safe and improves bone, function, and stature in postmenopausal women with low to very low bone mass: Novel early findings from the LIFTMOR trial. *Osteoporosis International, 26*(12), 2889–2894. https://doi.org/10.1007/s00198-015-3263-2.

Weaver, C. M., Teegarden, D., Lyle, R. M., McCabe, G. P., McCabe, L. D., Proulx, W., ... Johnston, C. (2001). Impact of exercise on bone health and contraindication of oral contraceptive use in young women. *Medicine and Science in Sports and Exercise, 33*(6), 873–880. https://doi.org/10.1097/00005768-200106000-00004.

Winters-Stone, K. M., Dobek, J., Nail, L. M., Bennett, J. A., Leo, M. C., Torgrimson-Ojerio, B., ... Schwartz, A. (2013). Impact + resistance training improves bone health and body composition in prematurely menopausal breast cancer survivors: a randomized controlled trial. *Osteoporosis International, 24*(5), 1637–1646. https://doi.org/10.1007/s00198-012-2143-2.

Xiong, J., & O'Brien, C. A. (2012). Osteocyte RANKL: New insights into the control of bone remodeling. *Journal of Bone and Mineral Research, 27*(3), 499–505. https://doi.org/10.1002/jbmr.1547.

Yakar, S., Rosen, C. J., Beamer, W. G., Ackert-Bicknell, C. L., Wu, Y., Liu, J.-L., ... LeRoith, D. (2002). Circulating levels of IGF-1 directly regulate bone growth and density. *Journal of Clinical Investigation, 110*(6), 771–781. https://doi.org/10.1172/JCI15463.

Yu, K., Sellman, D. P., Bahraini, A., Hagan, M. L., Elsherbini, A., Vanpelt, K. T., ... McGee-Lawrence, M. E. (2017). Mechanical loading disrupts osteocyte plasma membranes which initiates mechanosensation events in bone. *Journal of Orthopaedic Research.* https://doi.org/10.1002/jor.23665.

Zaman, G. Cheng, M. Z., Jessop, H. L., White, R., & Lanyon, L. E. (2000). Mechanical strain activates estrogen response elements in bone cells. *Bone, 27*(2), 233–239. https://doi.org/S8756-3282(00)00324-0 [pii].

Zanker, C. L., & Cooke, C. B. (2004). Energy balance, bone turnover, and skeletal health in physically active individuals. *Medicine and Science in Sports and Exercise, 36*(8), 1372–1381. https://doi.org/10.1249/01.MSS.0000135978.80362.AA.

Zhao, R., Zhao, M., & Zhang, L. (2014). Efficiency of jumping exercise in improving bone mineral density among premenopausal women: A meta-analysis. *Sports Medicine 44*(10), 1393–1402. https://doi.org/10.1007/s40279-014-0220-8.

8 Body image and the exercising female

Sarah Grogan

Introduction

This chapter provides a summary of the current multidisciplinary evidence base for research on body image in the exercising female, including considering how to improve body image in women who engage in sport and exercise. The chapter summarises research on relevant cultural and subcultural pressures to be slender, provides a critical review of relevant literature on body image in the exercising female, and makes recommendations for promoting positive body image in women engaged in sport and exercise.

Although there is some evidence that women who exercise for recreation or competition tend to have more positive body image than other women, cultural pressures to be slim, plus additional sport-related pressures to conform to particular body types, may lead to body dissatisfaction in exercising females. In this chapter, the effects of subcultural and societal pressures on body image among exercising females are analysed, and the impacts of sport and exercise environments are considered. Reducing internalisation of thin ideals and social comparison with unrealistic targets, raising self-esteem, encouraging a focus on body function and performance, and improving body appreciation and acceptance are evaluated as possible interventions for reducing body dissatisfaction. The importance of social support for a range of body shapes from within sport and exercise communities are also discussed.

Body-related cultural pressures, and resulting body dissatisfaction, are issues that exercising females are likely to encounter, either personally or in teammates, friends, and colleagues, and such issues are explored. Recommendations are also provided for how to optimise body image so that athletic success is not affected negatively by body dissatisfaction.

Aims of the chapter

The aims of the chapter are as follows:

1   To provide a review of relevant literature on body image with a specific focus on body image in the exercising female.

2   To make recommendations for promoting positive body image in women engaged in sport and exercise.

A consideration of the current evidence base

Defining body image

The definition of body image that will be taken in this chapter is adapted from Grogan (2016) and is: 'A woman's perceptions, thoughts, and feelings about her body'. This definition can be taken to include psychological concepts, such as perception and attitudes towards the body, as well as experiences of embodiment. It can also be taken to encompass both positive and negative aspects of body image. Body dissatisfaction relates to negative evaluations of body size, shape, muscularity/muscle tone, and weight, and it usually involves a perceived discrepancy between a woman's evaluation of her body and her ideal body.

Cultural pressures

Body image is a psychological phenomenon that is significantly affected by social factors. Body image pressures for exercising females come from mainstream expectations of slenderness and body tone, as well as specific sport and exercise-related pressures. In terms of mainstream pressures, media imagery may be particularly important in producing changes in the ways that the body is experienced and evaluated, depending on women's perception of the importance of those cues (Levine, 2012). For instance, it has been suggested that adolescent girls are especially vulnerable because body image is particularly salient while they undergo the significant physical and psychological changes of puberty (Ricciardelli & Yager, 2015). Pressure also comes from family, friends, and partners (Ordaz et al., 2018). Ideals for women's bodies tend to be a slender-but-curvy shape, which includes slenderness (associated with self-control, elegance, and youth; Bordo, 2003; Murray, 2016), a small waist (Grogan, Gill, Brownbridge, Kilgariff, & Whalley, 2013), and moderately large breasts (Reardon & Grogan, 2011; Swami, 2015). Muscle tone is also important, and the 21st century ideal is a firm-looking, toned body (Lupton, 2013), though high degrees of muscularity are generally not seen as culturally acceptable for women and may be seen as 'unfeminine' (Grogan, 2016; Krane, Choi, Baird, Amar, & Kauer, 2004). In certain types of sport, there are additional pressures. For instance, in sports with an aesthetic, antigravitational, or weight-category component, there is often pressure to be as lean as possible rather than slender-but-curvy (Petrie & Greenleaf, 2012). In other sports, such as body building, there is pressure to be muscular (Grogan, Evans, Wright, & Hunter, 2004). This puts exercising females under complex sets of social pressures: to be slender-but-curvy to conform to societal expectations, and also to conform to the performance-related body size requirements of their sport.

Body dissatisfaction

Researchers have concluded that the majority of women in Western cultures are dissatisfied with some aspect of their body weight and shape (Cash, 2012a; Grogan, 2016; Vartanian, 2012), and many are taking behavioural steps to try to change the look of their bodies such as using dieting and weight loss drugs, such as stimulants and laxatives, to lose weight (O'Dea & Cinelli, 2016; Petrie & Greenleaf, 2012). Interview studies tend to report that stomach, thighs, buttocks, and hips present most concern (e.g., Grogan, Gill, Brownbridge, Kilgariff, & Whalley, 2013; Grogan et al., 2017). These are areas of the body where women store fat, and also areas which are often the focus of media attention in advertisements for slimming products (Murray, 2016). Studies on body size estimation find that women tend to overestimate the size of their bodies (e.g., McCabe, Ricciardelli, Sitaram, & Mikhail, 2006), and showing women realistic images of their bodies, derived from three-dimensional, whole-body scans, has been shown to improve body satisfaction, possibly by reducing body size overestimation (Grogan et al., 2013).

Researchers have tended to find more positive body image in exercising females than those women who do not exercise. Hausenblas and Fallon (2007) reviewed 121 published and unpublished studies that examined the impact of exercise on body image. They concluded that exercising females had more positive body image than did non-exercisers, and that exercise intervention participants reported more positive body image post intervention compared to the non-exercising controls, concluding that exercise was associated with improved body image. Petrie and Greenleaf (2012) suggest that this clear link may be due to: (a) relatively greater focus on body performance rather than aesthetics in exercising females; (b) the fact that exercised bodies tend to be closer to the mainstream cultural ideal in terms of body fat levels and muscle tone, leading to fewer discrepancies with cultural ideals; and (c) the psychosocial benefits of sport, such as autonomy and competence that have been linked to more positive body image.

Although exercise has been linked with positive body image, this does not mean that exercising females do not have body image concerns. Mott and Griffiths (2014), summarising results from a survey by BT Sport, which included responses from 110 female athletes from 20 different sports, report that 80 per cent of respondents felt under pressure to look a certain way, with 66 per cent perceiving pressure from media, and 61 per cent from fellow athletes. Respondents reported social pressure from coaches and from sports' regulatory bodies. In response to body image pressures, 87 per cent had dieted, and 67 per cent of respondents thought the public and media valued how female athletes looked over what they achieved in sport. These data suggest that body image pressures impact negatively on large numbers of female athletes from a wide range of sports. Some women prioritised being thin over sport performance when choosing what to eat, suggesting that these body image pressures can affect sport performance as well as general well-being, with one woman saying, 'Sometimes it has meant my diet no longer is optimum for performance but becomes optimum for looking slimmer/thinner'.

In sports where low body weight may provide a competitive advantage, there is significant pressure to be as lean as possible. Women who exercise and engage in sport often spend time in environments that are highly regulated, especially at club and elite levels. Teammates and coaches may exert subtle, and not so subtle, messages about the importance of being slender (Mott & Griffiths, 2014). Weigh-ins and focus on diet and weight loss, requirements to wear revealing uniforms, and sport and exercise environments where body appearance is a key focus, can lead to significant pressures to be lean, which can lead to body dissatisfaction, disordered eating, and over-exercise to reduce weight (Mott & Griffiths, 2014; Petrie & Greenleaf, 2007, 2012).

Psychological factors predicting body image

As well as cultural factors, several psychological factors have been shown to predict body image in women such as: internalisation of the thin ideal, self-esteem, performance and body function, and body appreciation and acceptance.

Internalisation of the thin ideal

Women who internalise thin ideals may be particularly vulnerable to body dissatisfaction caused by self-ideal discrepancies (e.g., Ahern & Hetherington, 2006), and tendency to make comparisons to thin ideal imagery has been shown to increase body dissatisfaction in women (e.g., Slevec & Tiggemann, 2011). Yamamiya and colleagues (2005) showed that body dissatisfaction can be increased by as little as 5 min of exposure to thin and beautiful images in women high in thin-ideal internalisation, showing that social comparison with thin body ideals can produce particular risks for women who have internalised societal thin ideals. For exercising females, this may also lead to unhelpful body comparisons with other exercising females, resulting in reduced performance and avoidance of training (Pridgeon & Grogan, 2012; Wasilenko, Kulik, & Wanic, 2007).

Self-esteem

Women high in self-esteem tend to be most satisfied with their bodies (O'Dea, 2012), which has led to suggestions that raising women's self-esteem is key in improving body image (e.g., O'Dea & Cinelli, 2016).

Although finding that the two variables are linked does not necessarily demonstrate that self-esteem is the primary causal factor in determining body image, intervention studies have shown that raising self-esteem does tend to lead to an improvement in body image (e.g., O'Dea, 2012; Seekis, Bradley, & Duffy, 2017), suggesting that self-esteem may be the causal factor.

Performance and body function

Work on body function (performance rather than aesthetics) has shown that focusing on fitness and performance can promote body appreciation and reduce body dissatisfaction (Alleva Martijn, Van Breukelen, Jansen, & Karos, 2015). Many studies have shown that adult women who exercise for functional, health, and enjoyment reasons, rather than to improve appearance, tend to report higher body appreciation (e.g., Homan & Tylka, 2014), that activities such as yoga, which tend to promote awareness of body function rather than aesthetics, promote positive body image (Neumark-Sztainer, MacLehose, Watts, Pacanowski, & Eisenberg, 2018), and that women who focus on body function and fitness have more positive body image than those who focus on appearance (e.g., Frisen & Holmqvist, 2010).

Body appreciation and acceptance

Although body image research has a history of prioritising negative aspects of body image, a strong new focus within body image research is the move towards focusing on body appreciation and acceptance rather than body dissatisfaction. This approach is proving helpful in understanding how some women maintain body satisfaction in societies where the ideal is slender-but-curvy and their bodies do not correspond to this ideal. Tylka and Wood-Barcalow (2015) argue that if body image interventions reduce symptoms of negative body image without enhancing positive body image, they may merely enable people to tolerate their bodies, whereas enabling people to appreciate and accept their bodies may make interventions more effective and may enable maintenance of those gains.

Practical recommendations based on research

Various authors have suggested ways in which exercise cultures can be made more body-healthy, to promote positive body image in women. Petrie and Greenleaf (2012) suggest that it is important to create body-healthy sport and exercise environments so that women can be proud of what their bodies can do, satisfied with their appearance, and develop positive self-worth. A key factor identified by these authors is disconnecting the link between weight loss and improved performance. They argue that a positive way forward is to focus on health rather than weight. Arguing that weight loss can involve loss of fat-free muscle mass, and that dieting may reduce energy levels and reduce performance, they note that this cultural link between weight loss and performance is problematic and needs to be challenged. Normalising healthy eating, and focusing on attunement to nutritional needs, plus educating coaches about the possible damaging impacts of negative body image on health and well-being, as well as on performance, is also important. In addition, the research evidence noted in the previous section leads to suggestions for interventions based on psychological factors that may be helpful in promoting positive body image in women who exercise.

Interventions based on psychological factors

Reducing internalisation of the thin ideal

Psychologists have suggested that women can be made resistant to the negative effects of media imagery by changing the ways that they interpret incoming social information. A popular approach to resisting internalisation of the thin ideal is to use media-literacy programmes to teach women to reject media images as appropriate targets for comparison (e.g., Halliwell, Harcourt, & Easun, 2011). However, although successful in training women to be sceptical about media images, these kinds of interventions have not been very successful in reducing resulting body dissatisfaction in adults (e.g., Tiggemann, Slater, & Smyth, 2014). One alternative is to use feminist approaches to enable women to challenge the validity of the thin ideal (Murnen & Seabrook, 2012), and exposure to feminist theories may promote positive body image though raising perceived empowerment (Peterson, Grippo, & Tantleff-Dunn, 2010). Another approach that has enabled women to challenge the thin ideal and to rethink unrealistic body standards is cognitive behavioural therapy (Cash, 2012b). Cognitive restructuring and self-monitoring to change body-related thoughts such as internalisation of the thin ideal, have been extremely effective in promoting positive body image (Jarry & Ip, 2005).

Raising self-esteem

Research has shown that programmes designed to raise self-esteem in adolescents (O'Dea, 2012; Steese et al., 2006) and adults (Seekis et al., 2017) can be effective in improving body image. More work is needed to determine the effectiveness of programmes that aim to build self-esteem and resilience as a way of improving body image in adult exercising females, although existing work with more general groups of women is producing positive results.

Focusing on performance and body function

Women who engage in sport and exercise will necessarily have a focus on body performance and function, but coaches and others should be aware that conflicting pressures to focus on appearance may lead to unhelpful body critique. This may be reduced through acknowledging these pressures and encouraging refocusing on performance and body function rather than appearance (Homan & Tylka, 2014). In one study (Grogan et al., 2014), a dance movement, psychotherapy session, with a key focus on body function and appreciation, was effective in promoting body acceptance and reduced the importance that the 17-year-old participants placed on other people's opinions and attitudes towards their bodies. This finding shows that encouraging a focus on performance rather than appearance has promise as a means of promoting positive body image for young women.

Improving body appreciation and acceptance

Self-compassion has been defined in various ways, but broadly entails treating oneself in a caring and empathic way. Albertson, Neff, and Dill-Shackleford (2015) have shown that a three-week period of self-compassion focusing on body appreciation and acceptance significantly reduced body dissatisfaction and body shame in a multigenerational group of American women relative to wait-list controls. The authors suggest that self-compassion may be an effective way to improve body image in adult women. Most impressive, perhaps, is the fact that these improvements were maintained when the same women were assessed three months later, so benefits do not seem to be limited to the time period shortly after the intervention. This study did not specifically recruit exercising females, so results need to be replicated in samples of women targeted because they exercise, though results look promising.

Real-world examples

Two groups who tend to have generally positive views of their bodies are competition swimmers and bodybuilders. Given that mainstream Western cultures expect women's bodies not to take up space (e.g., Murray, 2016), women who swim competitively and those who body build are engaging in behaviours that place them outside mainstream norms of how much muscle is appropriate for women. Two studies (Grogan et al., 2004; Howells and Grogan, 2012) investigated how women experienced the reactions of those outside and also inside the confines of their sports, and what sources of social support these women used to enable them to maintain positive views of how their bodies looked. To investigate these factors, they ran interviews with adult women (over 18 years) and adolescent girls (under 18 years) who swam competitively (Howells & Grogan, 2012), and with adult women bodybuilders (Grogan et al., 2004). They found that all these factors were relevant in understanding how these women maintained positive body image.

Example 1: female swimmers

Although swimming has been categorised as a 'lean' sport as it requires lighter than normal weight (Robinson & Ferraro, 2004), it also enables the development of muscular bodies, and requires body exposure when in training and competition, which might be expected to lead to increased body awareness. In our interviews, both younger and older women reported that swimming had made them more muscular and that they were proud of their muscled shoulders and thighs when performing and training.

Responses when in non-sport and exercise contexts varied by age, and adolescent girls (who may be particularly sensitive to mainstream cultural pressures; O'Dea & Cinelli, 2016) were uncomfortable and wished to be thinner in non-sport contexts. This finding supports Krane and colleagues (2004) suggestions of a clash of body ideals in sport- and non-sport-related contexts. For instance, one interviewee said, when comparing how she felt in sport and non-sport settings:

> If we're all really competitive, like competitive athlete swimmers, we are all, we're all kind of the same because we all have the huge shoulders and huge thighs and are all flat chested, so we can walk round, but when I am with my friends I am really self-conscious cos like I'm built huge and they're like skinny and perfectly shaped.

Older women were comfortable and satisfied with their toned and muscular bodies both in and out of sport-related contexts, with one woman reporting, 'I really like swimming has given me a rather, a slightly more toned top part of my body' and another noting that, 'I quite like the fact that I've got big shoulders cos it evens me out'. These adult women linked increased muscularity with body function/strength, and had shifted their ideals to other women swimmers, with one woman noting, 'My idols, Carlin Pipes-Nelson, Dara Torres, all these swimmers, are fit and they have muscles'. The adult women noted that their muscular and toned bodies made them feel generally more confident, and that this confidence transferred into the rest of their lives outside swimming. Adult women swimmers showed high levels of focus on body function, had switched from idealising the bodies of thin models to elite women swimmers, appreciated their muscular bodies, and had high levels of self-esteem and confidence, which transferred outside the swimming context. Their stories showed how being muscular can lead to body satisfaction within this social and psychological context.

Example 2: female bodybuilders

Interviews were carried out with adult women bodybuilders who competed (or had competed in the past) in Physique (highly muscled) bodybuilding (see Grogan et al., 2004). Women said they were proud of their muscular bodies, and felt better about their bodies and about themselves generally than in their pre-bodybuilding days. For instance: 'Physically, I feel more sexy and sensual and umm better about myself trained'. One of the key factors was that they now felt in control of their bodies as they decided exactly how they wanted to look and worked towards that goal using nutrition and weight training. These women had also shifted their body ideals to more muscular figures, giving examples of elite competition bodybuilders as their ideals (rather than, for instance, magazine models). For instance: 'They're beautiful, and this is what people are looking for now. That athletic shape of the female'. The only people whose reactions concerned them were other body-builders and competition judges, and they trained in gyms where their trained bodies were appreciated and praised by other bodybuilders. They were unconcerned about the views of people from outside the bodybuilding community who may not find a hard and muscular body appealing. Focusing on body function/strength, they appreciated their muscular bodies and the muscular bodies of other women and made social comparisons to the bodies of other women bodybuilders, which were seen as aspirational rather than as a threat. All these factors enabled these women to feel physically and mentally strong, and raised their self-esteem, self-confidence, and body satisfaction. They presented accounts suggesting that resistance to internalising mainstream slender ideals, replacing with a sport-specific muscular ideal, and the significant support they received from within the bodybuilding community, enabled them to appreciate and be proud of their muscular bodies.

Summary

This chapter has provided a review of relevant literature on women's body image, with a specific focus on body image in exercising females. Key factors in promoting positive body image are creating body-healthy sport and exercise environments, reducing internalisation of thin ideals and social comparison with unrealistic targets, raising self-esteem, encouraging a focus on body function and performance, and improving body appreciation and acceptance. Having a strong and supportive sport and exercise community has been shown to enable positive body image in women swimmers and bodybuilders. Exercising females are under complex body-related pressures, and these may be particularly challenging for adolescents; however, social support from within sport and exercise communities, and a focus on body function/performance, appreciation, and acceptance, may promote positive body image in adult women who engage in sport and exercise.

References

Ahern, A. L., & Hetherington, M. M. (2006). The thin ideal and body image: An experimental study of implicit attitudes. *Psychology of Addictive Behaviours, 20*(3), 338–342. https://doi.org/10.1037/0893-164X.20.3.338.

Albertson, E. R., Neff, K. D., & Dill-Shackleford, K. E. (2015). Self-compassion and body dissatisfaction in women: A randomized controlled trial of a brief meditation intervention. *Mindfulness, 6*(3), 444–454. https://doi.org/10.1007/s12671-014-0277-3.

Alleva, J. M., Martijn, C., Van Breukelen, G. J. P., Jansen, A., & Karos, K. (2015). *Expand Your Horizon:* A programme that improves body image and reduces self-objectification by training women to focus on body functionality. *Body Image, 15*, 81–89. https://doi.org/10.1016/j.bodyim.2015.07.001.

Bordo, S. (2003). *Unbearable weight: Feminism, Western culture, and the body* (10th anniversary ed.). Berkeley, CA: University of California Press.

Cash, T. F. (Ed.). (2012a). *Encyclopedia of body image and human appearance.* London: Elsevier.

Cash, T. F. (2012b). Cognitive-behavioral perspectives on body image. In T. F. Cash (Ed.), *Encyclopedia of body image and human appearance* (pp. 334–342). London: Elsevier. https://doi.org/10.1016/B978-0-12-384925-0.00054-7.

Frisen, A., & Holmqvist, K. (2010). What characterises early adolescents with a positive body image? A qualitative investigation of Swedish girls and boys. *Body Image, 7*(3), 205–212. https://doi.org/10.1016/j.bodyim.2010.04.001.

Grogan, S. (2016). *Body image: Understanding body dissatisfaction in men, women and children* (3rd ed.). London: Routledge.

Grogan, S., Evans, R., Wright, S., & Hunter, G. (2004). Femininity and muscularity: Accounts of seven women bodybuilders. *Journal of Gender Studies, 13*(1), 49–63. https://doi.org/10.1080/0958923032000184970.

Grogan, S., Gill, S., Brownbridge, K., Kilgariff, S., & Whalley, A. (2013). Dress fit and body image: A thematic analysis of women's accounts during and after trying on dresses. *Body Image, 10*(3), 380–388. https://doi.org/10.1016/j.bodyim.2013.03.003.

Grogan, S., Siddique, M. A., Gill, S., Brownbridge, K., Storey, E., & Armitage, C. J, (2017). 'I think a little bit of a kick is sometimes what you need': Women's accounts of whole-body scanning and likely impact on health-related behaviours. *Psychology and Health, 32*(9), 1037–1054. https://doi.org/10.1080/08870446.2017.1329933.

Grogan, S., Williams, A., Kilgariff, S., Bunce, J., Heyland, S. J., Padilla, T., … Davies, W. (2014). Dance and body image: Young people's experiences of a dance movement psychotherapy session. *Qualitative Research in Sport, Exercise and Health, 6*(2), 261–277. https://doi.org/10.1080/2159676X.2013.796492.

Halliwell, E., & Dittmar, H. (2005). The role of self-improvement and self-evaluation motives in social comparisons with idealised female bodies in the media. *Body Image, 2*, 249–262. https://doi.org/10.1016/j.bodyim.2005.05.001.

Halliwell, E., Harcourt, D., & Easun, A. (2011). Body dissatisfaction: Can a short media literacy message reduce negative media exposure effects amongst adolescent girls? *British Journal of Health Psychology, 16*(2), 396–403. https://doi.org/10.1348/135910710X515714.

Hausenblas, H., & Fallon, E. (2006). Exercise and body image: A meta-analysis. *Psychology and Health, 21*(1), 33–47. https://doi.org/10.1080/14768320500105270.

Homan, K. J., & Tylka, T. L. (2014). Appearance-based exercise motivation moderates the relationship between exercise frequency and positive body image. *Body Image, 11*(2), 101–108. https://doi.org/10.1016/j.bodyim.2014.01.003.

Howells, K., & Grogan, S. (2012). Body image and the female swimmer: Muscularity but in moderation, *Qualitative Research in Sport, Exercise and Health*, 4(1), 98–116. https://doi.org/10.1080/2159676X.2011.653502.

Jarry, J. L., & Ip, K. (2005). The effectiveness of standalone cognitive-behavioural therapy for body image: A meta-analysis. *Body Image*, 2(4), 317–333. https://doi.org/10.1016/j.bodyim.2005.10.001.

Krane, V., Choi, P. Y. L., Baird, S. M., Aimar, C. M., & Kauer, K. J. (2004). Living the paradox: Female athletes negotiate femininity and muscularity. *Sex Roles*, 50(5–6), 315–329. https://doi.org/10.1023/B:SERS.0000018888.48437.4f.

Levine, M. P. (2012). Media influences on female body image. In T. F. Cash (Ed.), *Encyclopedia of body image and human appearance* (pp. 540–546). London: Elsevier. https://doi.org/10.1016/B978-0-12-384925-0.00085-7.

Lupton, D. (2013). *Fat*. London: Routledge.

McCabe, M. P., Ricciardelli, L. A., Sitaram, G., & Mikhail, K. (2006). Accuracy of body size estimation: Role of biopsychosocial variables. *Body Image*, 3(2), 163–173. https://doi.org/10.1016/j.bodyim.2006.01.004.

Mott, S., & Griffiths, R. (2014). *BT Sport body image survey results*. Retrieved from http://sport.bt.com.

Murnen, S. K., & Seabrook, R. (2012). Feminist perspectives on body image and physical appearance. In T. F. Cash (Ed.), *Encyclopedia of body image and human appearance* (pp. 438–443). London: Elsevier. https://doi.org/10.1016/B978-0-12-384925-0.00070-5.

Murray, S. (2016). *The 'fat' female body*. London: Palgrave.

Neumark-Sztainer, D., MacLehose, R. F., Watts, A. W., Pacanowski, C. R., & Eisenberg, M. E. (2018). Yoga and body image: Findings form a large population-based study of young adults. *Body Image*, 24, 69–75. https://doi.org/10.1016/j.bodyim.2017.12.003.

O'Dea, J. (2012). Body image and self-esteem. In T. F. Cash (Ed.), *Encyclopedia of body image and human appearance* (pp. 141–147). London: Elsevier. https://doi.org/10.1016/B978-0-12-384925-0.00021-3.

O'Dea, J., & Cinelli, R. L. (2016). Use of drugs to change appearance in girls and female adolescents. In M. Hall, S. Grogan, & B. Gough (Eds.), *Chemically modified bodies: The use of diverse substances for appearance enhancement* (pp. 51–76). London: Palgrave Macmillan. https://doi.org/10.1057/978-1-137-53535-1_4.

Ordaz, D. L., Schafer, L. M., Choquette, E., Scheler, J., Wallace, L., & Thompson, J. K. (2018). Thinness pressures in ethnically diverse college women in the United States. *Body Image*, 24, 1–4. https://doi.org/10.1016/j.bodyim.2017.11.004.

Peterson, R. D., Grippo, K. P., & Tantleff-Dunn, S. (2010). Empowerment and powerlessness: A closer look at the relationship between feminism, body image and eating disturbance. *Sex Roles*, 58(9), 639–648. https://doi.org/10.1016/j.bodyim.2013.08.001.

Petrie, T. A., & Greenleaf, C. (2007). Eating disorders in sport: from theory to research to intervention. In G. Tenenbaum & R. C. Eklund (Eds.), *Handbook of sport psychology*. (3rd ed., pp. 352–378). New Jersey: Wiley. https://doi.org/10.1002/9781118270011.ch16.

Petrie, T. A., & Greenleaf, C. (2012). Body image and sports/athletics. In T. F. Cash (Ed.), *Encylopedia of body image and human appearance* (pp. 160–165). London: Elsevier. https://doi.org/10.1016/B978-0-12-384925-0.00018-3.

Petrie, T. A., Greenleaf, C., Reel, J. J., & Carter, J. E. (2009). An examination of psychosocial correlates of eating disorders among female collegiate athletes. *Research Quarterly for Exercise and Sport, 80*, 621–632. https://doi.org/10.1080/027 01367.2009.10599601.

Pridgeon, L., & Grogan, S. (2012). Understanding exercise adherence and dropout: An interpretative phenomenological analysis of men and women's accounts of gym attendance and non-attendance. *Qualitative Research in Sport, Exercise and Health, 4*(3), 382–399. https://doi.org/10.1080/2159676X.2012.712984.

Reardon, R., & Grogan. S. (2011). Women's reasons for seeking breast reduction: A qualitative investigation, *Journal of Health Psychology, 16*(1), 31–41. https://doi.org/10.1177/1359105310367531.

Ricciardelli, L. A., & Yager, Z. (2015). *Adolescence and body image: From development to preventing dissatisfaction.* London: Routledge. https://doi.org/10.4324/97813 15849379.

Robinson, K., & Ferraro, F. (2004). The relationship between types of female athletic participation and female body type. *Journal of Psychology, 138*(2), 115–128. https://doi.org/10.3200/JRLP.138.2.115-128.

Seekis, V., Bradley, G. L., & Duffy, A. (2017). The effectiveness of self-compassion and self-esteem writing tasks in reducing body image concerns. *Body Image, 23*, 206–213. https://doi.org/10.1016/j.bodyim.2017.09.003.

Slevec, J., & Tiggemann, M. (2011). Media exposure, body dissatisfaction, and disordered eating in middle-aged women. A test of the sociocultural model of disordered eating. *Psychology of Women Quarterly, 35*(4), 617–627. https://doi.org/10.1177/0361684311420249.

Steese, S. Dollette, M., Phillips, W., Hossfeld, E., Matthews, G., & Taormina, G. (2006). Understanding girls' circle as an intervention on perceived social support, body image, self-efficacy, locus of control, and self-esteem. *Adolescence, 41*(161), 55–64.

Swami, V. (2015). Cultural influences on body size ideals: Unpacking the impact of Westernization and modernization. *European Psychologist, 20*(1), 44–51. https://doi.org/10.1027/1016-9040/a000150.

Tiggemann, M., Slater, A., & Smyth, V. (2014). 'Retouch free': The effect of labelling media images as not digitally altered on women's body dissatisfaction. *Body Image, 11*(1), 85–88. https://doi.org/10.1016/j.bodyim.2013.08.005.

Tylka, T., & Wood-Barcalow, N. (2015). A positive complement. *Body Image, 14*, 115–117. https://doi.org/10.1016/j.bodyim.2015.04.002.

Vartanian, L. R. (2012). Self-discrepancy theory and body image. In T. F. Cash (Ed.), *Encylopedia of body image and human appearance* (pp. 711–717). London: Elsevier. https://doi.org/10.1016/B978-0-12-384925-0.00112-7.

Wasilenko, K. A., Kulik, J. A., & Wanic, R. A. (2007). Effects of social comparisons with peers on women's body satisfaction and exercise behaviour. *International Journal of Eating Disorders, 40*(8), 740–745. https://doi.org/10.1002/eat.20433.

Yamamiya, Y., Cash, T. F., Melnyk, S. E., Posavak, H. D., & Posavac, S. S. (2005). Women's exposure to thin-and-beautiful media images: Body image effects of media-ideal internalisation and impact-reduction interventions. *Body Image, 2*(1), 74–80. https://doi.org/10.1016/j.bodyim.2004.11.001.

9 Exercise addiction in the exercising female

An interdisciplinary examination

Heather A. Hausenblas and Derek T. Y. Mann

Introduction

Although the physical, psychological, and social benefits of regular exercise are well documented, there is growing literature that a small proportion of the population may engage in excessive exercise, which can have negative health effects and manifest into an addiction. Exercise addiction is defined as a craving for leisure-time physical activity that progresses as excessive exercise behaviour and results in physiological (e.g., tolerance) and/or psychological (e.g., withdrawal) symptoms (Hausenblas & Symons Downs, 2002a). The incidence of high risk for exercise addiction is 0.3 to 0.5 per cent in the general population, while among regular exercisers it ranges between 1.9 and 3.2 per cent (Mónok et al., 2012). Although men and women are equally at risk for exercise addiction, it more often appears as a primary addiction in men and a secondary addiction in women.

Similar to other behavioural addictions, exercise addiction is a controversial concept (Starcevic & Khazaal, 2017). This controversy is reflected in its early designation as a 'positive addiction' (Glasser, 1979), because the excessive exercise was believed to have beneficial health effects. Since this time, research into the negative effects of excessive exercise has been conceptualised in a number of similar ways, including exercise addiction, exercise dependence, compulsive exercise, morbid exercise, exercise anorexia, exercise abuse, and obligatory exercise, to name just a few (Berczik et al., 2012; Davis, 2000; Hausenblas & Symons Downs, 2002a; Pasman & Thompson, 1988). Typically, the terms indicate pathological attitudes and excessive amounts of exercise in the context of addiction, commitment, and issues related to exercise. In a study of adult female exercisers, aside from a higher occurrence of recounted menstrual irregularities, the primary exercise dependence group was similar to the control group (Bamber, Cockerill, & Carroll, 2000). However, the secondary exercise dependence group, compared to the control group, reported higher levels of psychological illness, neuroticism, dispositional addictiveness and impulsiveness, lower self-esteem, and greater concern with body shape and weight as well as with the social, psychological, and aesthetic costs of not exercising. Given that exercise dependence is more likely classified as a secondary addiction in women, researchers and practitioners should consider screening women more so than men for related psychological comorbidities.

Currently, consensus has emerged that the term 'exercise addiction' best describes this compulsive exercise behaviour, because it contains both the elements of compulsion and dependence (Berczik et al., 2012). Thus, exercise addiction will be the term used throughout this chapter to represent this maladaptive excessive exercise behaviour. Embedded throughout this chapter is the science behind exercise addiction and how to differentiate between regular to committed to addicted exercise for the exercising female.

Aims of the chapter

The aims of the chapter are as follows:

1 To discuss the origins of exercise addiction research.
2 To provide operational clarity to exercise addiction in females.
3 To differentiate between primary and secondary exercise addiction.
4 To critically examine the correlates of exercise addiction.
5 To highlight the treatment of exercise addiction for the exercising female.

Operationalising exercise addiction

The operational definition that has received the most recognition for exercise addiction is based on the American Psychiatric Association's Diagnostic and Statistical Manual, 5th edition (DSM-5) criteria for substance dependence (American Psychiatric Association, 2013; Hausenblas & Symons Downs, 2002a; Veale, 1995). Using these criteria, exercise addiction is operationalised as a multidimensional, maladaptive pattern of physical activity, leading to significant impairment or distress, as manifested by three or more criteria from a list of seven (see Table 9.1). These criteria are described in more detail below.

First, for *tolerance*, the exerciser continually needs to increase her time spent exercising or the intensity of the workout to achieve the originally desired effect (such as being in a better mood or having more energy). The second criterion, *withdrawal*, refers to negative moods that are experienced when an addict is unable to exercise. The third criterion, *intention* effects, occurs when people exercise more than they had originally intended to. The fourth criterion is *loss of control* over the exercise behaviour. The worse an exercise addict's pathology becomes, the less of a handle she has over her thoughts, behaviour, and response to the gym. The fifth criterion, *time*, refers to huge amounts of time spent engaging in exercise or exercise-related activities. A large chunk of an exercise addict's time during the day is devoted to

Table 9.1 Exercise addiction criteria

Criteria	Description	Example
Tolerance	Need for increased exercise levels to achieve the desired effect, or diminished effects experienced from the same exercise level	Running 5 miles no longer results in improved mood
Withdrawal	Negative symptoms are evidenced with cessation of exercise, or exercise is used to relieve or forestall the onset of these symptoms	Anxiety, depression, and/or fatigue experienced when unable to exercise
Intention	Exercise is undertaken with greater intensity, frequency, or duration than was intended	Intended to run for 5 miles, but ran for 7 miles instead
Lack of control	Exercise is maintained despite a persistent desire to cut down or control it	Ran during lunch break despite trying to not exercise during work hours
Time	Considerable time is spent in activities essential to exercise maintenance	Vacations are exercise-related, such as skiing or hiking
Reduction in other activities	Social, occupational, or recreational pursuits are reduced or dropped because of exercise	Running rather than going out with friends for dinner
Continuance	Exercise is maintained despite the awareness of a persistent physical or psychological problem	Running despite shin splints

Sources: APA, 2013; Hausenblas and Symons Downs, 2002a; Veale, 1995.

physical activity. The sixth criterion, *conflict*, refers to non-fitness-related activities that fall by the wayside because they conflict with exercise. Time spent relaxing with friends or family is truncated to make more room for exercise. Finally, *continuance,* refers to continuing to exercise despite physical or psychological issues that should prevent the activity. Exercise addicts often push past pain, injury, and illness to finish a workout – even against their doctor's orders.

It is difficult to separate healthy exercise from obsessive or compulsive exercise. Meeting some of the above criteria does not directly indicate that a person is an exercise addict. A distinguishing indicator is when exercise becomes all consuming – when people start losing friends, forgoing social activities, or reneging work opportunities – that their workout schedule becomes a cause for concern. In other words, people addicted to exercise

continue to keep going despite injuries, mental issues, social/work obligations, and physical exhaustion. It is important to note that exercise addiction
is not included in the DSM-5 (American Psychiatric Association, 2013) as a
mental disorder. According to the American Psychiatric Association, all
other potentially addictive behaviours – not just exercise, but also sex, internet browsing, and shopping – require further research before unequivocally
being denoted as a uniquely diagnosable disorder.

Primary versus secondary exercise addiction

For many years, there was a misperception that exercise addiction was 'just
a symptom' of an eating disorder. However, Veale (1987, 1995) proposed
that exercise addiction is differentiated from an eating disorder by clarify-
ing the objective of the exercise. Primary exercise addiction is different
from excessive exercise present in eating disorder patients (also known as
secondary exercise addiction), in which the exercise represents a means to
control weight. Secondary exercise addiction is more compulsive while
primary exercise addiction is more addictive in nature. However, this dis-
tinction is not always easy because individuals with primary exercise addiction are often preoccupied with their weight, dieting, and body image, and
the primary motivation for exercising may not be clear. Thus, females suspected of exercise addiction should undergo further evaluation to determine if it is primary or secondary to ensure that the underlying symptoms
are properly addressed (Starcevic & Khazaal, 2017). Men and women are
equally at risk for exercise addiction – men being more susceptible to
primary exercise addiction and women to secondary exercise addiction
(Cunningham, Pearman, & Brewerton, 2016; Szabó, Griffiths, de la Vega
Marcos, Mervó, & Demetrovics, 2013). This gender difference is related to
the risk of eating disorders in the female population. We might consider
early socialisation and other norms that pertain to females having a significant influence in this regard (Meulemans, Pribis, Grajales, & Krivak,
2014). In the United States, eating disorders affect about 3 per cent of
girls and women and 1 per cent of boys and men. Those most at risk of
eating disorders are girls and women that participate in activities that are
concerned with maintaining low body weight and lean body image including track and field, gymnastics, diving, dancing, and figure skating (Hoek,
2006; National Eating Disorders Association, 2018).

Risk factors/correlates of exercise addiction

Alongside the growing interest in exercise addiction, both clinically and
empirically, researchers have begun to dig deeper into the aetiology of this
behavioural addiction. Of particular importance are physical self-concept and
exercise identity, perfectionism, and personality factors including those that
put female exercisers at a greater risk for secondary addiction.

Physical self-concept and exercise identity

Physical self-perception has been closely linked to positive and productive physical activity. For example, researchers considering the role of exercise across the lifespan have identified that participants who tend to be more physically active also report higher physical self-perception scores; meanwhile participants who identify with lower physical self-perception tend to engage in less physical activity and report a higher prevalence of obesity, eating disorders, and depression. Research has also supported a negative relationship between exercise dependence with physical self-perception, self-esteem (Hall, Hill, Appleton, & Kozub, 2009), and body satisfaction (Hausenblas & Fallon, 2002). In fact, some researchers have demonstrated meaningfully different trends in the relationship between physical self-concept and exercise dependence in men and women. Specifically, as males reported more physical activity, appearance and esteem were strongly correlated with symptoms of exercise dependence and this relationship was further strengthened by the presence of lower self-esteem. Conversely, in female athletes, perceived ability and physical activity levels were more closely related to exercise dependence symptomology. Thus, the underlying motives linking physical activity and dependence may, in fact, be different between men and women.

To this point, Murray, McKenzie, Newmann, and Brown (2013) proposed the relationship between exercise identity and exercise dependence. According to the identity theory, role and identity become intertwined, with the individual becoming preoccupied with the behaviours most closely related to their perceived role (Cook et al., 2015; Stets & Burke, 2000). As a result, physical self-perception or self-concept becomes the catalyst for future exercise behaviour in an effort to maintain one's self-perception. Unfortunately, those with a high exercise identity or physical self-perception are likely to engage in exercise behaviour despite negative consequences such as injury, excessive time commitment, or interpersonal loss (Murray et al., 2013). Of particular importance here is the relationship between exercise identity and secondary exercise dependence, which is sufficiently more prevalent in women than men. Furthermore, those who strongly identify themselves as an exerciser coupled with above average reporting of social physique anxiety are at greater risk for exercise dependence (Cook et al., 2015). In both cases, the comorbidity is more prevalent in women than men, placing women at greater risk.

Personality

Personality can be defined as individual differences in characteristic patterns of thinking, feeling, and behaving (American Psychiatric Association, 2013). Although there are two distinct approaches towards advancing our measurement and understanding of personality (i.e., type and trait), the trait-based approach is characterised by the five-factor model of personality. The five-factor model is affectionately known as the prevailing framework for assessing personality. Although there are several derivatives of the five-factor model along with several assessments, there is a universal acceptance of factors that comprise the model. The five factors include: neuroticism (a measure of proneness to stress, anxiety, and emotional instability); extraversion (a measure of the individual's energy directed towards the external, social world); openness (one's willingness and eagerness to seek out new things and experiences); agreeableness (a measure of one's orientation towards others, concern for cooperation, and social harmony); and conscientiousness (measure of one's actions and attitudes towards organisation, persistence, control, and goal-directed behaviour). Although each dimension encompasses several unique facets that allow for distinct insights into one's patterns of thinking, feeling, and behaving, much of the research relating personality with exercise dependence has focused on the relationship between the overarching factors at the expense of the facets (i.e., personality subscale of each of the five factors) and the behaviours associated with exercise addiction.

Given that personality traits are believed to be stable across situations and are representative of individual differences in thinking, feeling, and acting, the exploration of the relationship between personality and exercise addiction sought to unveil the specific personality characteristics that separate adaptive exercise behaviour from the excessive, even compulsive, behaviours associated with exercise addiction. The relationship between personality and exercise addiction has been explored using a variety of research designs often yielding a common result with the exception of the tenuous relationship between neuroticism and exercise addiction. In the early work of Jibaja-Rusth (1989), a positive relationship was found between exercise addiction and neuroticism, a finding that was later supported by Andreassen et al. (2013). However, several authors have reported a negative relationship (Davis & Fox, 1993; Hausenblas & Giacobbi, 2004) between exercise dependence and neuroticism, while some have reported no relationship (Spano, 2001). However, a positive relationship between extraversion, facets of conscientiousness, narcissism (Miller & Mesagno, 2014), and agreeableness have been more consistently reported (Hausenblas & Giacobbi, 2004). In addition, in early research conducted by Coen and Ogles (1993) a positive relationship was reported between perfectionism, trait anxiety, and exercise addiction. In studies of runners, a positive relationship between anxiety and a negative relationship between self-esteem and social physique anxiety have been evidenced with exercise addiction (Cook et al., 2015).

Perfectionism

An extension of the personality research recently discussed is perfectionism, a multidimensional personality trait that necessitates the actual or perceived need to perform perfectly, which has also been linked to exercise addiction (Hewitt & Flett, 2002). Exercise addiction, not unlike other behavioural outlets, is often used as a means of escape from the unpleasant psychological experience that the exerciser is trying to avoid (Korolenko, 1991). However, for those with perfectionistic tendencies, we might consider the interactive effects of the individual and the environment/situational factors. In the case of the perfectionist, we must consider the perfectionist belief that is held. According to the multidimensional perfectionism framework (Hewitt & Flett, 1996), perfectionism is comprised of perfectionistic self-expectations and perfectionistic interpersonal dynamics that result in three distinct personality traits (Hewitt & Flett, 2002). These traits include: self-oriented perfectionism (SOP: considered to require perfection of oneself); other-oriented perfectionism (involving unrealistic expectations or judgements of others); or socially-prescribed perfectionism (SPP: maintaining the perception that others are demanding perfection of oneself). In line with multi-dimensional perfectionism, perfectionism not only includes an embedded personal belief and self-perception (e.g., failure is not an option), it also involves personal motives or drives (e.g., pursuit of perfection) and the resultant actions or behaviours that are the manifestation of the beliefs and motives (e.g., expecting others to strive for perfection; Sherry, Hewitt, Flett, & Harvey, 2003). The origin of perfectionism can have a profound effect on perception and functioning both adaptive and maladaptive. Recent research suggests that both men and women are adversely affected by perfectionistic strivings and these strivings may be indicative of a strong link between eating disorders and exercise dependence in women (Costa, Hausenblas, Oliva, Cuzzocrea, & Larcan, 2016).

The fact that some individuals engage in exercise behaviours beyond what is customary for health benefits, or even beyond that which might be expected of one with a mastery orientation, is the result of a shift in belief or perception of self that results in a maladaptive pattern of exercise behaviour to overcome or suppress the psychological distress being experienced. As a result, maladaptive coping strategies are likely, and, in exercisers, this may result in excessive or even compulsive exercise (Flett & Hewitt, 2005). For example, Coen and Ogles (1993) identified a clear link between neurotic perfectionists and obligatory runners, while Hagan and Hausenblas (2003) reported that those in the high exercise dependence group reported a higher need to excel and be the best, a belief aligned with SOP. Individuals who are exceedingly absorbed in their perfectionist tendencies are more inclined to worry about public perception and body image and tend to be more self-conscious and have greater levels of trait anxiety (Flett & Hewitt, 2005; Hausenblas & Fallon, 2002). In fact, the seminal work of Flett, Pole-Langdon, and Hewitt (2003) with regular exercisers supports the contention that SOP and SPP are intimately connected with compulsive exercise. Most recently, Miller and Mesagno (2014) reported that exercise addiction was positively related to SOP and SPP as well as the personality trait, narcissism.

In fact, the combination of narcissism and SOP proved to be a unique and powerful predictor of exercise addiction. Although SOP is highly motivating and even rewarding, SOP may also increase one's susceptibility to other psychological difficulties, especially when under stress (Flett & Hewitt, 2005). The real challenge, however, lies with SPP, which has been linked to various clinical outcomes, including depression and even suicidal ideation (O'Connor, 2007). In fact, research exploring the mediating relationship of maladaptive perfectionism, associated with the conditional social support tied to unrealistic standards established by others, fully mediates the relationships between perfectionism, exercise dependence, and eating disorders in women (Costa et al., 2016).

Treatment of exercise addiction

The literature examining the treatment of exercise addiction is scant. Given the lack of awareness in professional and lay communities about exercise addiction, coupled with the common belief that more exercise results in improved health, health care professionals may not recognise the signs of exercise addiction even when its adverse health consequences are apparent (e.g., overuse injuries, interpersonal dysfunction) or when it is comorbid with other conditions (e.g., eating disorders, other addictions). As with most behavioural addictions, cognitive behavioural therapy is recommended to restructure maladaptive beliefs about exercise and manage mood disturbances (Hausenblas, Schreiber, & Smoliga, 2017). Since regular exercise is a desired behaviour of health promotion and maintenance, efforts should be redirected to maintaining an active lifestyle while rebalancing the role that exercise plays (Jee, 2016). The goal of treatment is not to prevent the person from working out, but to help her recognise the addictive behaviour and reduce her exercise routine rigidity. Early identification can enable prompt management before compulsive exercise leads to other health issues such as an eating disorder or physical pathologies associated with excessive exercise such as injuries. Moreover, given that women are less likely to report primary exercise dependence and more likely to report secondary exercise dependence, it is essential for clinicians and practitioners to explore other psychological comorbidities to better understand the motive for excessive exercise behaviour.

Treating the exercise addict, therefore, necessitates a multipronged approach. Practically speaking, the first step is to clarify for the exercise addict whether or not she is experiencing a primary or secondary diagnosis, differentiating between the addictive psychological, physiological, and behavioural outcomes associated with the addiction, rather than emphasising the secondary compulsive behaviours that are often associated with a secondary diagnosis. An exercise specialist should then determine the female's state of health, including physical and emotional well-being. Motivational interviewing (Hettema, Steel, & Miller, 2005), in addition to the use of the

Exercise Dependence Scale (Hausenblas & Symons Downs, 2002b), may prove useful for gaining insight into the factors that drive the exercise addiction. Further analyses from nutritionists, psychologists, and kinesiology/exercise science specialists should focus on the person's dietary habits, motivation for recovery, redirection of exercise goals, and capacity for the implementation of coping strategies. Treatment therapies for exercise addicts should also include the development of healthy eating habits, strategies for improving and maintaining a healthy self-esteem and body image, gradual incorporation of healthy alternative recreational pursuits, and the monitoring of progress. Furthermore, in the event the exercise addict is motivated to mask physiological sensations as a result of psychological hardship, biofeedback training coupled with other forms of cognitive behavioural therapy may prove effective by increasing the ability of the exercise addict to gain awareness and control of the very sensations they attempt to replace with excessive exercise behaviour. Even as the research into treatment efficacy progresses, individual counselling and monitoring will remain critical to achieving recovery from exercise addiction.

Real-world example

Carla

Carla grew up in a household where the importance of fitness was heavily stressed, and a regular exercise regimen was strongly encouraged. Struggling with low self-esteem, Carla delighted in the changes brought about to her body by running on her high school track team. Running granted Carla a sense of empowerment. Wanting more relief, she convinced her parents to let her join a gym close to her school and began running four to five miles each day on the treadmill before classes – even on days she had track practice. This doubled physical activity still didn't satisfy Carla. In response to a nagging sense that she had to do more, she increased her physical activity levels. Whereas she'd previously woken at 5:30 a.m. to run before school, she now felt the need to lace up her running shoes at 4:00 a.m., just to get in enough.

Deprived and exhausted, Carla's compulsive thought patterns raced out of control. Her menstrual cycle ceased, she battled severe insomnia, she experienced constant physical pain, and she began losing her hair. Emotionally, she cycled between depression and numbness. Carla's identity and self-worth were so enmeshed in how many miles she logged and how thin she appeared that she lost hold on who she was apart from exercise. Like most exercise addicts, Carla withdrew from most social activities, declining invitations to dinners or evening events, for fear that staying out too late might throw off her morning routine. She was continuously tired and barely able to focus. As a consequence of her self-destruction, her academic performance began suffering almost as much as her health.

She eventually enrolled herself in an intensive outpatient programme. One of Carla's biggest challenges was resisting the urge to run every morning at 5:00 a.m. Carla never wrote off exercise entirely. She continues to run about four miles several times each week. Though she still admits feeling 'a bit over-regimented and rigid about exercise', she's able to successfully cut herself off when she hears that compulsive voice in her head urging her to push past her limits. 'I'm better able now to talk myself out of the guilt or anxiety I feel if I miss a day or don't do "enough"'. Carla recognises the challenges of overcoming exercise addiction. Unlike kicking a habit with substance abuse, 'you can't walk away from exercise – you have to practice moderation. You don't have a choice to be abstinent'. This case study was adapted from Schreiber and Hausenblas (2016).

Summary

People with exercise addiction experience loss of control such that exercise becomes an obligation and excessive. Although exercise addiction is not officially classified as a mental health disorder, it is characterised by similar negative effects on emotional and social health as other addictions. Primary exercise addiction differs from excessive exercise seen in people with eating disorders (also known as secondary exercise addiction), in which exercise represents a means to control weight. Ongoing research continues to be conducted across the globe and mental health professionals are becoming increasingly cognisant of an all-too-easy to mask issue that plagues a select segment of the exercising female population. Furthermore, researchers and practitioners must continue to better understand the unique mediators differentiating male and female exercisers.

References

American Psychiatric Association. (2013). *Diagnostic and statistical manual of mental disorders* (5th ed.). Arlington VA, USA: American Psychiatric Association. https://doi.org/10.1176/appi.books.9780890425596.

Andreassen, C. S., Griffiths, M. D., Gjertsen, S. R., Krossbakken, E., Kvam, S., & Pallesen, S. (2013). The relationships between behavioral addictions and the five-factor model of personality. *Journal of Behavioral Addictions, 2,* 90–99. https://doi.org/10.1556/JBA.2.2013.003.

Bamber D., Cockerill, I. M., & Carroll, D. (2000). The pathological status of exercise dependence. *British Journal of Sports Medicine, 34,* 125–132. https://doi.org/10.1136/bjsm.34.2.125.

Berczik, K., Szabó, A., Griffiths, M. D., Kurimay, T., Kun, B., Urbán, R., & Demetrovics, Z. (2012). Exercise addiction: Symptoms, diagnosis, epidemiology, and etiology. *Substance Use Misuse, 47,* 403–417. https://doi.org/10.3109/10826084.2011.639120.

Coen, S., & Ogles, B. (1993). Psychological characteristics of the obligatory runner: A critical examination of the anorexia analogue hypothesis. *Journal of Sport & Exercise Psychology, 15,* 338–354. https://doi.org/10.1123/jsep. 15.3.338.

Cook, B., Karr, T. M., Zunker, C., Mitchell, J. E., Thompson, R., Sherman, R., … Crosby, R. D. (2015). The influence of exercise identity and social physique anxiety on exercise dependence. *Journal of Behavioral Addictions, 4*, 195–199. https://doi.org/10.1556/2006.4.2015.020.

Costa, S., Hausenblas, H. A., Oliva, P., Cuzzocrea, F., & Larcan, R. (2016). Maladaptive perfectionism as mediator among psychological control, eating disorders, and exercise dependence symptoms in habitual exerciser. *Journal of Behavioral Addictions, 5*, 77–89. https://doi.org/10.1556/2006.5.2016.004.

Cunningham, H. E., Pearman, S., & Brewerton, T. D. (2016). Conceptualizing primary and secondary pathological exercise using available measures of excessive exercise. *International Journal of Eating Disorders, 49*, 778–792. https://doi.org/10.1002/eat.22551.

Davis, C. (2000). Exercise abuse. *International Journal of Sport Psychology, 31*, 278–289.

Davis, C., & Fox J. (1993). Excessive exercise and weight preoccupation in women. *Addiction Behavior, 18*, 201–211. https://doi.org/10.1016/0306-4603(93)90050-j.

Egorov, A. Y., & Szabó, A. (2013). The exercise paradox: An interactional model for a clearer conceptualization of exercise addiction. *Journal of Behavioral Addictions, 2*, 199–208. https://doi.org/10.1556/JBA.2.2013.4.2.

Flett, G. L., & Hewitt, P. L. (2005). The perils of perfectionism in sports and exercise. *Current Direction in Psychological Science, 14*, 14–18. https://doi.org/10.1111/j.0963-7214.2005.00326.x.

Flett, G. L., Pole-Langdon, L., & Hewitt, P. L. (2003). *Trait perfectionism and perfectionistic self-presentation in compulsive exercise.* Unpublished manuscript, York University, Toronto, Ontario, Canada.

Glasser, W. (1976). *Positive addiction.* New York: Harper & Row.

Hagan, A. L., & Hausenblas, H. A. (2003). The relationship between exercise dependence symptoms and perfectionism. *American Journal of Health Studies, 18*(2–3), 133–137.

Hall, H. K., Hill, A. P., Appleton, P. R., & Kozub S. A. (2009). The mediating influence of unconditional self-acceptance and labile self-esteem on the relationship between multidimensional perfectionism and exercise dependence. *Psychology of Sport and Exercise, 10*, 35–44. https://doi.org/10.1016/j.psychsport.2008.05.003.

Hausenblas, H. A., & Fallon, E. A. (2002). Relationship among body image, exercise behavior, and exercise dependence symptoms. *International Journal of Eating Disorders, 32*, 179–185. https://doi.org/10.1002/eat.10071.

Hausenblas, H. A., & Giacobbi, P. R., Jr. (2004). Relationship between exercise dependence symptoms and personality. *Personality and Individual Differences, 36*, 1265–1273. https://doi.org/10.1016/s0191-8869(03)00214-9.

Hausenblas, H. A., Schreiber, K., & Smoliga, J. M. (2017). Exercise addiction. *British Medical Journal, 26*, 357. https://doi.org/10.1136/bmj.j1745.

Hausenblas, H. A., & Symons Downs, D. (2002a). Exercise dependence: a systematic review. *Psychology of Sport and Exercise, 3*, 89–123. https://doi.org/10.1016/S1469-0292(00)00015-7.

Hausenblas, H. A., & Symons Downs, D. (2002b). How much is too much? The development and validation of the Exercise Dependence Scale. *Psychology and Health: An International Journal, 17*, 387–404. https://doi.org/10.1080/0887044022000004894.

Hettema, J., Steele, J., & Miller, W. R. (2005). Motivational interviewing. *Annual Review of Clinical Psychology, 1*, 91–111. https://doi.org/10.1146/annurev.clinpsy.1.102803.143833.

Hewitt, P. L., & Flett, G. L. (2002). Perfectionism and stress processes in psychopathology. In G. L. Flett & P. L. Hewitt (Eds.), *Perfectionism: Theory, research, and treatment* (pp. 255–284). Washington, DC: American Psychological Association. https://doi.org/10.1037/10458-000.

Hoek, H. W. (2006). Incidence, prevalence and mortality of anorexia nervosa and other eating disorders. *Current Opinion in Psychiatry, 19*, 389–394. https://doi.org/10.1097/01.yco.0000228759.95237.78.

Jee, Y-S. (2016). Exercise addiction and rehabilitation. *Journal of Exercise Rehabilitation, 12*, 67–68. https://doi.org/10.12965/jer.1632604.302.

Jibaja-Rusch, M. L. (1989). *The development of a psycho-social risk profile for becoming an obligatory runner* (Unpublished doctoral dissertation). University of Houston, Texas.

Korolenko, T. P. (1991) Addictive behavior: Total characteristics and laws of development. *History of Psychiatric and Medical Psychology, 1*, 8.

Meulemans, S., Pribis, P., Grajales, T., & Krivak, G. (2014). Gender differences in exercise dependence and eating disorders in young Adults: A path analysis of a conceptual model. *Nutrients, 6*, 4895–4905. https://doi.org/10.3390/nu6114895.

Miller, K. J., & Mesagno, C. (2014). Personality traits and exercise dependence: Exploring the role of narcissism and perfectionism. *International Journal of Sport and Exercise Psychology, 12*, 368–381. https://doi.org/10.1080/1612197X.2014.932821.

Mónok, K., Berczik, K., Urbán, R., Szabó, A., Griffiths, M. D., Farkas, J. ... Demetrovics, Z. (2012). Psychometric properties and concurrent validity of two exercise addiction measures: A population wide study. *Psychology of Sport and Exercise, 13*, 739–746. https://doi.org/10.1016/j.psychsport.2012.06.003.

Murray, A. L., McKenzie, K., Newman, E., & Brown, E. (2013). Exercise identity as a risk factor for exercise dependence. *British Journal of Health Psychology, 18*, 369–382. https://doi.org/10.1111/j.2044-8287.2012.02091.

National Eating Disorders Association. (2018). *Statistics and research on eating disorders.* Retrieved from www.nationaleatingdisorders.org/statistics-research-eating-disorders.

O'Connor R. C. (2007). The relations between perfectionism and suicidality: A systematic review. *Suicide and Life-Threatening Behavior, 37*, 698–714. https://doi.org/10.1521/suli.2007.37.6.698.

Pasman, L., & Thompson, J. K. (1988). Body image and eating disturbance in obligatory runners, obligatory weightlifters, and sedentary individuals. *International Journal of Eating Disorders, 7*, 759–769. https://doi.org/10.1002/1098-108X(198811)7:6759::AID-EAT22600706053.0.CO;2-G.

Schreiber, K., & Hausenblas, H. A. (2016). *The truth about exercise addiction. Understanding the dark side of thinspiration.* Lanhan, Maryland: Rowman & Littlefield.

Sherry, S. B., Hewitt, P. L., Flett, G. L., & Harvey. M. (2003). Perfectionism dimensions, perfectionistic attitudes, dependent attitudes, and depression in psychiatric patients and university students. *Journal of Counseling Psychology, 50*, 373–386. https://doi.org/10.1037/0022-0167.50.3.373.

Spano, L. (2001). The relationship between exercise and anxiety, obsessive-compulsiveness, and narcissism. *Personality and Individual Differences, 30*, 87–93. https://doi.org/10.1016/s0191-8869(00)00012-x.

Starcevic, V., & Khazaal, Y. (2017). Relationships between behavioural addictions and psychiatric disorders: What is known and what is yet to be learned? *Frontiers in Psychiatry, 8*. https://doi.org/10.3389/fpsyt.2017.00053.

Stets, J. E., & Burke, P. J. (2000). Identity theory and social identity theory. *Social Psychology Quarterly, 63*, 224–237. https://doi.org/10.2307/2695870.

Szabó, A., Griffiths, M. D., de la Vega Marcos, R., Mervó, B., & Demetrovics Z. (2015). Methodological and conceptual limitations in exercise addiction research. *Yale Journal of Biology and Medicine, 88*, 303–308. https://doi.org/10.1556/jba.2.2013.4.9.

Veale, D. (1995). Does primary exercise dependence really exist? In J. Annett, B. Cripps, & H. Steinberg (Eds.), *Exercise addiction: Motivation for participation in sport and exercise* (pp. 1–5). Leicester, UK: British Psychological Society.

Veale, D. M. (1987). Exercise dependence. *British Journal of Addiction, 82* 735–740. https://doi.org/10.1111/j.1360-0443.1987.tb01539.x.

10 Immune function and the exercising female

Judith Allgrove and Glen Davison

Introduction

The area of exercise immunology research originated from anecdotal reports of athletes experiencing increased incidence of upper respiratory illness following heavy training and competition. This research initiated a number of important studies investigating the relationship between exercise, immunity, and infection risk. The relationship can be modelled into a J-shaped curve, where moderate exercise can reduce the risk above sedentary levels and intense exercise can increase the risk. It is known that prolonged, strenuous exercise can temporarily depress some components of the immune system for between 3 and 72 hr, leaving an open window for infection. Immune function can be affected by sex differences, and females respond to pathogens with stronger innate and adaptive immune responses, which may reduce susceptibility to infections but may also increase the risk of autoimmune diseases. Noticeable differences in the immune response to exercise in females and across the menstrual cycle have been observed, yet the clinical significance of these has not yet been established. In this chapter, what is known about the immune response to exercise and infection risk is examined. The first section gives a general overview of the area, based on the original studies where differences between females and males in many of these responses were not considered, before later sections specifically consider how these effects may vary in females (and/or throughout the menstrual cycle). Recommendations are given on how to minimise immune system changes and infection risk to preserve exercise performance and health for the exercising female.

Aims of the chapter

The aims of the chapter are as follows:

1. To appreciate the relationship between exercise and infection risk.
2. To understand the effect of exercise on the immune system.
3. To understand the effect of exercise on the immune system and infection risk in exercising females compared with males.

4   To identify practical recommendations to minimise immune system changes and infection risk.

Exercise and infection risk in athletes

Interest in the relationship between exercise, immunity, and infection originated from a series of anecdotal reports of athletes contracting higher than 'normal' rates of infection during periods of heavy training and competition. These anecdotes prompted a number of epidemiological studies during the 1980s and 1990s assessing the link between exercise training 'load', immunity, and illness. These studies were typically survey-based using self-reported symptoms, but did confirm the original anecdotal reports, that those with the highest training loads tended to be more susceptible to upper respiratory tract infections (URTI, e.g., the common cold and influenza) or the associated symptoms (upper respiratory symptoms, URS). This relationship is best described by the J-shaped model of exercise training load and illness (Nieman, 1994), where moderate exercise training is associated with a reduced risk but strenuous exercise and high training loads are associated with an increased risk. Malm (2006) later suggested that in order to achieve the highest level/elite status, athletes must be resistant to regular illness despite high training loads, and strenuous training and competition, and hence proposed an S-shaped rather than a J-shaped model. Malm (2006) suggested that the elite level athletes do not follow the J-shaped trend, but instead have an immune system that is not perturbed by high training loads/intensive training, suggesting this is a prerequisite to achieving elite level. This proposed explanation, however, does not adequately consider the many other factors that may explain the lower URTI/URS incidence rates in elite athletes. That is, it is highly likely that elite/professional athletes will have considerable support (such as financial, medical, sports science, and medicine) that will contribute to reducing illness risks rather than their immune system per se being naturally able to withstand strenuous training.

Since the early survey-type studies, many researchers have sought to better understand the relationship between exercise and the immune system, and have attempted to identify the underpinning mechanisms, with acute and/or chronic exercise-induced changes in immune function being the most logical. There is now a strong body of evidence demonstrating that moderate amounts of exercise improve immune system functions, whereas athletes engaged in regular, prolonged, and/or intensive training may experience periods when immune function is (clinically normal, but) 'suboptimal' (Gleeson, 2007; Gleeson & Walsh, 2012; Nieman, 1994; Pedersen & Ullam, 1994). This immunodepression is particularly apparent in endurance athletes such as cyclists, runners, swimmers, and triathletes, but any athletes with a high training load and/or suboptimal recovery may be at increased risk. Such infections can compromise training and/or competition performance (Pyne,

Hopkins, Batterham, Gleeson, & Fricker, 2005). Also, overtraining or training with insufficient recovery between sessions can exacerbate these effects. Infections may be increased, because many components of the immune system are temporarily reduced (immunodepression) after strenuous and/or prolonged bouts of exercise. This exercise-induced immunodepression typically lasts between 3 and 72 hr, depending on the nature and frequency of the exercise. If the next training bout is commenced too soon, before the immune system has fully recovered, then the immunodepressive effects may build up, resulting in further increased infection risk. Periods of depressed immunity have been termed as 'open windows' during which athletes are more susceptible to picking up an infection. Intensified training periods and training camps are also associated with increased risk. Indeed, the way training is distributed or periodised is of key importance. In support of this idea, Svendsen, Taylor, Tønnessen, Bahr, and Gleeson (2016) have recently shown that rapid changes in training load (i.e., increasing too quickly) are better predictors of URS risk than total load alone, and hence may be more informative than simply considering total training loads or volumes. However, a direct link between changes in immunity and infection risk is difficult to confirm in a sport and exercise context. One of the difficulties is due to the known redundancy in the immune system (where there are compensatory mechanisms, meaning that a deficiency in any one component can be compensated by other components so that 'overall' defence is not compromised). This redundancy is why studies, in which one (or few) isolated immune marker has been investigated, may be inappropriate or may lead to incorrect conclusions. It is important (from both research and applied perspectives) to select clinically relevant markers, such as symptoms and actual infection incidence, and *in vivo* (whole-body integrated response) immune markers, which are 'clinically relevant' (see Albers et al., 2013 for a detailed overview). Nevertheless, exercise has been shown to affect most areas of the immune system (in men and women) in some way and it is well accepted that athletes participating in regular intensive training, especially endurance athletes, may be more susceptible to URTI, as discussed earlier. From a practical perspective, although depressed immune function may increase the chances of picking up an infection, whether or not an athlete contracts an infection is also dependent on their exposure to pathogens, which may be beyond their control. Factors like having contact with lots of other people (i.e., crowded places, work, and travel), increased ventilation during exercise, skin abrasions, and environmental factors may also increase the exposure to or entry of pathogens into the body. Many of these factors are difficult (if not impossible) to control, but it is possible, to limit or minimise some (e.g., exposure) in order to reduce risk of contracting an infection during periods of increased susceptibility.

It has recently become apparent that not all reports of illness in athletes are necessarily caused by an infection. Some athletes may present with symptoms (e.g., sore throat, runny nose), but this might not necessarily be a true infection. Strenuous exercise may be associated with acute inflammation in the upper airways (possibly caused by factors such as increased ventilation, especially of cold dry air during training or the switch from nose to mouth breathing during harder exercise), which may cause some symptoms when there is, in fact, no infection. It is often difficult to distinguish between true infection and other causes of URTI-type symptoms. In one study, Spence and colleagues (2007) suggested that the self-reported URS did match the J-shaped curve when studying recreational, sub-elite, and elite athletes ($n = 83$ cyclists and triathletes, 47 per cent female); however, in addition to self-reports, this study included physician examination along with nasal and throat swabs to screen for known URTI-causing pathogens. They observed that only 30 per cent of reported illnesses were confirmed by identification of common respiratory pathogens. It is worthy to note, however, that only specific pathogens were tested, so it remains possible that a true infection was present that was caused by known pathogens not tested for, unknown pathogens, and/or new strains of viruses that were yet to be identified (Bermon, 2007). It must be emphasised, therefore, that this finding does not rule out infectious causes for these cases, as such diagnostics procedures do have inherent limitations in identifying causative agents from an evolving diverse pool of pathogens (e.g., ~200 common cold viruses) (Eccles, 2005; Heikkinen & Järvinen, 2003). Furthermore, in a more recent (albeit smaller) study based in the UK during the winter months (i.e., typical URTI season), it was observed that a much higher proportion (82 per cent) of reported illnesses were confirmed by identification of URTI-causing pathogens (Hanstock et al., 2016). In this study, 40 recreational level athletes were recruited (35 per cent female), of which 33 completed the study, which included a three-week monitoring period. During this monitoring period, 11 participants (six females) reported URS using the daily Jackson common cold questionnaire. Of these 11 participants, URTI-causing pathogens were detected in nine (all were positive for Rhinovirus and one was concurrently positive for Coronavirus). It is clear that symptoms can be caused by infection or non-infective causes, but both could negatively influence the athlete. An infective cause is more serious, typically persisting for longer (>2 days) and presenting additional risks if not managed appropriately (see practical recommendations' section).

Exercise and the immune system

Immunity is the ability to defend against infection and disease. The immune system is comprised of a variety of cells, tissues, and molecules that function in a highly orchestrated manner to mount an immune response. This system is able to protect the body from pathogens (e.g., viruses, bacteria, fungi, and parasites). It also has an important role in the removal of damaged or old 'self' cells and tissue components. The immune system is generally classified into two main 'arms': innate (non-specific) and adaptive (specific and acquired), but all components work synergistically. The innate arm (e.g., involving phagocytes, natural killer [NK] cells) can respond very quickly but lacks specificity (i.e., the same response to all challenges), whereas the adaptive response (e.g., involving T and B lymphocytes) has both antigen specificity and 'memory' properties, but takes much longer to develop on initial exposure to an infectious agent. The adaptive response, however, increases in speed and magnitude with subsequent exposures (which is the basis for vaccinations). A comprehensive overview of the immune system is beyond the scope of this short chapter, but the interested reader, wanting to explore this topic further, is directed to the comprehensive reviews of Walsh and colleagues (2011) and Gleeson (2007).

Acute and chronic effects

The response of the immune system to both acute and chronic exercise has been extensively researched and reported in the exercise immunology literature. The influence of exercise on immune function depends largely on the nature of the exercise (in terms of intensity and duration). When prolonged and/or strenuous exercise is repeated with insufficient recovery, the acute effects may cumulate in a state of chronically lowered immune function (i.e., even at rest), presenting a more prolonged open window. The nature of the acute effects of exercise is of key importance and intricately related to the chronic effects. Hence, a lot of attention in the exercise immunology literature has been devoted to characterising and quantifying the acute effects. These acute changes are sometimes described as being similar to the responses induced by infection, which is true to some extent, but there are also important differences in the magnitude and temporal responses (Shephard, 2001, 2002). The relationship between acute and/or chronic exercise is very specific to the individual athlete (and will vary with training status and training phase), so it is difficult to identify specific exercise intensities, durations and loads associated with increased risk. However, prolonged (>90 min) exercise at ~55–75 per cent maximal aerobic capacity is frequently suggested as the 'tipping point'.

Some of the typical exercise-induced changes may include:

- Increases in the plasma concentrations of various substances that are known to influence leucocyte functions, including:

  - Some cytokines, such as tumour necrosis factor alpha (TNFα), interleukin (IL)-1 IL-6, IL-10, and IL-1 receptor antagonist (IL-1ra).
  - Several hormones that are known to have immunomodulatory effects, including catecholamines and cortisol (stress hormones).

- A transient increase in the number of circulating leucocytes (primarily neutrophils; there is also an initial increase of circulating lymphocytes followed by a significant decrease below resting values).

- An effect on the function of many immune cells:

  - Neutrophil functions are often seen to be decreased.
  - Natural killer cell cytotoxic activity (NKCA) may increase immediately after exercise but soon decreases below resting values for up to 6 hr.
  - A number of monocyte/macrophage functions may be decreased following prolonged exercise, including toll-like receptor expression and function and antigen-presenting functions.
  - A number of lymphocyte functions may be diminished, including mitogen-stimulated lymphocyte proliferation and cytokine production, and B-lymphocyte production of immunoglobulins.

- A decrease in the concentration and secretion of mucosal secretory immunoglobulin (sIgA and sIgM).

Mechanisms of exercise-induced immunodepression

Many of the depressive effects of exercise on immune functions are thought to be largely mediated, either directly or indirectly, by: increased levels of hypothalamic-pituitary-adrenal (HPA) axis stress hormones (particularly glucocorticoids and catecholamines) and some cytokines; metabolic factors and substrate availability; leucocyte redistribution; and possibly oxidative stress. For example, glucocorticoids, like cortisol, may have a direct inhibitory effect on some immune cell functions and catecholamines, and glucocorticoids may also act indirectly by inducing leucocyte redistribution. Increased IL-6 release may contribute to exercise-induced leucocyte redistribution and induce an increase in cortisol secretion. Saliva flow and immunoglobulin secretion is also under neural control, so the stress response has been implicated in the effects of exercise on mucosal immunity. The leucocyte redistribution effects may influence overall immune function due to the premature release of immune cells from the bone marrow. These functionally immature cells have a reduced capacity to function (and may persist in the circulation in place of older/mature cells at a later stage, thus reducing immune defence). Lymphocyte numbers can decrease (by as much as 50 per cent) after prolonged/strenuous exercise. Although the actual clinical significance of this exercise-induced lymphocytopenia is unknown (blood lymphocyte counts are usually restored after 24 hr of recovery), it may contribute to the open window for opportunistic infections. Decreases in substrate availability and increases in oxidative stress during exercise have also been implicated. Detailed further discussion of each mechanism that may contribute to exercise-induced immunodepression is beyond the scope of this chapter, but interested readers can find further discussion in the comprehensive review of Walsh and colleagues (2011).

Psychological stress

Psychological stress may also cause or add to the effects of exercise on the immune system (Perna, Schneiderman, & LaPerriere, 1997; Clow & Huckelbridge, 2001). Psychological stress is known to induce stress responses (i.e., increase stress hormones), which could have both direct and indirect effects on immunity and resistance to infection (Cohen et al., 1991). Athletes are also known to be exposed to additional stressors related to serious training or competition (e.g., competitive stress and anxiety, and pressures associated with selection, performance expectations, media, and personal life) that can be experienced concomitantly with the physical and physiological stress of their sport. It is possible, therefore, that the immunodepressive effects of exercise would be exacerbated under these conditions of additional/psychological stress.

Females and the immune response (sex differences)

An understanding of the role that sex differences play in the immune response is important for interventions to treat infections and prescribe practical recommendations to minimise the immune response and infection risk. Under non-exercising conditions, several differences have been observed between men and women, and immunity is influenced by the menstrual cycle and pregnancy. In general, females exhibit a stronger innate and adaptive immune response to pathogens. Women have a higher percentage of T lymphocytes (from the total pool of lymphocytes), and a higher phagocytic activity of neutrophils and macrophage number is observed (Gillum, Kuennen, Schneider, & Moseley, 2011). Differences in cytokine production (pro- and anti-inflammatory) have been observed, and women exhibit increased T helper cytokine responses, specifically Th2 responses (IL-4, IL-10), which are heightened during the follicular phase when oestrogen levels are high (Pennell et al., 2012). Moreover, the numbers of circulating T-regulatory cells also fluctuate during the menstrual cycle, which tend to be higher during the follicular phase (Arruvito, Sanz, Banham, & Fainboim, 2007), and females tend to have higher humoral immune response with increased levels of B cell immunoglobulin antibody production compared with males.

The sex differences in immune function are typically attributed to the sex hormones oestrogen, progesterone, and androgens, which bind to specific receptors on immune cells. Oestrogen receptors (ERα or ERS1) and ERβ (ERS2) are expressed on various immune cells including T and B cells, dendritic cells (DCs), macrophages, neutrophils, and NK cells, indicating key immunoregulatory functions. Activation of their cognate receptors by progesterone and androgens also modulates the functions of NK cells, macrophages, DCs, and T and B cells (Klein et al., 2016). It is suggested that oestrogen typically enhances immune responses, while progesterone and androgens (which occur in higher concentrations in post pubertal men compared to women) typically suppress immunity (Oertelt-Prigione, 2012). Thus, hormonal changes during the menstrual cycle, menopause, and pregnancy could significantly affect the immune response.

Sex-based immunological differences are also attributed to sex chromosomes. Many genes on the X chromosome, with its ~1000 genes, regulate immune function and play a role in the development of immune-related diseases. The presence of the additional X chromosome in females influences immune function. As males possess XY chromosome and females XX, any damaging mutations or polymorphisms relating to X-linked genes are more likely to have an impact on the immune response in males compared with females, and some X-linked diseases relating to immune responses can invoke severe phenotypes in males, with females being relatively unaffected. The X chromosome also codes for crucial microRNAs, which regulate immune responses, notably high in inflammatory cells, and thus influence sex-based differences in immunity.

As a result of the observed immune differences, females of reproductive age tend to have a more active immune system than do age-matched males. Females appear less susceptible to respiratory diseases, viral, and some bacterial infections and sepsis, and have a greater vaccine efficacy; however, they are more susceptible to autoimmune diseases and have a greater immunoreactivity to particular pathogens (Fragala et al., 2011). For example, the female-to-male susceptibility ratio is 9:1 for systemic lupus erythematosus; 3:1 for multiple sclerosis; 4:1 for rheumatoid arthritis; and 9:1 for Sjogren's syndrome (Fragala et al., 2011). Other factors that could affect the infection risk between sexes would be social and behavioural.

Females and the immune response to exercise (sex differences)

Understanding sex differences in response to exercise have implications for understanding sex-specific adaptations to exercise for the exercising female. Although research is limited, the immune response to exercise appears to be similar between sexes in immune cell counts and functions, plasma cytokine levels, and lymphocyte apoptosis, when menstrual cycle or the use of oral contraceptives (OCs) are not controlled for at the time of testing (Northoff et al., 2008). However, when menstrual phase and OCs are controlled for, marked differences in certain aspects of the immune response have been observed (Gillum et al., 2011). In one study, leucocytosis of exercise was affected by menstrual cycle and triphasic OC use. Ninety min of cycling at 65 per cent maximal aerobic power demonstrated that female OC users had higher numbers of circulating neutrophils, monocytes, and lymphocytes during the luteal phase (day 20) of the menstrual cycle than they did during the follicular phase (day 8), and these responses were also greater than those occurring in men (Timmons, Hamadeh, Devries, & Tarnopolsky, 2005).

Neutrophil responses were also greater during the luteal phase in OC versus non-OC users, and the exercise-induced changes in IL-6 were 80 per cent greater in non-OC versus OC users during the follicular phase. Greater NK cell responses to exercise were observed in adolescent eumenorrhoeic girls compared with boys after 60 min of cycling at 70 per cent maximal aerobic power (Timmons, Tarnopolsky, & Bar-Or, 2006a). Furthermore, exercise-induced increases in lymphocyte and NK cells were greater in older girls versus older boys, but no differences were observed between young girls and young boys (Timmons Tarnopolsky, Snider, & Bar-Or, 2006b). These findings of age-specific differences in immunity between sexes suggest that female sex hormones may be an important determinant of the observed responses.

The inflammatory response to exercise appears to be influenced by sex and menstrual cycle. Edwards, Burns, Ring, and Carroll (2006) demonstrated an increased IL-6 response to maximal exercise in females compared with males. A 1-hr run at 90 per cent above the individual's anaerobic threshold was associated with differences in the expression of pro- and anti-inflammatory genes between menstrual phases and sexes. For example, expression of IL-6 at the transcriptional level was lower in women in the luteal phase and higher in the follicular phase (Northoff et al., 2008). Furthermore, sex differences in the immunological response to exhaustive exercise (a half marathon) were examined using microarrays to assess the genome-wide transcriptional responses (notably inflammatory genes TNIP-1, TNIP-3, IL-6, HIVEP1, CXCL3, CCR3, IL-8 and CD69) of whole blood with lipopolysaccharide stimulation as a model of *in vivo* infection. There was a bias towards less anti-inflammatory activation in luteal phase women compared with men (Abbasi et al., 2016). These findings suggest that the immune system demonstrates sex-specific responses to high-intensity exercise, which are greater in females during the luteal phase of the menstrual cycle and more pro-inflammatory.

In contrast, a lesser immune response – leucocytosis and lymphocytosis – to a maximal incremental swimming test was observed in well-trained female swimmers, who reported regular menstrual cycles and were not on OCs, compared with males, and these changes were not influenced by menstrual status (Morgado et al., 2014). Furthermore, a weaker neutrophil (oxidative damage; carbonyl index) and lymphocyte (antioxidant defence; glutathione peroxidase) response to 1 hr of swimming at 75–80 per cent maximal capacity was observed in adolescent females compared with males (Ferrer, Tauler, Sureda, Tur, & Pons, 2009), although there was no account for the menstrual cycle. These findings were suggested to relate to a lower stress hormone response (e.g., catecholamines and cortisol) and possibly oestrogen and testosterone (Fragala et al., 2011), which can influence immune function. It was also suggested that males, as a consequence of higher levels of immunosurveillance, may be at a lower risk of infection (Morgado et al., 2014), although the clinical relevance of these differences have yet to be fully determined.

Data examining the effects of exercise between men and women on the mucosal immune response are mixed. Rutherfurd-Markwick, Starck, Dulson, and Ali (2017) demonstrated a greater response to steady-state cycling exercise stress in recreationally active females compared with males, where a significant increase in sIgA with exercise was observed. These findings were related to the increased stress response with exercise in females, coupled with an increase in alpha-amylase activity (a surrogate marker of sympathetic nervous system activity), heart rate, and ratings of perceived exertion. There was also a trend for an increase in cortisol in females. In contrast, no differences in the mucosal immune response to exercise were reported between men and women with swimming (Gleeson et al., 2002), cycling (Allgrove Geneen, Latif, & Gleeson, 2009), and running (Nieman et al., 2002), with no differences in the stress response between sexes being reported. Significantly lower levels of sIgA in exercising females compared with males, however, were observed at rest in recreational cyclists (Allgrove et al., 2009) and elite swimmers (Gleeson et al., 1999). Lower sIgA at rest in females contrast the findings of sex differences in immune variables in the general population, since B cell immunoglobulins are reported to be enhanced by oestrogen, and suggest a possible negative effect of exercise training on mucosal immunity in females. It is noteworthy that menstrual cycle was not controlled for in these studies. A previous study, however, observed no fluctuations in sIgA over the menstrual cycle in endurance-trained females (Burrows, Bird, & Bishop, 2002). The differences in the findings between studies may be related to differences in the training status of the athletes, the type of exercise performed, or exercise stress experienced, the timing of the sample (rest versus post-exercise), and the method of expressing sIgA (i.e., whether the saliva flow rate was controlled for).

The mechanisms for the differences in the immune response to exercise among men and women are typically attributed to sex hormones, notably oestrogen; however other factors could be involved. Stress hormone responses with exercise, including cortisol and catecholamines, which can affect immune function, may also be responsible. Changes in stress hormones may reflect the different relative or absolute intensity of exercise performed. Indeed, an altered level of stress response in females has been noted in some studies with exercise (Rutherfurd-Markwick et al., 2017) and with OC use, and females possess a greater density of lymphocyte beta-adrenergic receptors (Timmons et al., 2005). A greater IL-6 response in females with exercise has been related to increased adiposity (Edwards et al., 2006), which is involved in IL-6 release. Furthermore, overall training status or training phase may also be a factor. Clearly, the mechanisms responsible for the immune response to exercise in men and women are multifactorial in nature and the role they play will depend on the specific type of exercise performed, menstrual phase, population studied, and immune parameter measured.

There are limited data examining the immune response and infection risk relating to exercise in both males and females. Animal models have shown that male and female mice had similar morbidity rates (sickness symptoms) after infection with herpes simplex virus-1 as a model of respiratory infection, and repeated exercise stress, but females appeared to recover to a greater extent and had a lower mortality (were ultimately protected from death) (Brown et al., 2004). These effects were attributed, in part, to ovarian function and possibly oestrogen (Brown et al., 2007), and to a greater macrophage, antiviral resistance to the infection in females than males at rest and following exercise (Brown et al., 2006). Moderate repeated exercise increased resistance whereas exhaustive exercise decreased resistance in these studies. In human studies, in a cohort of 80 endurance athletes examined over 4 months, no differences between sexes were observed in infection incidence, duration, and symptom severity, despite lower sIgA secretion rates, B cell and NK cell numbers in the female group compared with males (Gleeson et al., 2011). In one more recent study, the epidemiology of acute illness in elite athletes during competition was assessed. It showed that in shorter duration (<4 weeks) major international games and tournaments, 6–7 per cent of athletes suffered from an illness episode, with a higher incidence proportion in females compared with males (Schwellnus et al., 2016). The findings from these studies are opposite to what is found in the general population and highlight the difficulty in directly linking individual immune markers to URTI outcome/reports; other factors may also be important (i.e., social, and behavioural).

Practical recommendations

Minimising risks

Although an appropriately structured and periodised training programme can go some way to minimising the risks, many athletes must train intensively if they are to be successful, and are consequently at an increased risk for considerable periods of time. Therefore, taking measures to maximise the immune system (and minimise controllable factors and exposure to infection) will be particularly beneficial to such individuals. One major factor is exposure to other people. People with URTIs such as the common cold are most contagious in the first few days when they have the early symptoms such as a runny nose and sneezing. The pathogens that cause these infections can also be spread via contact (e.g., shaking hands) or by touching contaminated surfaces (e.g., door handles), so good personal hygiene is always recommended. Other factors including stress and lack of sleep may add to the effects of exercise on the immune system. Employing effective management strategies to help minimise such effects will, therefore, be beneficial. Psychological stress (if related directly to sports, such as competitive anxiety leading up to important events, or otherwise) may exacerbate immunodepression, and if athletes suffer with this, it may be worth working with a sport psychologist to help manage such stress.

Training when ill

Exercising females are often reluctant to reduce or stop training when ill; however, this can cause more serious problems and/or increase the chances of developing secondary infections. Indeed, such complications could result in more lost training days and loss of fitness in the long term (and/or more serious health consequences). Hence, appropriate management of the exercising female during this period can also allow quicker recovery and return to training. There are some general recommendations about exercising when you have symptoms – the 'above the neck' rule, for example. That is, if symptoms are localised to above the neck only, then it is okay to continue with light training, otherwise training should be stopped until the illness has passed; more specific details on this are provided by Gleeson and Walsh (2011) and Ronsen (2005).

Real-world example

Acute illness incidence proportion (percentage) was studied among athletes at major competitive events lasting 9–18 days (Schwellnus et al., 2016) (Table 10.1). The data showed that 6–17 per cent of registered athletes were likely to suffer an illness episode, which was higher in females compared with males, greater in winter games compared with summer games, and that Paralympic athletes appeared to have a higher illness incidence proportion than those athletes competing in the Olympic Games.

Summary

Exercise can have profound effects on the immune system, driven by stress hormone, and cytokine release, which may leave individuals more susceptible to infection. Females tend to have stronger innate and adaptive immunity compared with males, which may reduce the susceptibility to infectious agents (viruses, bacteria, fungi, and parasites) in the general population. However, females are more susceptible to autoimmune diseases. Females demonstrate marked differences to males in the immune response to exercise and across the menstrual cycle, which may relate to female sex hormones and stress hormones; however, the clinical significance of these differences in terms of infection risk is unclear at present. Infection risk may also relate to exposure to pathogens, and thus, highlights the difficulty in directly linking individual immune markers to URTI reports. Several practical recommendations have been proposed to minimise infection risk in the exercising female, which include managing exposure to pathogens, hygiene, stress levels, and sleep.

Table 10.1 Illness incidence proportion (per cent) among athletes at major competitive events

Games/competition	Season	Illness duration (days)	Athletes (n)[1]	Males (n)[1]	Females (n)[1]	All athletes (%)	Males (%)	Females (%)	Respiratory (% total)
Paralympics 2014	Winter	12	547	418	129	17.4	17.0	18.6	50
Olympics 2014	Winter	18	2780	1659	1121	8.9	7.3	10.9	64
Paralympics 2012	Summer	14	3565	2347	1218	14.2	17.6	20.1	34
Olympics 2012	Summer	17	10,568	5892	4676	7.2	5.3	8.6	41
Youth Olympics 2012	Winter	10	1021	562	459	8.4	6.0	11.0	61
IAAF 2011	Summer	9	1851	971	880	6.8	7.1	7.7	39
Olympics 2010	Winter	17	2567	1522	1045	7.2	5.2	8.7	63
IAAF[2] 2009	Summer	9	1979	1082	897	6.8	5.6	8.4	36
FINA[3] 2009	Summer	18	2318	1306	1012	6.6	5.1	7.9	50

Source: Adapted by permission from BMJ Publishing Group Limited (Schwellnus et al., 2016).

Notes

1 n: number of registered athletes.
2 IAAF: International Athletics Federation.
3 FINA: Fédération Internationale de Natation.

References

Abbasi, A., de Paula Vieira, R., Bischof, F., Walter, M., Movassaghi, M., Berchtold, N. C., … Northoff, H. (2016). Sex-specific variation in signalling pathways and gene expression patterns in human leukocytes in response to endotoxin and exercise. *Journal of Neuroinflammation, 13*(1), 289. https://doi.org/10.1186/s12974-016-0758-5.

Albers, R., Bourdet-Sicard R., Braun, D., Calder, P. C., Herz, U., Lambert, C., … van Loveren, H., & Sack, U. (2013). Monitoring immune modulation by nutrition in the general population: identifying and substantiating effects on human health. *British Journal of Nutrition, 110*(S2), S1–S30. https://doi.org/10.1017/S0007114513001505.

Allgrove, J. E., Geneen, L., Latif, S., & Gleeson, M. (2009). Influence of a fed or fasted state on the s-IgA response to prolonged cycling in active men and women. *International Journal of Sport Nutrition and Exercise Metabolism, 19*(3), 209–221. https://doi.org/10.1123/ijsnem.19.3.209.

Arruvito, L., Sanz, M., Banham, A. H., & Fainboim, L. (2007). Expansion of CD4+CD25+and FOXP3+ regulatory T cells during the follicular phase of the menstrual cycle: implications for human reproduction. *Journal of Immunology, 178*(4), 2572–2578. https://doi.org/10.4049/jimmunol.178.4.2572.

Bermon, S. (2007). Airway inflammation and upper respiratory tract infection in athletes: is there a link? *Exercise Immunology Review, 13*, 6–14.

Brown, A. S., Davis, J. M., Murphy, E. A., Carmichael, M. D., Carson, J. A., Ghaffar, A., & Mayer, E. P. (2006). Gender differences in macrophage antiviral function following exercise stress. *Medicine and Science in Sport and Exercise, 38*(5), 859–863. https://doi.org/10.1249/01.mss.0000218125.21509.cc.

Brown, A. S., Davis, J. M., Murphy, E. A., Carmichael, M. D., Carson, J. A., Ghaffar, A., Mayer, E. P. (2007). Susceptibility to HSV-1 infection and exercise stress in female mice: role of estrogen. *Journal of Applied Physiology, 103*(5), 1592–1597. https://doi.org/10.1152/japplphysiol.00677.2007.

Brown, A. S., Davis, J. M., Murphy, E. A., Carmichael, M. D., Ghaffar, A., & Mayer, E. P. (2004). Gender differences in viral infection after repeated exercise stress. *Medicine and Science in Sport and Exercise, 36*(8), 1290–1295. https://doi.org/10.1249/01.MSS.0000135798.72735.B3.

Burrows, M., Bird, S. R., & Bishop, N. (2002). The menstrual cycle and its effect on the immune status of female endurance runners. *Journal of Sport Sciences, 20*(4), 339–344. https://doi.org/10.1080/026404102753576116.

Clow, A., & Hucklebridge, F. (2001). The impact of psychological stress on immune function in the athletic population. *Exercise Immunology Review, 7*, 5–17.

Cohen, S., Tyrrell, D. A., & Smith, A. P. (1991). Psychological stress and susceptibility to the common cold. *New England Journal of Medicine, 325*, 606–612. https://doi.org/10.1056/NEJM199108293250903.

Eccles, R. (2005). Understanding the symptoms of the common cold and influenza. *Lancet Infectious Diseases, 5*(11), 718–725. https://doi.org/10.1016/S1473-3099(05)70270-X.

Edwards, K. M., Burns, V. E., Ring, C., & Carroll, D. (2006). Individual differences in the interleukin-6 response to maximal and submaximal exercise tasks. *Journal of Sport Sciences, 24*(8), 855–862. https://doi.org/10.1080/02640410500245645.

Ferrer, M. D., Tauler, P., Sureda, A., Tur, J. A., & Pons, A. (2009). Antioxidant regulatory mechanisms in neutrophils and lymphocytes after intense exercise. *Journal of Sport Sciences, 27*(1), 49–58. https://doi.org/10.1080/02640410 802409633.

Fragala, M. S., Kraemer, W. J., Denegar, C. R., Maresh, C. M., Mastro, A. M., & Volek, J. S. (2011). Neuroendocrine-immune interactions and responses to exercise. *Sports Medicine, 41*(8), 621–639. https://doi.org/10.2165/11590430-000000000-00000.

Gillum, T. L., Kuennen, M. R., Schneider, S., Moseley, P. (2011). A review of sex differences in immune function after aerobic exercise. *Exercise Immunology Review, 17*, 104–121.

Gleeson, M. (2007). Immune function in sport and exercise. *Journal of Applied Physiology, 103*(2), 693–699. https://doi.org/10.1152/japplphysiol.00008.2007.

Gleeson, M., Bishop, N., Oliveira, M., McCauley, T., & Tauler, P. (2011). Sex differences in immune variables and respiratory infection incidence in an athletic population. *Exercise Immunology Review, 17*, 122–135.

Gleeson, M., McDonald, W. A., Pyne, D. B., Cripps, A. W., Francis, J. L., Fricker, P. A., & Clancy, R. L. (1999). Salivary IgA levels and infection risk in elite swimmers. *Medicine and Science in Sport and Exercise, 31*(1), 67–73. https://doi.org/10.1097/00005768-199901000-00012.

Gleeson, M., Pyne, D. B., Austin, J. P., Lynn Francis, J., Clancy, R. L., McDonald, W. A., & Fricker, P. A. (2002). Epstein-Barr virus reactivation and upper-respiratory illness in elite swimmers. *Medicine and Science in Sport and Exercise, 34*(3), 411–417. https://doi.org/10.1097/00005768-200203000-00005.

Gleeson, M., Walsh, N. P., & British Association of Sport and Exercise Sciences. (2012). The BASES expert statement on exercise, immunity, and infection. *Journal of Sports Sciences, 30*(3), 321–324. https://doi.org/10.1080/02640414.2011. 627371.

Hanstock, H. G., Walsh, N. P., Edwards, J. P., Fortes, M. B., Cosby, S. L., Nugent, A., ... Yong, X. H. A. (2016). Tear fluid SIgA as a noninvasive biomarker of mucosal immunity and common cold risk. *Medicine and Science in Sport and Exercise, 48*(3), 569–577. https://doi.org/10.1249/MSS.0000000000000801.

Heikkinen, T., & Järvinen, A. (2003). The common cold. *The Lancet, 361*(9351), 51–59. https://doi.org/10.1016/S0140-6736(03)12162-9.

Klein, S. L. & Flanagank, K. L. (2016). Sex differences in immune responses. *Nature Reviews Immunology, 16*(10), 626–638. https://doi.org/10.1038/nri.2016.90.

Malm, C. (2006). Susceptibility to infections in elite athletes: The S-curve. *Scandinavian Journal of Medicine and Science in Sports, 16*(1), 4–6. https://doi.org/10.1111/ j.1600-0838.2005.00499.x.

Morgado, J. P., Monteiro, C. P., Matias, C. N., Alves, F., Pessoa, P., Reis, J., ... Laires, M. J. (2014). Sex-based effects on immune changes induced by a maximal incremental exercise test in well-trained swimmers. *Journal of Sports Science and Medicine, 13*(3), 708–714.

Nieman, D. C. (1994). Exercise, infection, and immunity. *International Journal of Sports Medicine, 15*, S131–S141. https://doi.org/10.1055/s-2007-1021128.

Nieman, D. C., Henson, D. A., Fagoaga, O. R., Utter, A. C., Vinci, D. M., Davis, J. M., & Nehlsen-Cannarella, S. L. (2002). Change in salivary IgA following a competitive marathon race. *International Journal of Sports Medicine, 23*(1), 69–75. https://doi.org/10.1055/s-2002-19375.

Northoff, H., Symons, S., Zieker, D., Schaible, E. V., Schäfer, K., Thoma, S., ... Fehrenbach, E. (2008). Gender- and menstrual phase dependent regulation of inflammatory gene expression in response to aerobic exercise. *Exercise Immunology Review, 14*, 86–103.

Pedersen, B. K., & Ullum, H. (1994). NK cell response to physical activity: possible mechanisms of action. *Medicine and Science in Sport and Exercise, 26*(2), 140–146. https://doi.org/10.1249/00005768-199402000-00003.

Perna, F. M., Schneiderman, N., & LaPerriere, A. (1997). Psychological stress, exercise and immunity. *International Journal of Sports Medicine, 18*(Suppl 1), S78–S83. https://doi.org/10.1055/s-2007-972703.

Pyne, D. B., Hopkins, W. G., Batterham, A. M., Gleeson, M., & Fricker, P. A. (2005). Characterising the individual performance responses to mild illness in international swimmers. *British Journal of Sports Medicine, 39*(10), 752–756. https://doi.org/10.1136/bjsm.2004.017475.

Ronsen, O. (2005). Prevention and management of respiratory tract infections in athletes. *New Studies in Athletics, 20*, 49–56.

Rutherfurd-Markwick, K., Starck, C., Dulson, D. K., & Ali, A. (2017). Salivary diagnostic markers in males and females during rest and exercise. *Journal of the International Society of Sports Nutrition, 14*, 27. https://doi.org/10.1136/s12970-017-0185-8.

Schwellnus, M., Soligard, T., Alonso, J. M., Bahr, R., Clarsen, B., Dijkstra, H. P., ... Engebretsen, L. (2016). How much is too much? (Part 2) International Olympic Committee consensus statement on load in sport and risk of illness. *British Journal of Sports Medicine, 50*(17), 1043–1052. https://doi.org/10.1136/bjsports-2016-096572.

Shephard, R. J. (2001). Sepsis and mechanisms of inflammatory response: is exercise a good model? *British Journal of Sports Medicine, 35*(4), 223–230. https://doi.org/10.1136/bjsm.35.4.223.

Shephard, R. J. (2002). Cytokine responses to physical activity, with particular reference to IL-6: sources, actions, and clinical implications. *Critical Reviews in Immunology, 22*(3), 165–182. https://doi.org/10.1615/CritRevImmunol.v22.i3.10.

Spence, L., Brown, W. J., Pyne, D. B., Nissen, M. D., Sloots, T. P., McCormack, J. G., ... Fricker, P. A. (2007). Incidence, etiology, and symptomatology of upper respiratory illness in elite athletes. *Medicine and Science in Sports and Exercise, 39*(4), 577–586. https://doi.org/10.1249/mss.0b013e31802e851a.

Svendsen, I. S., Taylor, I. M., Tønnessen, E., Bahr, R., & Gleeson, M. (2016). Training-related and competition-related risk factors for respiratory tract and gastrointestinal infections in elite cross-country skiers. *British Journal of Sports Medicine, 50*(13), 809–815. https://doi.org/10.1136/bjsports-2015-095398.

Timmons, B. W., Hamadeh, M. J., Devries, M. C., & Tarnopolsky, M. A. (2005). Influence of gender, menstrual phase, and oral contraceptive use on immunological changes in response to prolonged cycling. *Journal of Applied Physiology, 99*(3), 979–985. https://doi.org/10.1152/japplphysiol.00171.2005.

Timmons, B. W., Tarnopolsky, M. A., & Bar-Or, O. (2006a). Sex-based effects on the distribution of NK cell subsets in response to exercise and carbohydrate intake in adolescents. *Journal of Applied Physiology, 100*(5), 1513–1519. https://doi.org/10.1152/japplphysiol.01125.2005.

Timmons, B. W., Tarnopolsky, M. A., Snider, D. P., & Bar-Or, O. (2006b). Immunological changes in response to exercise: influence of age, puberty, and gender.

Medicine and Science in Sports and Exercise, 38(2), 293–304. https://doi.org/10.1249/01.mss.0000183479.90501.a0.

Walsh, N. P., Gleeson, M., Shephard, R. J., Woods, J. A., Bishop, N. C., … Simon, P. (201_). Position statement. Part one: Immune function and exercise. *Exercise Immunology Review, 17*, 6–63.

11 Musculoskeletal injury and the exercising female

Mimi Zumwalt

Introduction

Gender differences between males and females have been evident since ancient times, stemming from societal perception of whether or not female athletes should exercise, or even be permitted to compete in sports/athletic activity. In fact, the Greeks actively banned women/girls from watching the Olympic Games, and publicly punished those few brave females who dared try to participate! In modern contemporary countries, cultural roles have definitely changed, and continue to slowly evolve over time for the better. 'You've come a long way, baby. It's a woman thing', is a historical campaigning slogan for a lifestyle product – Virginia Slims cigarette brand, which is appropriate for females becoming more of age in terms of exercising and athletic competition. Gradually over time, more females started exercising, and eventually competing in sports previously only offered to males. This surge of ongoing female athletic participation sprouted a myriad of gender-related musculoskeletal trauma. Subsequently, researchers started studying epidemiological characteristics of injuries, which are more prevalent in exercising females, while trying to delineate various reasons for this sex difference, in order to find ways of counteracting deleterious consequences. In this chapter, the anatomical, physical, hormonal/physiological, biomechanical, and neuromuscular differences between males and females, which can contribute to injury risk accompanying those exercising/participating in recreational activities or athletic competitions, are explored. Scientific/research studies are also critically reviewed, along with identifying alternative methods of physical training to help prevent future injuries in the exercising female, for enhancing athletic performance to succeed recreationally or competitively while engaged in sports.

Aims of the chapter

The aims of the chapter are as follows:

1   To describe the history, background, and evolution of exercising females.
2   To explain anatomical/physiological and biomechanical differences between males and females.

3   To delineate various factors contributing to sex differences in muscu-
    loskeletal injuries of exercising females.
4   To review research on different types of athletic activities causing musc-
    uloskeletal injury in exercising females.
5   To debate which sports/physical manoeuvres cause more prevalent kinds
    of musculoskeletal injuries in exercising females.
6   To evaluate/implement representative training regimens that have been
    scientifically shown to decrease anterior cruciate ligament (ACL) injury
    risk in exercising females.

History

Gender separation between females and males in sports existed since
Ancient Greece, dating back to the Archaic period (800 BC) up until the
Roman period (AD 400) (Spears, 1984). Females not only were discouraged
from athletic participation, but prohibited by law, and threatened to be
punished by death for attending the male only Olympic Games! Gender
differentiation of male/masculinity continued onward, even when female
athletes were finally allowed to participate in athletic competitions. Specifically, the same sporting events were modified to be 'easier' for females,
giving them a 'handicap' compared to males, since women were viewed as
extremely inferior to men back then regarding athletic skills (Kemp,
2009). Although gender segregation still exists, the gap between male and
female athletic events/representation is narrowing, especially in the past
century within certain North American countries. Most recently, since the
early 1970s (after Title IX in the US), more and more women are entering
organised physical competitions alongside men. In fact, the number of
female athletes involved with sports participation has exceeded beyond 10
times in the last four decades; with that accompanies an explosive rise in
certain musculoskeletal injuries at an alarmingly higher rate in exercising
females (Chinurum, Ogunjimi, & O'Neill, 2014; Hewett, Myer, Ford,
Paterno, & Quatman, 2016; Manfreda, Teodori, Rinonapoli, & Caraffa,
2017; Stracciolini et al., 2015; Wick, 2014).

Epidemiology

In the past decade, data gathered by North American researchers stratified
the prevalence of musculoskeletal injuries according to age groups, types of
athletic activity, and anatomical region. According to Murphy, Connolly,
and Beynnon (2003), and Patel, Yamasaki, and Brown (2017), the incidence
of sports-related trauma was estimated to be one out of ten children per year,
more often during competition than practice. The highest rates were found
in males between five and 14 years old while participating in basketball, track/
field events, American football, softball, football (soccer), and gymnastics.
Other physical exercises contributing to injury risk in the younger population

include roller sports (field hockey), swimming/diving, cycling, trampolining, and negotiating on playground equipment. The most common injuries were found in the lower more than upper extremity, and least in the head/neck areas. Females tend to injure their pelvic/hip and/or knee joints more so than males. Water sports such as swimming/diving appeared to have the lowest risk of musculoskeletal trauma (Patel et al., 2017). As per the Centers for Disease Control and Prevention (CDC), college-aged males sustained most athletic injuries while playing American football and wrestling, whereas the most athletic injuries in females occurred during football (soccer) and gymnastics (Kerr et al., 2015). As for sex differences in specific injury patterns, exercising females seemed to sustain more stress fractures, shoulder (instability), foot/ankle, plus knee (patellofemoral), and especially ACL tears (2–10 times higher than sustained in males), with the highest risk during the adolescent period, peaking at 16 years old (Hewett et al., 2016; Myer et al., 2009; Sigward, Pollock, & Powers, 2012; Smith & Smith, 2002; Stracciolini et al., 2015; Tenan & Griffin, 2013; Wick, 2014; Willis et al., 2017; Wolf, Cannada, Heest, O'Connor, & Ladd, 2015; Voskanian, 2013). The ACL injury occurs extremely rapidly (within 30–100 ms) primarily (70–80 per cent) due to a non-contact mechanism, when young female athletes are playing multidirectional sports with high velocity such as skiing, volleyball, football, basketball, and handball, while their lower extremity is performing landing/pivoting/twisting/side-cutting joint motions. It appears that teenage females sustain a higher number of lower limb injuries involving mostly the knee joint (especially ACL tears) more frequently than do young males while participating in gymnastics and football (Donnell-Fink et al., 2015; Duncan, Chopp-Hurley, & Maly, 2016; Hewett et al., 2016; Johnsen et al., 2017; Kaux, Delvaux, Forthomme, Crielaard, & Croisier, 2013; Khayambashi, Ghoddosi, Straub, & Powers, 2015; Myer et al., 2009; Stracciolini et al., 2015; Voskanian, 2013; Wolf et al., 2015).

Anatomy/physiology/biomechanics

Anatomy

Males and females are inherently different, not only in the musculoskeletal structure morphology, but also in the endocrine system (especially during adolescence) and neuromuscular control while participating in athletic activity. Even though all these factors add to the risk of musculoskeletal injuries, neuromuscular control causes more problems in females, since it affects how limbs are directed in space, i.e., balance and proprioception of the lower extremities while engaging in physical exercise. This biomechanical variation, in turn, contributes to the propensity towards different traumatic conditions involving certain joints especially upon single leg landing, affecting more females than males (Figure 11.1) (Anderson, Browning, Urband, Kluczynski, & Bisson, 2016; Kaux et al., 2013; Wick, 2014).

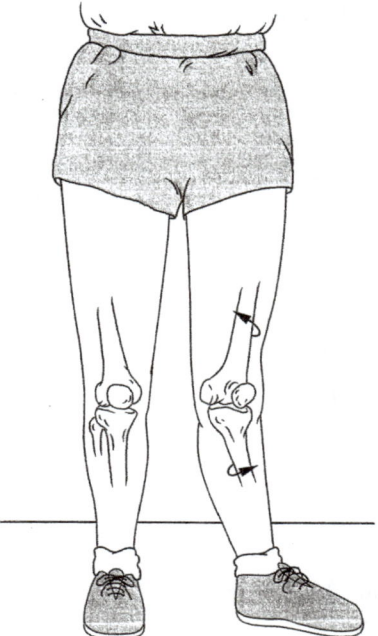

Figure 11 1 Risky limb landing attitude.

Anatomically, during formation of bodily skeletal structure/shape, females differ from males more in the lower versus the upper extremity. Specifically, women naturally possess broader pelvic brims to allow for eventual potential childbearing (Figure 11.2). This, in turn, results in their hips being wider apart, further accentuated by being 'knocked knee' (genu valgum). This morphological phenomenon originating at the hips causes dysfunction in joints below (i.e., the knees and ankles) due to non-linear vector forces; the phenomenon is described as increased Q angle or 'miserable malalignment syndrome' (Figure 11.3) (Wick, 2014). As a result, females with a higher Q angle are more prone to lateral maltracking of the patella, contributing to anterior knee/patellofemoral pain experienced by active young women. Additionally, patellar subluxation or dislocation can also occur while females are participating in athletic activity (Smith & Smith, 2002; Tenan & Griffin, 2013; Wolf et al., 2015). Alternately, research is conflicting about the other potential traumatic risk factor within the knee joint regarding shape/size of the intercondylar notch, which appears to be more narrowed in women, along with housing a smaller/weaker ACL (Anderson et al., 2016; Murphy et al., 2003; Smith & Smith, 2002; Voskanian, 2013; Wolf et al., 2015).

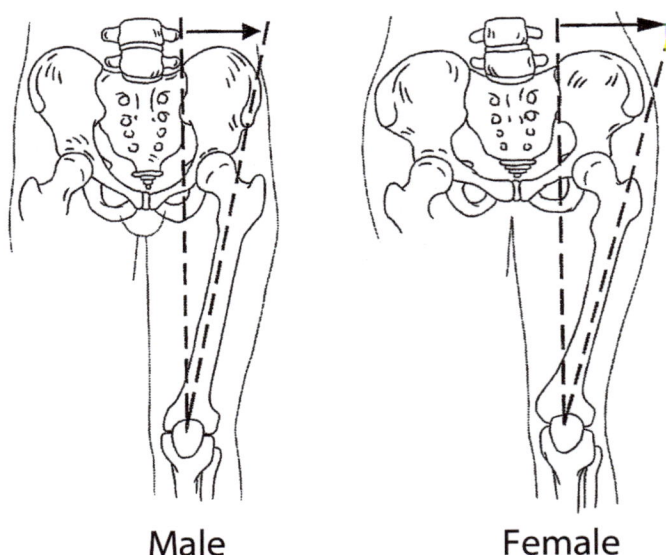

Male   Female

Figure 11.2 Hip/knee angular difference.

The ankle is another articulation where injuries frequently occur, about two times more in female athletes, while participating in high school and collegiate sports. One plausible explanation is that women tend to have looser surrounding ligaments than men, resulting in a higher rate of ankle sprains with subsequent chronic instability (Wolf et al., 2015). Similarly, the shoulder is one main upper extremity joint affecting more exercising females resulting in muscular/articular injuries (Wolf et al., 2015). The reason lies in men naturally having greater upper limb strength, stronger rotator cuff and periscapular muscles as compared to women. Females are, therefore, more prone to injuring their rotator cuff muscles from relatively weak supporting soft tissues. In addition, similar to the lower extremity ankle joint, female athletes inherently possess more laxity of adjacent soft tissue structures in the upper body, which compounds the problem by putting them more at risk for other shoulder girdle injuries and glenohumeral instability (especially in sports involving overhead movements such as softball, volleyball, and swimming) (Wick, 2014; Wolf et al., 2015). Interestingly, but also unfortunately, if and when exercising females eventually need to undergo surgery (e.g., arthroscopic stabilisation procedures) for persistent shoulder instability, they tend to end up with less successful outcomes as well (Wolf et al., 2015).

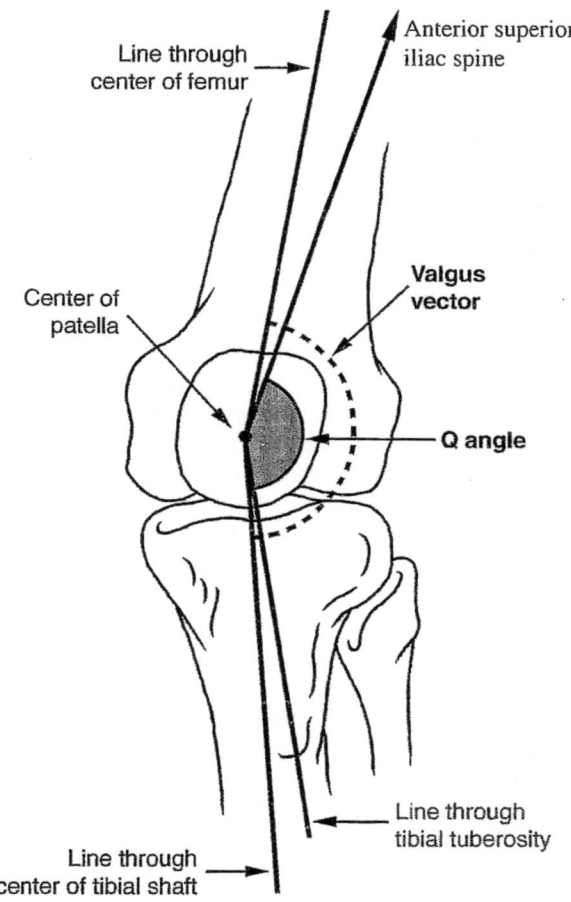

Figure 11.3 Alignment/forces across the knee joint.

Physiology

Physiologically, cyclical alterations in the hormonal milieu, i.e., reproductive hormone fluctuations of oestrogen/progesterone circulating in the bloodstream during certain phases of the menstrual cycle of exercising females, can contribute to generalised ligament/tendon laxity, adding another risk factor for musculoskeletal injury. Specifically, more traumatic episodes have occurred in the first half of menses (days one and two having the highest ACL rupture rates), during the pre/ovulatory phase accompanied by peaking of oestrogen (due to decreased knee stiffness/increased looseness), versus fewer joint injuries happening during the follicular phase when the level of this female sex-specific hormone drops (Anderson et al., 2016; Smith & Smith, 2002; Stracciolini et al., 2015; Wolf et al., 2015). However, in another article (Tenan & Griffin, 2013), it was stated that during the luteal phase of the menstrual cycle when oestrogen levels are high, minimal change was found in the mechanical property of tendons and ligaments. Furthermore, these same researchers have investigated and concluded that females may already naturally possess more 'lax' joints or less stiff soft tissues compared to those of males, which may contribute to the higher risk of ACL tears, but, thus far, evidence remains inconclusive (Tenan & Griffin, 2013). At the molecular level, however, the ACL possesses receptors for relaxin and the male sex-specific hormone, androgen, in addition to oestrogen/progesterone. Relaxin levels are higher in the circulatory system of a pregnant woman, but also normally found in both men and women. Interestingly, relaxin levels have been discovered to rise in the serum of female athletes who have sustained ACL tears as well, demonstrating a possible relationship between this hormone and its role in 'relaxing' soft tissues, which subsequently adds to ligamentous laxity and thus further raises knee injury risk (Anderson et al., 2016; Smith & Smith, 2002; Stracciolini et al., 2015; Wolf et al., 2015). Similarly, for females who are taking oral contraceptives, which act to stabilise hormonal levels and regulate the cyclical timing of menstruation, if coupled with appropriate neuromuscular training, dynamic knee stability may be aided (Anderson et al., 2016).

Additional research on sex hormones has indicated a possible link of female sex-specific hormones to the musculoskeletal system via the central nervous system (Tenan & Griffin, 2013). Both oestrogen and progesterone are lipid soluble, thus can easily cross the blood-brain barrier and influence the neuromuscular system. During the midluteal menstrual phase when progesterone level peaks, neural inhibition increases from activation of gamma-aminobutyric acid (GABA) receptors. Conversely, central neural stimulation occurs in response to oestrogen peaking during the late follicular phase. Both of these hormonal actions could potentially influence peripheral muscular recruitment/contraction by neuro control during exercise or athletic activity, thus altering susceptibility of the knee joint to trauma (Tenan & Griffin, 2013).

Biomechanics

Regarding the neuromuscular system, disparities between males and females also exist involving strength/balance of the hip/thigh muscle groups. Due to the male sex hormone androgen or testosterone, men inherently possess more muscle mass/strength in the lower limbs compared to that of women (Smith & Smith, 2002). Specifically, the anterior quadriceps muscle group is more dominant for knee stabilisation in females (much more so in the pubescent stage), rather than the posterior hamstring muscles, the latter being stronger in males (co-contraction of both muscle groups lends protection for the knee joint). In effect, the imbalance between knee extensors (stronger) versus knee flexors (weaker) in women naturally causes more anterior shear force on the tibia as the quadriceps muscle group contracts, which then places more strain on the ACL, and ultimately contributes to stretching and/or complete rupture during athletic activity (Anderson et al., 2016; Hewett et al., 2016, Kaux et al. 2013; Myer et al., 2009; Sigward et al., 2012; Smith & Smith, 2002).

Mechanism/aetiology

Using the US as an example, each year seven million student athletes participate in high school team sports, with 3–11 per cent continuing at the collegiate level. Of all musculoskeletal injuries occurring more frequently in young exercising females, knee joint trauma comprises 10–25 per cent (Donnell-Fink et al., 2015). ACL tears constitute the highest rate of injury (the most often ligament injured in at least 50 per cent of knee traumatic episodes), especially between the ages of 12 and 18, during the pubescent period of rapid development and growth (Khayambashi et al., 2015; Sigward et al., 2012; Stracciolini et al., 2015; Staurowsky et al., 2015). This knee injury is also extremely disabling, affecting the exercising female for the rest of her life (through increased risk of subsequent meniscal/chondral damage and early degenerative joint disease), along with placing a tremendous financial strain on the economy (Hewett et al., 2016; Manfreda et al., 2017; Staurowsky et al., 2015). Indeed, in the US, 5 per cent of all varsity, high school, female athletes tear their ACLs and ~100–250,000 ACL injuries occur annually, plus possibly 350,000 total tears occurring in the world (Hewett et al., 2016, Xia, Zhang, Wang, Sun, & Fu, 2017).

Risk factors for adolescent female athletes incurring more ACL injuries than males involve both intrinsic and extrinsic components (Murphy et al., 2003). Specifically, intrinsic risk factors contributing to higher rate of ACL tears in young active females include: body type/composition from genetic inheritance of the Collagen type I alpha 1 (COLIA1) gene (identified after ACL ruptures); height; body mass index; knee joint morphology (increased lateral tibial plateau posterior slope); stenotic intercondylar notch; ACL size/shape; pelvic to foot alignment/structural morphology; generalised/specific knee joint laxity; dynamic genu valgum landing attitude; and thigh muscles' differential extensor/flexor activation pattern (Anderson et al., 2016, Sigward et al., 2012). Additionally, during the 'growth spurt', anthropometric proportions of the body are modified, with acceleration of height velocity, expansion of femur/tibia length and magnification of body mass. The centre of mass is, therefore, altered along with lengthy long bone lever arms, which, in turn, affect core stability. This structural shift in body frame/skeletal structures is not equally compensated for by a simultaneous increase of hip/trunk muscle strength and recruitment in adolescent females, thus putting the lower limbs at higher risk for knee/ACL trauma. In addition, females strike the ground flatter with their midfoot, contributing to less energy absorption (Hewett et al., 2016; Sigward et al., 2012; Stracciolini et al., 2015). As for extrinsic factors causing ACL ruptures, researchers have found that shoe-surface interaction along with playing position in certain sports, plus increased frictional forces, seem to affect unanticipated side-stepping manoeuvres, resulting in higher ACL injury risk (Anderson et al., 2016). Furthermore, in research by the National Collegiate Athletic Association, it was shown that artificial turf caused more (up to 1.5 times higher) non-contact knee injuries compared to when practising/playing sports on grass surfaces (Staurowsky et al., 2015).

To reiterate, a multitude of risk factors (intrinsic and extrinsic) contribute to the several times higher incidence of ACL tears in exercising adolescent females as compared to males (Murphy et al., 2003). Unfortunately, most intrinsic factors cannot be modified. However, one extrinsic factor, which has received much attention from researchers, clinicians, physiotherapists, and athletic trainers alike involves the neuromuscular system, which seems to respond to potential preventative training methods (Voskanian, 2013). The following will explain the difference in landing biomechanics of the lower extremity in young active females, which puts them more at risk for non-contact ACL ruptures versus males. By studying details of gender-specific lower limb characteristics, training can then be adapted to address neuro deficits/weak points in the exercising females' musculature, enabling them to maximise practising in such a manner to minimise, and hopefully avoid, future knee injury (Hewett et al., 2016).

To elaborate, neuromuscular control can be defined as, 'unconscious activation of dynamic phenomena that surround a joint in response to sensory stimuli' (Kaux et al., 2103). In other words, neural input from the brain exerts action on muscles to contract, causing joint motion, which then effects a reflexive reaction/movement of the involved extremity. The neuromuscular reflex influences how athletes perform during sporting activities, and is an important component of the 'risky' landing position in exercising females (Kaux et al., 2013, Sigward et al., 2012). Individual fitness level also affects muscular endurance and specifically targets the lower limbs while athletes are performing impact activity or participating in team sports such as football (soccer) and basketball (Murphy et al., 2003). This muscular fatigue concept, in addition to the strength imbalance between hamstrings and quadriceps in females, along with anterior thigh muscles activating before the posterior muscle group, act in concert to pull the tibia anterior to the femur as the knee extends, resulting in a shear damaging force on the ACL. Furthermore, knee joint stiffness reacting to collateral or torsional forces of low magnitude is also lessened, adding to the already reduced protective mechanism. It appears that under repeated bouts of exercise to fatiguing levels, pelvis and trunk muscles take over to keep the body less upright, at the expense of imparting more load to the lower extremities (Kaux et al., 2013, Myer et al., 2009). However, this concept was found, in one study, not to have much gender differences when analysing single leg landing (Weeks, Carty, & Horan, 2015).

The aforementioned 'sport fatigue' is the other extrinsic factor, which affects the neuromuscular system upon excessive exercising. Not only is the body physically worn out, the central nervous system also gets 'tired', and the rate of neural input to muscles slows down. As a result, muscular contraction is delayed and proprioception (sense of limb position in space) is altered. Motor control is lessened, which, in turn, negatively affects the reflexive/protective mechanism of the lower extremity contacting the surface below, possibly contributing to more musculoskeletal injury since landing biomechanics is changed (though the resultant effect on how the entire body physically reacts has been challenged by one researcher) (Xia et al., 2017). Compounding the problem is the fact that reaction forces associated with impact activity upon the feet striking the ground can reach up to ten times bodyweight (Xia et al., 2017). This ground reaction force at landing is dangerously 20 per cent higher in athletes who have injured their ACL (Hewett et al., 2016). In some research studies, in which the 'posture' or lower limb attitude of young female athletes upon landing from a jump or cutting manoeuvres has been analysed, the following less erect body position observed in non-contact ACL injuries has been revealed (this dynamic phenomenon being most marked after puberty): knee less flexed (from increased extensor activation; reduced hip extension; more valgus/adducted moment (5 times that of males), resulting in greater frontal plane loading of the knee joint, putting an extra traumatic force on the ACL (Figure 11.4). The differentiating

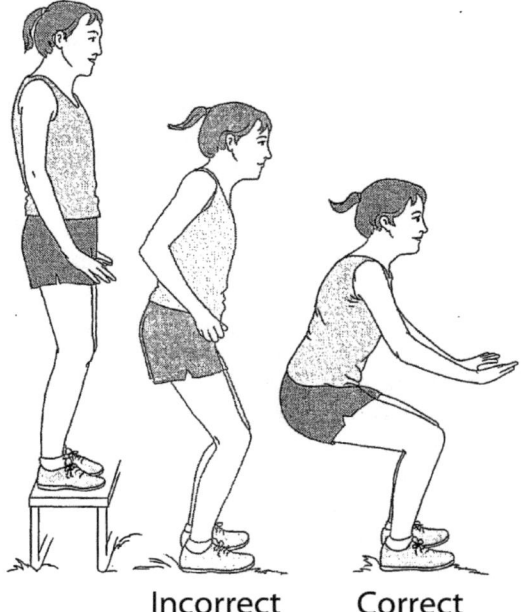

Incorrect   Correct

Figure 11.4 Risky versus safe landing positions.

effect is that males, versus active adolescent females, tend to recruit posterior thigh/hip musculature to a larger extent (2 to 3 times greater), which helps to protect the knee joint by decelerating the energy of impact more in the sagittal plane for better shock absorption (Myer et al., 2009, Sigvard et al., 2012). Additionally, truncal control is lost and cannot be centralised, thus the upper body moves laterally in either direction to the side and/or forward to the front, causing a shift in the lever arm (Hewett et al., 2016). In other words, teenage female athletes 'stick' a fairly 'stiff' inward lower limb landing attitude during sporting activity (hip/knee adduction/internal rotation), while males land in a less flexed/frontal body position with greater hip extension/abduction-knee flexion, which helps to protect the ACL from traumatic rupture (Hewett et al., 2016, Willis et al., 2017, Xia et al., 2017).

Treatment/prevention

A healthy exercising female has 1/60th to 1/100th chance of tearing her ACL (Figure 11.5); however, after being torn, risk of another similar knee injury on the same or opposite side increases significantly (by 15–25 times) once returning to sports (~25 per cent), and the post traumatic sequelae is extremely debilitating regarding painful/dysfunctional symptoms, not to mention the tremendous costs incurred for treatment (Hewett et al., 2016, Murphy et al., 2003; Taylor, Waxman, Richter, & Shultz, 2013; Willis et al., 2017). As compared to males, injured females are at four times greater risk of suffering another ipsilateral ACL rupture, and six times more likely to tear their contralateral ACL! One-half to all of these female athletes will experience pain, functional limitations, and signs of knee osteoarthrosis (40–80 per cent) 12–20 years, or earlier, post trauma (Hewett et al., 2016; Taylor et al., 2013). Management options for ACL ruptures include physical activity modification, bracing for knee support, avoidance of impact/pivoting manoeuvres, physiotherapy rehabilitation exercises, and/or replacement/reconstruction surgery. Again, research has shown that at least 50 per cent and up to 100 per cent of female patients who sustain an ACL rupture will experience symptomatic and radiographic signs of early post traumatic degenerative arthritis within one or two decades after the initial traumatic episode (Hewett et al., 2016). In fact, the chance of knee arthrosis occurring in the ACL-injured athlete is 10–100 times exceeding those without knee trauma (Duncan et al., 2016; Hewett et al., 2016)!

Regarding definitive management after ACL ruptures, in the US, out of 250,000 ACL tears, which occur yearly, 80–100,000 surgical procedures are performed on these injured athletes (Donnell-Fink et al., 2015). Since 1980, at least 1.5 million ACL reconstructions have been done to restore joint stability (costing more than three billion dollars), in hopes of preventing further knee degeneration (Hewett et al., 2016). In Norway, the overall rate of ACL reconstruction is ~40 per 100,000 person-years, more than three times higher in level I (involving more advanced skills and/or vigorous physical

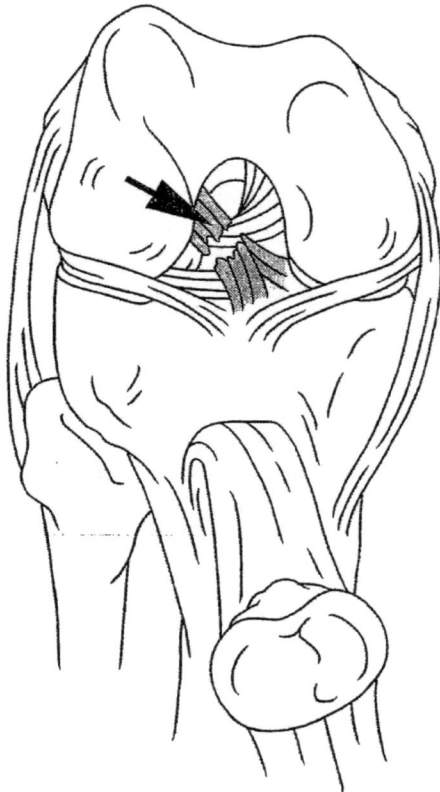

Figure 11.5 Anterior cruciate ligament tear.

activity) as compared to level II or III (less advanced) sporting events. The number of surgical procedures for ACL tears is four times greater in adolescent girls participating in athletic competitions, versus those who do not compete in sports (Johnsen et al., 2017). Unfortunately, those athletes who undergo ACL surgery will still have residual neuromuscular deficits, and favour their uninjured extremity (putting the contralateral limb at risk of trauma due to asymmetric loading) for up to two years after or even longer (Hewett et al., 2016). Furthermore, minimal if any correlation has been found between surgical fixation of knee joint laxity and subsequent functional outcome, especially painful symptoms of arthritis. Even after surgery, 23–28 per cent of injured athletes already have radiographic signs of moderate to severe knee osteoarthrosis within 8–10 years, with 2.4–4.7 times higher in those reconstructed versus native ACL. It appears that irreparable damage to the articular cartilage has already happened at initial trauma, and seems to worsen progressively over time. Thus, there has been a great push towards preventative measures to hopefully help minimise the chance that young exercising females will sustain ACL injuries (Anderson et al., 2016; Duncan et al., 2016; Hewett et al., 2016).

Since frontal and transverse plane kinematics differ between the sexes during athletic performance involving lower body balancing activities, which lead to higher rates of knee/ACL injuries, numerous studies have concentrated on training exercises to assist in lowering this risk in exercising females. Studies have shown that a preseason six weeks' duration of strength and conditioning programme, consisting of 10–20-min warm-up exercise routines targeting truncal/core muscles and lower limb muscle groups, can decrease knee injury rate by ~40 to 75 per cent and up to ~90 per cent; these regimens consist of neuromuscular movements including plyometrics, designed to train athletes' technique of deceleration, landing plus push off with the body in the correct position, while maintaining balance, control, and proprioception (Anderson et al., 2016; Manfreda et al., 2017; Thorlund, Culvenor, & Ratzlaff, 2014; Voskanian, 2013; Willis et al., 2017). Furthermore, other researchers have described that weak proximal hip muscles are predictive of future ACL trauma, by contributing to increased dependence of thigh muscles to absorb more forces on impact, thus putting the knee at higher risk of injury; therefore, targeting strengthening exercises focused on the gluteus maximus (which affects hip extension/external rotation), will assist in 'unloading' the knee joint by relying less on the quadriceps muscles for load absorption upon landing, thereby reducing injury risk (Hewett et al., 2016; Khayambashi et al., 2015; Manfreda et al., 2017; Powers, 2010). As previously explained, exercising females tend to be 'quadriceps dominant' (quadriceps overpowering hamstrings), thus at greater risk of ACL rupture compared to males, who have more balanced muscle groups (hamstrings before quads recruitment) (Hewett et al., 2016). It has been shown that neuromuscular/proprioceptive training can protect the knee joint by decreasing risk of trauma by >25 per cent, and can reduce ACL tears by 40–50 per cent (Donnell-Fink et al., 2015; Manfreda et al., 2017).

Practical recommendation based on research

Since ACL tears are devastating injuries with predictable short- and long-term sequelae regardless of treatment (especially early post traumatic arthrosis), measures to assist and protect these young exercising females from initial knee trauma are extremely important. In order to design injury prevention programmes, one must first analyse causable mechanism(s) and address the multiplanar contribution towards potential bodily harm. The underlying cause of knee injury or most 'at risk' posture by adolescent female athletes in sustaining non-contact ACL tears has been previously delineated (Figure 11.1) (Hewett et al., 2016; Myer et al., 2009). Isolated resistance training protocols for only muscular strength are ineffective for reducing injury risk; thus, for ~20 years, researchers have investigated specific components of different training regimens that are most successful in ACL injury prevention (Donnell-Fink et al., 2015; Myer et al., 2009; Noyes & Westin, 2011; Taylor et al., 2013; Voskanian, 2013). Four neuromuscular/functional deficits have been identified, all of which must be addressed and modified/ retrained for effective injury prevention. The first two involve limb dominance, including imbalances in neurological input for ligament protection, along with asymmetry of thigh muscle extensor/flexor strength. The third is 'leg dominance' i.e., differences in both lower extremities regarding control/ coordination. The final deficiency is 'trunk dominance' or 'core dysfunction', whereby central stabilising muscles cannot adjust to overcome perturbation in inertial moments on the body. A comprehensive plyometric/balance/ resistance training regimen focusing on power, proprioception plus agility, in addition to strengthening truncal abdominal/spinal and hip abductor muscles, tends to result in better stability of single-limb attitude upon landing. The end result is teaching these athletes how to reflexively land with their body in a safer position (Figure 11.4) (Hewett et al., 2016; Manfreda et al., 2017; Voskanian, 2013). Plyometrics and strength training were found to be more significant than dynamic balancing exercises; and 15–20 min (Prevent Injury and Enhance Performance [PEP]; http://smsmf. org/smsf-programs/pep-program) or 1–2-hr (Sportsmetrics; http://sports-metrics.org) sessions 3 days a week seem to have the best results for injury reduction and performance enhancement, though compliance may be an issue due to the lengthy duration of the latter regimen (Noyes & Westin, 2011).

Timing of introducing integrative fitness training into young exercising females' exercise programme is still under debate. Ideally, incorporation prior to 18 years old or completion of adolescence, preferably right around the start of puberty, is ideal, to induce the 'neuromuscular spurt' (Anderson et al., 2016; Hewett et al., 2016). Frequency and duration of training regimens may vary, but participation should start in preseason and continue during in-season athletic activity, at least one session weekly for at least six weeks. By following this regimen, exercising females can stay strong in both muscular strength and endurance, thereby preparing them to perform their very best (Anderson et al., 2016).

Real-world example

A 15-year-old, Hispanic, active female involved in school competitive athletics initially injured her right knee at 13 years of age. She fell after being tripped by a boy, and felt a 'pop' with pain and swelling. After staying out of sports for two weeks, she reinjured the same knee when it buckled during basketball practice. After referral to me, I ordered magnetic resonance imaging (MRI) scan confirming ACL and meniscal tears found on her knee exam. After several weeks of physiotherapy, the patient continued to experience painful instability. I performed right-knee arthroscopy two months post initial injury, debrided the meniscus but did not reconstruct the ACL since she was still skeletally immature. She recovered quickly after surgery. After a few months of physical rehabilitation exercises and passing a functional test, I cleared her to play basketball wearing a brace. She returned to my clinic two years later after sustaining another traumatic episode to her right knee during basketball. After a repeat MRI and a month of physiotherapy rehabilitation, she underwent right ACL reconstruction to address persistent knee instability. Her knee joint already showed signs of early osteoarthrosis arthroscopically. She is currently undergoing formal physiotherapy and will continue for at least six months. I will allow her to return to basketball eight to ten months post operatively after right-knee functional testing and learning how to land safely.

This young female athlete is a prime example of injuring her knee/ACL while participating in multidirectional sport. The patient and her parents have been forewarned about potential repeat trauma to the same and/or opposite knee once she goes back to playing basketball, since she is already at higher risk of re-injury.

Summary

In conclusion, male and female athletes differ, not only in anatomy, physiology, and biomechanics, but also in neuromuscular recruitment patterns involving the lower limbs especially upon entering puberty. This sex disparity becomes most notable in exercising females competing in multidirectional team sports, since they tend to injure their ACLs several-fold more than those of males, by inherent risky landing position. The neuromuscular system is one identified extrinsic factor that can be modified to aid in knee trauma prevention. Of the different training regimens developed, two strength and conditioning programmes have been found to provide the best chance to reduce ACL injury risk: Sportsmetrics and PEP. Both conditioning programmes focus on changing patterns of motor skills through core stabilisation and lower extremity strengthening, also incorporating plyometric movements for maximising muscle power. Through education and feedback about body mechanics and correcting neuromuscular deficiencies, female athletes are able to practice and train to land more safely. The resultant positive effects on reflex mechanisms of the body during training eventually translate into improving functional movements, and ultimately transferring to sports competition and athletic performance. Ideally, preventing ACL injuries in young female athletes will help to decrease incidence of early post traumatic degenerative joint disease, which, in turn, reduce the economic burden on society, plus improving quality of life in the years to come!

References

Anderson, M. J., Browning, W. M., Urband, C. E., Kluczynski, M. A., & Bisson, L. J. (2016). A systematic summary of systematic reviews on the topic of the anterior cruciate ligament. *Orthopaedic Journal of Sports Medicine, 4*(3), 1–23. https://doi.org/10.1177/2325967116634074.

Chinurum, J., Ogunjimi, L. O., & O'Neill, C. B. (2014). Gender and sports in contemporary society. *Journal of Educational and Social Research, 4*(7), 25–30. https://doi.org/10.5901/jesr.2014.v4n7p25.

Donnell-Fink, L. A., Klara, K., Collins, J. E., Yang, H. Y., Goczalk, M. G., Katz, J. N., & Losina, E. (2015). Effectiveness of knee injury and anterior cruciate ligament tear prevention programs: A meta-analysis. *PLoS One, 10*(12), 1–17. https://doi.org/10.1371/journal.pone.0144063.

Duncan, K. J., Chopp-Hurley, J. N., & Maly, M. R. (2016). A systematic review to evaluate exercise for anterior cruciate ligament injuries: Does this approach reduce the incidence of knee osteoarthritis? *Open Access Rheumatology: Research and Reviews, 8*, 1–16. https://doi.org/10.2147/oarrr.s81673.

Hewett, T. E., Myer, G. D., Ford, K. R., Paterno, M. V., & Quatman, C. E. (2016). Mechanisms, prediction, and prevention of ACL injuries: Cut risk with three sharpened and validated tools. *Journal of Orthopaedic Research, 34*(11), 1843–1855. https://doi.org/10.1002/jor.23414.

Johnsen, M. B., Guddal, M. H., Småstuen, M. C., Moksnes, H., Engebretsen, L., & Zwart, J. A. (2016). Sport participation and the risk of anterior cruciate ligament reconstruction in adolescents: A population-based prospective cohort study (The Young-HUNT study). *American Journal of Sports Medicine, 44*(11), 2917–2924. https://doi.org/10.1177/0363546516643807.

Kaux, J. F., Delvaux, F., Forthomme, B., Crielaard, J. M., & Croisier, J. L. (2013). The risk factors for rupture of the anterior cruciate ligament of the knee: The neuromuscular state. *OA Sports Medicine, 1*(1), 9, 1–5. https://doi.org/10.13172/2053-2040-1-1-687.

Kemp, M. (2009). *Ancient Greek women in sport.* Retrieved from https://faculty.elmira.edu/dmaluso/sports/greece/greecewomen.html.

Kerr, Z. Y., Marshall, S. W., Dompier, T. P., Corlette, J., Klossner, D. A., & Gilchrist, J. (2015). College sports-related injuries – United States, 2009–10 through 2013–14 academic years. *Morbidity and Mortality Weekly Report, 64*(48), 1330–1336. https://doi.org/10.15585/mmwr.mm6448a2.

Khayambashi, K., Ghoddosi, N., Straub, R. K., & Powers, C. M. (2015). Hip muscle strength predicts noncontact anterior cruciate ligament injury in male and female athletes. *The American Journal of Sports Medicine, 44*(2), 355–361. https://doi.org/10.1177/0363546515616237.

Manfreda, F., Teodori, J., Rinonapoli, G., & Caraffa, A. (2017). Strategies for prevention of ACL injuries in sportive females. *Juniper Online Journal of Case Studies, 2*(4), 1–3. https://doi.org/10.19080/JOJCS.2017.02.555593.

Murphy, D. F., Connolly, A. J., & Beynnon, B. D. (2003). Risk factors for lower extremity injury: A review of the literature. *British Journal of Sports Medicine, 37*(1), 13–29. https://doi.org/10.1136/bjsm.37.1.13.

Myer, G. D., Ford, K. R., Foss, K. D., Liu, C., Nick, T. G., & Hewett, T. E. (2009). The relationship of hamstrings and quadriceps strength to anterior cruciate ligament injury in female athletes. *Clinical Journal of Sport Medicine, 19*(1), 3–8. https://doi.org/10.1097/JSM.0b013e318190bddb.

Noyes, F. R. & Westin, S. D. (2011). Anterior cruciate ligament injury prevention training in female athletes: A systematic review of injury reduction and results of athletic performance tests. *Sports Health: A Multidisciplinary Approach, 4*(1), 36–46. https://doi.org/10.1177/1941738111430203.

Patel, D. R., Yamasaki, A., & Brown, K. (2017). Epidemiology of sports-related musculoskeletal injuries in young athletes in United States. *Translational Pediatrics, 6*(3), 160–166. https://doi.org/10.21037/tp. 2017.04.08.

Powers, C. M. (2010). The influence of abnormal hip mechanics on knee injury: A biomechanical perspective. *Journal of Orthopaedic & Sports Physical Therapy, 40*(2), 42–51. https://doi.org/10.2519/jospt.2010.3337.

Sigward, S. M., Pollard, C. D., & Powers, C. M. (2012). The influence of sex and maturation on landing biomechanics: Implications for anterior cruciate ligament injury. *Scandinavian Journal of Medicine & Science in Sports, 22*(4), 502–509. https://doi.org/10.1111/j.1600-0838.2010.01254.x.

Smith, F. W., & Smith, P. A. (2002). Musculoskeletal differences between males and females. *Sports Medicine and Arthroscopy Review, 10*(1), 98–100. https://doi.org/10.1097/00132585-200210010-00014.

Spears, B. (1984). A perspective of the history of women's sport in ancient Greece. *Journal of Sport History, 11*(2), 32–47.

Staurowsky, E. J., DeSousa, M. J., Miller, K. E., Sabo, D., Shakib, S., Shakib, S., ... Williams, N. (2015). The Women's Sports Foundation Report Brief: Her life depends on it III & female athletes and knee injuries. *Sport, physical activity, and the health and well-being of American girls and women.* https://doi.org/10.13140/RG.2.1.3660.6880.

Stracciolini, A., Stein, C. J., Zurakowski, D., Meehan, W. P., Myer, G. D., & Micheli, L. J. (2015). Anterior cruciate ligament injuries in pediatric athletes presenting to sports medicine clinic. *Sports Health: A Multidisciplinary Approach, 7*(2), 130–136. https://doi.org/10.1177/1941738114554768.

Taylor, J. B., Waxman, J. P., Richter, S. J., & Shultz, S. J. (2013). Evaluation of the effectiveness of anterior cruciate ligament injury prevention programme training components: A systematic review and meta-analysis. *British Journal of Sports Medicine, 49*(2), 79–87. https://doi.org/10.1136/bjsports-2013-092358.

Tenan, M. S., & Griffin, L. (2013, September). Effects of sex hormones on incidence of knee pain. *Lower Extremity Review.* Retrieved from http://lermagazine.com/article/effect-of-sex-hormones-on-incidence-of-knee-pain.

Thorlund, J. B., Culvenor, A. G., & Ratzlaff, C. (2014). Down on one knee: Soft tissue knee injuries across the lifespan. *Arthritis Research & Therapy, 16*(6), 1–2. https://doi.org/10.1186/s13075-014-0499-8.

Voskanian, N. (2013). ACL injury prevention in female athletes: Review of the literature and practical considerations in implementing an ACL prevention program. *Current Reviews in Musculoskeletal Medicine, 6*(2), 158–163. https://doi.org/10.1007/s12178-013-9158-y.

Weeks, B. K., Carty, C. P., & Horan, S. A. (2015). Effect of sex and fatigue on single leg squat kinematics in healthy young adults. *BMC Musculoskeletal Disorders, 16*(271), 1–9. https://doi.org/10.1186/s12891-015-0739-3.

Wick, J. Y. (2014, 16 June). *Sports injuries: Are women more at risk?* Retrieved from www.pharmacytimes.com/publications/issue/2014/june2014/sports-injuries-are-women-more-at-risk.

Willis, B. W., Razu, S., Baggett, K., Jahandar, A., Gray, A. D., Skubic, M., ... Guess, T. M. (2017). Sex differences in frontal and transverse plane hip and knee kinematics during the modified star excursion balance test. *Human Movement,* *18*(3), 26–33. https://doi.org/10.1515/humo-2017-0028.

Wolf, J. M., Cannada, L., Heest, A. E., O'Connor, M. I., & Ladd, A. L. (2015). Male and female differences in musculoskeletal disease. *Journal of the American Academy of Orthopaedic Surgeons, 23*(6), 339–347. https://doi.org/10.5435/jaaos-d-14-00020.

Xia, R., Zhang, X., Wang, X., Sun, X., & Fu, W. (2017). Effects of two fatigue protocols on impact forces and lower extremity kinematics during drop landings: Implications for noncontact anterior cruciate ligament injury. *Journal of Healthcare Engineering, 2017*, 1–8. https://doi.org/10.1155/2017/5690519.

12 Breast health and the exercising female

Jenny Burbage, Michelle Norris, Brogan Horler, and Tim Blackmore

Introduction

Research into breast biomechanics has increased exponentially over the past 15 years. During this time, the first procedure to establish dynamic breast movement in three dimensions has been published (Scurr, White, & Hedger, 2009), and this procedure has continually been developed and then applied to determine the effectiveness of varying designs of breast support (e.g., Scurr, White, & Hedger, 2011). By increasing our understanding of how the breast moves during exercise, the information generated is able to inform sports bra design.

Alongside an increasing knowledge of breast biomechanics, a wealth of literature has also been published on breast health issues, such as: breast pain, bra fit, the breast as a barrier to exercise, and breast education initiatives. It is of growing importance to understand issues, which may prevent females from taking part in exercise, and research has shown that the breast is a barrier to 17 per cent of the general female population, increasingly so for larger-breasted female exercisers. However, wearing a well-fitting and supportive bra can reduce breast motion and pain, and may encourage more females to exercise.

This chapter starts by exploring the problem of breasts; this includes their anatomy, breast ptosis (sag), breast size, and movement-induced breast pain. Research is then presented on breast biomechanics and specifically the parameters that are measured to assess breast motion (e.g., breast displacement, velocity, and acceleration). Information is provided on the types of breast support available and for whom they are best suited, including a discussion on the need for sports-specific breast support. Finally, this chapter discusses recent research into how the breast may affect an exercising female, in terms of how breast health issues can be a barrier to exercise participation, and also whether performance can be improved by wearing a supportive bra.

Aims of the chapter

The aims of the chapter are as follows:

1   To present the problems associated with the healthy adult female breast, such as breast anatomy, breast ptosis, breast size, and breast pain.
2   To discuss research into breast biomechanics and parameters that have been assessed during exercise, such as breast displacement, velocity, acceleration, and skin strain.
3   To provide information on the breast support options available to exercising females and to discuss the efficacy of sports-specific breast support.
4   To debate whether wearing an unsupportive sports bra can lead to negative performance effects and present research into how the breast can be a barrier to taking part in exercise.

The problem

This section will introduce the fundamental topics related to the healthy adult female breast, including breast anatomy, breast ptosis, breast size, and breast pain. The female adult breast is located on the superior anterior aspect of the chest wall, and while the area of the chest surface that is covered by breast tissue varies, in general it extends vertically from the level of the second rib to the level of the sixth rib, while spreading laterally to the midaxillary line and into the axillary region (Gefen & Dilmoney, 2007; Page & Steele, 1999). The breast is composed of three major components: fibrous (connective), glandular (mammary), and adipose (fat) tissue. These components are interspersed with blood vessels, nerves, and lymphatics (McCool, Stone-Condry, & Bradford, 1998). The fibrous tissue in the breast is termed the Cooper's ligaments, and is often described as a supporting structure for the breast (Gefen & Dilmoney, 2007; Page & Steele, 1999). However, the Cooper's ligaments are not thought to be true ligamentous tissue, rather, thin sheets of fibrous bands located in the superficial fascia of the breast, which separates the breast's lobules. No experimental data are available for the mechanical properties of the Cooper's ligaments (Gefen & Dilmoney, 2007), but they can most likely offer only limited anatomical support to the breast due to their attachment to the deep fascia, which, in turn, overlays the pectoralis major muscle (Page & Steele, 1999). Additional support to the breast is provided by the skin.

Breast skin provides a thin (1 to 2 mm) elastic layer across the surface of the breast (Page & Steele, 1999) and has been suggested to provide the most support to limit breast movement (Hindle, 1991). However, research suggests that both elasticity and skin thickness reduce with age as a result of hormonal changes such as the reduction of oestrogen (Ulger, Erdogan, Kumanlioglu, & Unur, 2003) and the degradation of elastic fibres in the skin (Coltman et al., 2017a). Interestingly, changes in skin elasticity across the breast surface are not uniform, with the superior and medial quadrants deteriorating the most (Coltman, Steele, & McGhee, 2017b). These findings agree with reported changes in breast shape associated with ageing, whereby, due to the force of gravity acting downward on the breast, the breast moves inferiorly and laterally with increasing age (Coltman et al., 2017a; Machida & Nakadate, 2015), commonly termed breast ptosis, or breast sag.

As the breast has limited internal anatomical support, even minor displacement of the body's centre of mass results in associated breast movement, thus emphasising the need for some level of external support (Page & Steele, 1999). This need for external support is exacerbated during sport and exercise, where repeated loading of the weak supporting structures of the breast may lead to irreparable damage of these structures (Mason, Page, & Fallon, 1999; Page & Steele, 1999) and may contribute towards accelerated breast ptosis. Breast ptosis characterises the location of the nipple, relative to the inframammary fold, and, typically, clinical assessment of ptosis is based on Regnault's (1976) adapted method (Li et al., 2016). This method is assessed on a 4-point grading system (Table 12.1) from 0 to 3, where 0 represents a breast absent of ptosis, and 3 represents a breast with extreme ptosis (Regnault, 1976). A number of risk factors have been significantly associated with the development of breast ptosis, including increasing age, history of weight loss ($> \sim 22.5\,\mathrm{kg}$), larger body mass index (BMI), pregnancy, smoking, and breast size (Rinker, Veneracion, & Walsh, 2010).

There is a large variation in the anatomical presentation and development of breasts, and healthy female breasts are often asymmetrical in both size and shape (McCool et al., 1998). Breast size has been strongly linked to body composition (Brown et al., 2012; Page & Steele, 1999), with larger-breasted women having a greater fat mass and BMI when compared to their smaller-breasted counterparts (Brown et al., 2012), while also reporting higher incidences of breast pain (Brown, White, Brasher, & Scurr, 2014b) and postural issues (Findikcioglu, Findikcioglu, Ozmen, & Guclu, 2007). The average breast size is difficult to identify as the majority of data is available from

Table 12.1 Regnault's system for the grading of breast ptosis

Ptosis grade	Description
0	*Pseudoptosis:* The nipple lies above the inframammary fold; the breast is not ptotic
1	*Stage 1 ptosis:* Nipple is level with inframammary fold
2	*Stage 2 ptosis:* Nipple lies below the level of the fold but remains above the lower contour of the breast
3	*Stage 3 ptosis:* Nipple lies below the fold and at the lower contour of the breast

Source: Regnault, 1976.

lingerie retailers, which is confounded by women wearing the wrong size bra and the lack of an industry standard (Brown & Scurr, 2016a). However, we do know that breast size is reported to be increasing (Brown & Scurr, 2016a). Using the UK as an example, research suggests that the average bust circumference has increased by 6.3 cm between 1951 and 2002, at a rate of +0.12 cm per year (Brown & Scurr, 2016a). Brown and Scurr (2016a) suggest that the observed increase in breast circumference may be related to the obesity epidemic, which would see an increase in the proportion of adipose tissue in the breast and thus an increase in breast size.

Between-person variation in the contribution of adipose and glandular tissue to breast mass results in a variation in breast mass-density (mass per unit volume), the effects of which are largely under-researched due to the difficulties associated with assessing this *in vivo*. Recent advances in medical imaging have led to the development of semi-automated methods to help segregate breast tissue in regions where adipose and glandular tissue are interspersed, thus improving accuracy (Sanchez, Mills, & Scurr, 2016). Due to the inextricable link between the mass-density (of the breast) and Newton's laws of motion, a better understanding of this relationship has the potential to help explain the variation observed in breast motion (due to changes in inertia) and shape, and is an area that is highlighted as a focus for future research.

Due to the limited intrinsic support within the breast, excessive breast motion during sport and exercise can lead to breast pain (Page & Steele, 1999). It is common for exercising females to experience breast pain, with it being reported by 32 per cent of marathon runners (Brown et al., 2014b), 40 per cent of horse riders (Burbage & Cameron, 2017), and 72 per cent of general exercising females (Lorentzen & Lawson, 1987). Exercise-related breast pain increases as breast size increases (Brown, White, Brasher, & Scurr, 2014a; Burbage & Cameron, 2017) and is greater during vigorous-, compared to moderate-intensity sport and exercise (Brown et al., 2014b; Burnett, White, & Scurr, 2015). Although exercise-related pain is proposed to be associated with stretch in the breasts' anatomical structures (Mason et al., 1999), the exact source of breast pain is surprisingly unknown and recent research into breast biomechanics has been investigating possible links between breast pain and breast displacement, velocity, acceleration, and skin strain.

Breast biomechanics

To date, the primary parameters investigated in relation to breast movement during sport and exercise are breast displacement, breast velocity, breast acceleration, and breast skin strain, with these parameters providing information, which can inform both an understanding of breast pain during exercise and sports bra design.

Lorentzen and Lawson (1987) provided some of the first quantitative data on breast movement during running by utilising video footage of 59 women running on a treadmill bare-breasted and in various sports bras to offer recommendations on breast support. Lorentzen and Lawson (1987) focused on the vertical displacement of the breast relative to the body and, while this provided an initial indication of the amount of breast movement possible (8 cm vertical breast displacement), more recently, advances in technology have allowed researchers to investigate the three-dimensional (3D) movement of the breast both in sports bras, and bare-breasted. Scurr, White, and Hedger (2009) investigated the 3D displacement of the breast during running and walking using 3D motion capture, with retro-reflective markers placed on the left and right nipples, clavicles, and anterior superior iliac spine. Scurr et al. (2009) identified that the unsupported breast moved ~1 cm and ~7 cm vertically during walking and running, respectively. Scurr and colleagues (2009) also emphasised the importance of understanding 3D breast movement as they identified that, while 56 per cent of overall breast displacement occurs in the vertical direction during walking and running, the remainder of this (44 per cent) consists of the combined anterior-posterior and mediolateral breast displacements. This supports the figure of eight breast trajectory first proposed by Gehlsen and Albohm (1980) (representative figure of eight trajectory, Figure 12.1) and emphasises the requirement of understanding 3D breast movement.

Additionally, Scurr and colleagues (2009) emphasised the importance of assessing breast movement relative to the torso, identifying that absolute breast displacement calculation resulted in increased values, possibly due to the influence of shoulder rotation during running. While this can be easily accounted for using torso markers when collecting 3D motion capture, Mills, Loveridge, Milligan, and Scurr (2015) outlined that the axes convention utilised to calculate relative breast displacement can also impact calculations, and suggested utilising the 'stable' longitudinal axes convention. To date, values of unsupported breast displacement across sport and exercise have ranged from 1 cm vertically in walking (Mason et al., 1999), through 15.2 cm during running (Scurr et al., 2011), to 18.7 cm during a two-step star jump (Bridgman, Scurr, White, Hedger, & Galbraith, 2010), and this large range of breast displacement occurs due to factors such as activity choice and the breast size of participants.

Not only is the magnitude of breast displacement important when understanding how the breast moves, but the velocity and acceleration at which the breast moves are also key. McGhee, Power, and Steele (2007) and Shivitz (2001) identified that the breast moves at an absolute velocity of between 50 and 100 cm/s, with the downward movement of the breast generally towards the higher velocity (100 cm/s). McGhee and colleagues (2007) suggested that this downward speed of movement may contribute to the displeasure of women when running bare-breasted, possibly due to the breasts 'slapping against the chest wall' (Haycock, Shierman, & Gillette, 1978), causing discomfort. In terms of breast acceleration, Haake, Milligan, and Scurr, (2013) identified that the breast vertically accelerates at a maximal rate of nearly

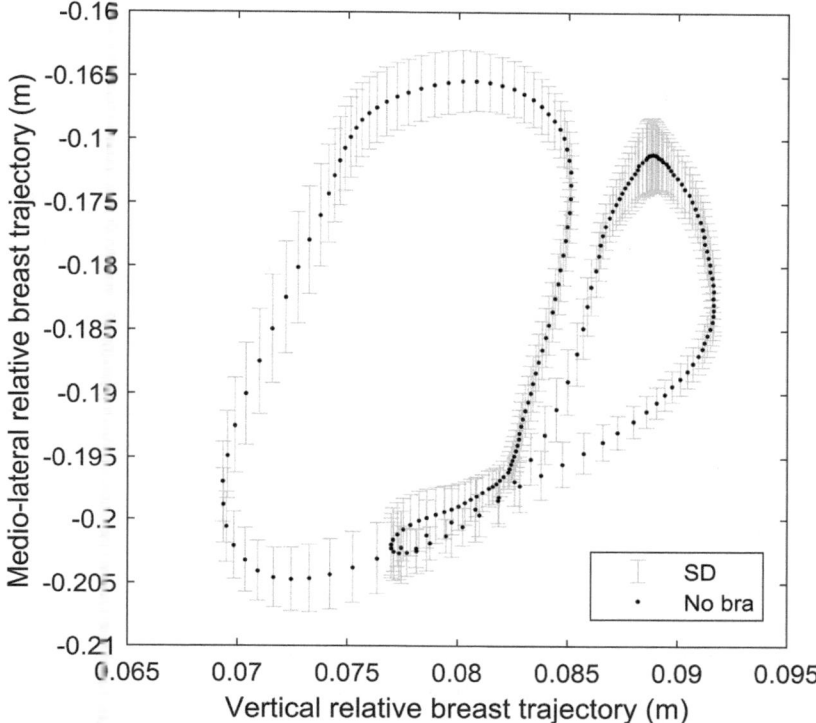

Figure 12.1 Representative figure of eight breast trajectory for a 34D female over five gait running cycles.

$5g$ ($g = 9$ 81 m/s^2) during running in women with larger breasts and this was related to participant discomfort. Interestingly, this vertical rate of breast movement was reduced to $1.3g$ during a two-step star jump in women with a D cup size and was negatively associated with participant discomfort (as breast acceleration increased, participant discomfort increased). Nolte, Burgoyne, Nolte, Van der Meulen, and Fletcher (2016) suggested that perhaps breast acceleration is not a sensitive enough measure to assess breast discomfort during jumping, and it may also be that a one-off bout of breast movement, such as that of a single jump, does not inflict as much discomfort on participants as the repetition of breast movement observed during running.

Lastly, researchers have also begun to look at breast skin strain during sport and exercise with Haake and Scurr (2011) identifying the neutral breast position (*Lo*) (the position where the upper and lower tissues of the breast are neither in compression or tension) utilising a 'lift and drop' breast method. Utilising this neutral position, they then calculated the vertical strain of the breast (ε) as a percentage,

$$\varepsilon \frac{\delta}{Lo} = \frac{d - Lo}{Lo} = \frac{d}{Lo} - 1$$

where δ represents the viscoelastic extension of the skin and d represents the linear distance between the suprasternal notch and the nipple. Haake and Scurr (2011) not only identified that wearing a bra reduced breast skin strain levels during walking and running, but strain was also related to breast discomfort in running, and this increased with breast size (Haake et al., 2013).

While the biomechanical parameters previously mentioned (breast displacement, velocity, acceleration, and strain) have all been discussed in relation to unsupported breast movement during sport and exercise, numerous research has been conducted on the use of high and low support sports bras, and their impact on breast movement. To date, high support sports bras have effectively reduced multidirectional breast displacement during running (Scurr, White, & Hedger, 2010), plyometrics (Nolte et al., 2016), and horse riding (Burbage, Cameron, & Goater, 2016), compared to both bare-breasted and/or low support conditions. Additionally, while breast velocity has displayed similar results to displacement with an addition of breast support (i.e., an increase in breast support results in a decrease in breast velocity), this is not necessarily the case with breast acceleration. Scurr and colleagues (2010) identified no significant changes in breast acceleration in all directions, despite the use of an everyday bra (low support) and a sports bra (high support) when compared to bare-breasted, during running. Therefore, it was suggested that breast acceleration may not be the best parameter to inform sports bra design.

Overall the knowledge, which we have accumulated in relation to both unsupported and supported breast movement during sport and exercise, has led to research strongly recommending the appropriate use of sports bras for women. However, it is well known that, on a daily basis, women are still wearing inappropriate breast support garments during sport and exercise, and this may be impacting both their quality of life and ability to perform.

Breast support

The first sports bra was patented in 1977, with the aim of supporting the breast and limiting breast movement during exercise. Currently, among the designs on the market, there are three distinct styles: *compression*, *encapsulation*, and *combination*.

Compression sports bras aim to reduce breast movement by compressing the breast tissue to the chest wall (Page & Steele, 1999). They are most commonly constructed from one piece of strong, elastic material to create the compressive element. Research suggests that compression sports bras are more suitable for smaller-breasted women (<D cup) (Page & Steele, 1999). Encapsulation sports bras contain two moulded cups with a centre gore to

separate the breasts, with the aim of limiting breast movement by individually lifting and holding the breasts in place (Page & Steele, 1999). Encapsulation-style sports bras are promoted for larger-breasted women (>D cup) to reduce breast movement (Page & Steele, 1999). Combination sports bras incorporate both compressive and encapsulating features; however, the contribution of these elements can vary depending on the bra. Some combination sports bras may have fully encapsulating cups with an outer layer of fabric covering the front of the bra to add compression to the design, whereas, some combination sports bras may be largely compressive with some added structuring to the cups in the form of seams, panels, or underwire, to incorporate some encapsulation. There is currently little evidence to confirm if one particular style is more successful at limiting breast movement during exercise than another. This may be due to the wide range of components that sports bras are comprised such as differences in shoulder strap configuration, adjustability options, and the variable levels of structuring in the cups.

The under band of a sports bra can vary depending on the sports bra design; it may be wide, narrow, adjustable, non-adjustable, firm, or elastic, with various combinations of these features. The under band should provide the primary support for the breasts so that the breast mass is not being held solely by the shoulder straps of the bra. This is so the pressure on the shoulders (from the shoulder straps) is reduced to prevent pain and potential injury in this area (Ryan, 2000). Therefore, the under band should be a secure fit to anchor the bra to the chest and support the breasts, but without causing discomfort. Bowles, Steele, and Munro (2012) identified that under-band tightness was a deterrent for Australian women to wear sports bras during exercise. It is, therefore, suggested that an adjustable under band may increase comfort and, in turn, increase the wearing of sports bras for exercise.

Shoulder straps of sports bras can be positioned in various configurations within sports bra design and many can be adjusted to offer more than one orientation within the same bra (e.g., vertical straps to crossed straps). It has been reported that a vertical strap orientation with a wide strap width (4.5 cm) is preferable in terms of comfort and bra-strap pressure on the shoulders (Coltman, McGhee, & Steele, 2015); however, in terms of support, when comparing this orientation to a crossed back strap design, there were no differences found in the amount of breast movement that was reduced by the bra. Therefore, when selecting a sports bra, personal preference towards shoulder strap type and the comfort experienced are sensible gauges. Many sports bras feature a racer-back design where the straps are made from fabrics with highly elastic properties and no adjustability. In these cases, the elastic straps may stretch with the movement of the breasts during exercise reducing the amount of breast support the bra can provide. It is advised that these types of sports bras are more suitable for lower impact activities such as yoga and Pilates, where excessive breast bounce is less likely to occur.

The neckline of a sports bra can vary considerably depending on the style of the bra. Currently, it is suggested that the most supportive sports bras are those with a higher neckline. A neckline is considered to be high when it reaches the upper boundary of the breast tissue and the front of the bra encases all of the breast tissue within the fabric or cups (Zhou, Yu, & Ng, 2013). A high neckline has a greater opportunity to reduce the movement of the breasts particularly by preventing upward movement as all the breast tissue is held within the bra (Zhou et al., 2013).

The cups of a sports bra can incorporate a number of different features such as padding, underwire, structured panels, and seams to aid support. Initially, the inclusion of padding to a cup was first thought to protect the breasts during sporting activity (Page & Steele, 1999); however, there is evidence to suggest that a cup with padding also increases the breast support the bra can provide (Parthasarathi, Priya, Sivaranjani, & Dhivya, 2016), which may be due to the greater rigidity and compression added to the cup. The underwire is also a component of sports bras used to hold the breast in place during exercise. However, there has been some concern shown towards the discomfort that underwire can cause during exercise due to rubbing and digging in (Bowles et al., 2012; Parthasarathi et al., 2016). As an alternative, sports bra cups are often designed with structured seams and panels to create shape and reduce breast movement. It has been found that inelastic panels within a sports bra are effective at supporting the breast during running, particularly when positioned horizontally at the upper breast boundary to reduce upward breast movement (Zhou et al., 2013).

In terms of sport- or activity-specific sports bras, there is evidence to suggest that different activities have different breast support requirements (Risius, Milligan, Mills, & Scurr, 2014). Sports bra brands have arranged their products in various ways to exhibit the levels of breast support their sports bras may provide and their suitability towards certain activities. Sports bras are often grouped into low-, medium-, and high-impact/support levels, where each category may reference which sports are suitable. For example, a high-impact/support sports bra may be more suitable for running, whereas a low-impact/support sports bra may be more suitable for yoga. However, little is known about what *scientifically* has informed these impact levels and the sports associated with them, and more importantly what makes one bra a high-impact sports bra over another.

Effects of the breast on exercising females

If a well-fitting and highly-supportive sports bra can reduce breast motion, pain, and embarrassment, this may lead to increased self-confidence and subsequently exercise engagement, benefiting exercising females. There is a need to understand and address perceived barriers to exercise, as sedentary lifestyles established in youth can track into adulthood and are a predisposing factor to chronic disease (Robbins, Pender, & Kazanis, 2003). The breast has been found to be a barrier to exercise participation by 17 per cent of the general population (Burnett et al., 2015) and 25 per cent of a horse riding population (Burbage & Cameron, 2017). Larger-breasted women, in particular, may refrain from exercise due to breast pain, embarrassment caused by excessive breast motion, their breast size, and not being able to find an appropriate sports bra (Bowles et al., 2012; Burbage & Cameron, 2017; Burnett et al., 2015; Page & Steele, 1999).

Of particular interest to the exercising female may be whether negative consequences related to the breast have an effect on their performance. Research in this area is in its infancy; however, there have been some relevant recent studies that have started to explore this notion. The impact of breast mass on marathon performance was investigated by Brown and Scurr (2016b); larger-breasted runners had greater BMIs, completed fewer marathons and had slower marathon finish times (316 ± 48 min) compared to smaller-breasted runners (281 ± 51 min), with 25 per cent less larger-breasted runners finishing in the fastest quartile. This finding suggests that breast size may be a factor that negatively affects running performance and warrants further investigation.

In addition to breast size effects, research has now been conducted into whether wearing increased breast support (i.e., a high support 'sports' bra versus a low support 'everyday' bra) can impact biomechanical and physiological parameters, which may infer performance effects. For example, when runners wore low breast support, this has led to increased muscle activation in the pectoralis major, anterior and medial deltoid, proposed to be due to increased tension within these muscles induced by the greater breast pain experienced (Milligan, Mills, & Scurr, 2014). Furthermore, low breast support has been found to lead to a less economical upper body running profile (Milligan, Mills, Corbett, & Scurr, 2015), increased ground reaction forces (White, Scurr, & Smith, 2009), and a lower breathing frequency (White, Lunt & Scurr, 2011). However, research has also concluded that level of breast support does not affect performance variables, such as running gait, ground reaction forces, or muscle activity (Risius, Milligan, Berns, Brown, & Scurr, 2016; White, Mills, Ball, & Scurr, 2015), highlighting the need for further research into possible performance effects due to breast support level. This possible performance effect may be of particular importance to an elite sportswoman where even very small positive changes can impact outcomes significantly.

Practical recommendations based on research

There are some clear practical recommendations for exercising females from the breast health and breast biomechanics literature. Excessive breast motion during exercise leads to negative effects such as breast pain, embarrassment, and negative performance outcomes, therefore a well-fitting, and highly-supportive bra is recommended for exercising females of all breast sizes. A compression sports bra may, however, be more appropriate for exercising females with smaller breasts, yet an encapsulation or combination style sports bra is likely to provide superior support for the larger-breasted female. The bra should also be appropriate to the level of activity being undertaken (i.e., low-impact activities like yoga have a different support requirement to that of running) and features such as adjustable shoulder straps and a high neckline will help to improve the level of support given.

Real-world example

An elite female rower approached researchers after suffering from costo-chrondritis (inflammation of the cartilage in the ribcage), with a concern this was related to their breast support choice. Pain had reduced substantially following a rest period and change in activities (to cycling), yet the athlete sought help identifying appropriate breast support for rowing that would not aggravate this issue or inhibit their performance. Biomechanical and physiological testing took place to explore whether introducing a high support bra would affect their rowing performance. The athlete completed a 12-min rowing ergometry test consisting of a 3-min warm-up, then 3 min of light-, moderate-, and high-intensity exercise in their own bra (low compression support) and in a high support bra. During light- and moderate-intensity rowing there were no changes in technique or physiological demand. However, during high-intensity rowing the athlete had less trunk extension (less backwards lean) and pulled the oar handle higher, leading to a more vertical arm position when wearing the high support bra. Pulling their arms back by ~10° more on each stroke, in a lower position, may have had benefits for their stroke performance. Ventilation (153 vs. 142.3 L/min), oxygen uptake (3933 vs. 3882 ml/min), and carbon dioxide output (4641 vs. 4294 ml/min) were all lower in the high support bra compared to their own bra in the high-intensity trial. These differences were minimal and could reflect natural unavoidable variation; however, the data indicate that the high support bra did not negatively affect their physiological performance. The biomechanical results also support the notion that wearing this high support bra does not negatively affect rowing performance and could actually produce some small positive performance outcomes. This case study highlights the need for further investigation into how breast support may affect the exercising female.

Summary

In this chapter, we have presented the problems associated with the healthy adult female breast, such as: breast anatomy, breast ptosis, breast size, and breast pain. Research into breast biomechanics (the assessment of breast displacement, velocity, acceleration, and skin strain) has been discussed. Information has been provided on the breast support options available to exercising females and whether sports-specific breast support is necessary. The notion that wearing a low support bra during exercise can lead to bio-mechanical and physiological changes, which may lead to a negative per-formance effect, has been debated. And finally, research into how the breast can be a barrier for females to take part in exercise has been presented. Research into breast health issues and breast biomechanics is still relatively novel, and it is hoped that, as general awareness of participating in exercise as part of a healthy lifestyle increases, further research in these areas will help to support and encourage more females to take part in exercise.

References

Bowles, K.-A., Steele, J., & Munro, B. (2012). Features of sports bras that deter their use by Australian women. *Journal of Science and Medicine in Sport, 15*(3), 195–200. https://doi.org/10.1016/j.jsams.2011.11.248.

Bridgman, C., Scurr, J., White, J., Hedger, W., & Galbraith, H. (2010). Three-dimensional kinematics of the breast during a two-step star jump. *Journal of Applied Biomechanics, 26*(4), 465–472. https://doi.org/10.1123/jab.26.4.465.

Brown, N., & Scurr, J. (2016a). Breasts are getting bigger. Where is the evidence? *Journal of Anthropological Sciences, 94*, 1–8. https://doi.org/10.4436/jass.94020.

Brown, N., & Scurr, J. (2016b). Do women with smaller breasts perform better in long-distance running? *European Journal of Sport Science, 16*(8), 965–971. https://doi.org/10.1080/17461391.2016.1200674.

Brown, N., White, J., Brasher, A., & Scurr, J. (2014a). An investigation into breast support and sports bra use in female runners of the 2012 London Marathon. *Journal of Sports Sciences, 32*(9), 801–809. https://doi.org/10.1080/02640414.2013.844348.

Brown, N., White, J., Brasher, A., & Scurr, J. (2014b). The experience of breast pain (mastalgia) in female runners of the 2012 London Marathon and its effect on exercise behaviour. *British Journal of Sports Medicine, 48*(4), 320–325. https://doi.org/10.1136/bjsports-2013-092175.

Brown, N., White, J., Milligan, A., Risius, D., Ayres, B., Hedger, W., & Scurr, J. (2012). The relationship between breast size and anthropometric characteristics. *American Journal of Human Biology, 24*(2), 158–164. https://doi.org/10.1002/ajhb.22212.

Burbage, J., & Cameron, L. (2017). An investigation into the prevalence and impact of breast pain, bra issues and breast size on female horse riders. *Journal of Sports Sciences, 35*(11), 1091–1097. https://doi.org/10.1080/02640414.2016.1210818.

Burbage, J., Cameron, L., & Goater, F. (2016). The effect of breast support on ver-tical breast displacement and breast pain in female riders across equine simulator gaits. *Journal of Veterinary Behavior: Clinical Applications and Research, 15*, 81. https://doi.org/10.1016/j.jveb.2016.08.020.

Burnett, E., White, J., & Scurr, J. (2015). The influence of the breast on physical activity participation in females. *Journal of Physical Activity and Health, 12*(4), 588–594. https://doi.org/10.1123/jpah.2013-0236.

Coltman, C. E., McGhee, D. E., & Steele, J. R. (2015). Bra strap orientations and designs to minimise bra strap discomfort and pressure during sport and exercise in women with large breasts. *Sports Medicine – Open, 1*(1), 21. https://doi.org/10.1186/s40798-015-0014-z.

Coltman, C. E., McGhee, D. E., & Steele, J. R. (2017a). Three-dimensional scanning in women with large, ptotic breasts: Implications for bra cup sizing and design. *Ergonomics, 60*(3), 439–445. https://doi.org/10.1080/00140139.2016.1176258.

Coltman, C. E., Steele, J. R., & McGhee, D. E. (2017b). Effect of aging on breast skin thickness and elasticity: Implications for breast support. *Skin Research and Technology, 23*(3), 303–311. https://doi.org/10.1111/srt.12335.

Findikcioglu, K., Findikcioglu, F., Ozmen, S., & Guclu, T. (2007). The impact of breast size on the vertebral column: A radiologic study. *Aesthetic Plastic Surgery, 31*(1), 23–27. https://doi.org/10.1007/s00266-006-0178-5.

Gefen, A., & Dilmoney, B. (2007). Mechanics of the normal woman's breast. *Health Care, 15*(4), 259–271.

Gehlsen, G., & Albohm, M. (1980). Evaluation of sports bras. *The Physician and Sportsmedicine, 8*(10), 89–96. https://doi.org/10.1080/00913847.1980.11948653.

Haake, S., Milligan, A., & Scurr, J. (2013). Can measures of strain and acceleration be used to predict breast discomfort during running? *Proceedings of the Institution of Mechanical Engineers, Part P: Journal of Sports Engineering and Technology, 227*(3), 209–216. https://doi.org/10.1177/1754337112456799.

Haake, S., & Scurr, J. (2011). A method to estimate strain in the breast during exercise. *Sports Engineering, 14*(1), 49–56. https://doi.org/10.1007/s12283-011-0071-6.

Haycock, C. E., Shierman, G., & Gillette, J. (1978). The female athlete–does her anatomy pose problems. In *Proceedings of the American Medical Association 19th Conference on the Medical Aspects of Sports* (pp. 1–8).

Hindle, W. (1991). The breast and exercise. In R. W. Hale (Ed.), *Caring for the exercising woman.* (pp. 83–92). New York: Elsevier Science Publishing.

Li, D., Cheong, A., Reece, G. P., Crosby, M. A., Fingeret, M. C., & Merchant, F. A. (2016). Computation of breast ptosis from 3D surface scans of the female torso. *Computers in Biology and Medicine, 78*, 18–28. https://doi.org/10.1016/j.compbiomed.2016.09.002.

Lorentzen, D., & Lawson, L. (1987). Selected sports bras: A biomechanical analysis of breast motion while jogging. *The Physician and Sportsmedicine, 15*(5), 128–139. https://doi.org/10.1080/00913847.1987.11709355.

Machida, Y., & Nakadate, M. (2015). Breast shape change associated with aging. *Plastic and Reconstructive Surgery – Global Open, 3*(6), e413. https://doi.org/10.1097/GOX.0000000000000289.

Mason, B. R., Page, K.-A., & Fallon, K. (1999). An analysis of movement and discomfort of the female breast during exercise and the effects of breast support in three cases. *Science and Medicine in Sport, 2*(2), 134–144. https://doi.org/10.1016/S1440-2440(99)80193-5.

McCool, W. F., Stone-Condry, M., & Bradford, H. M. (1998). Breast health care. A review. *Journal of Nurse-Midwifery, 43*(6), 406–430. https://doi.org/10.1016/S0091-2182(98)00065-2.

McGhee, D. E., Power, B. M., & Steele, J. R. (2007). Does deep water running reduce exercise-induced breast discomfort? *British Journal of Sports Medicine, 41*(12), 879–883. https://doi.org/10.1136/bjsm.2007.036251.

Milligan, A., Mills, C., Corbett, J., & Scurr, J. (2015). The influence of breast support on torso, pelvis and arm kinematics during a five kilometer treadmill run. *Human Movement Science, 42*, 246–260. https://doi.org/10.1016/j.humov.2015.05.008.

Milligan, A. Mills, C., & Scurr, J. (2014). The effect of breast support on upper body muscle activity during 5km treadmill running. *Human Movement Science, 38,* 74–83. https://doi.org/10.1016/j.humov.2014.06.001.

Mills, C., Loveridge, A., Milligan, A., & Scurr, J. (2016). Trunk marker sets and the subsequent calculation of trunk and breast kinematics during treadmill running. *Textile Research Journal, 86*(11), 1128–1136. https://doi.org/10.1177/00405 1751560S257.

Nolte, K., Burgoyne, S., Nolte, H., Van der Meulen, J., & Fletcher, L. (2016). The effectiveness of a range of sports bras in reducing breast displacement during treadmill running and two-step star jumping. *The Journal of Sports Medicine and Physical Fitness, 56*(11), 1311–1317.

Page, K.-A. & Steele, J. (1999). Breast motion and sports brassiere design. Implications for future research. *Sports Medicine, 27*(4), 205–211. https://doi.org/10.2165/00007256-199927040-00001.

Parthasarathi, D. V, Priya, T. R., Sivaranjani, S., & Dhivya, A. (2016). Design and development of sports intimate apparel: A review. *International Journal Online of Sports Technology & Human Engineering, 3,* 1–9.

Regnault, P. (1976). Breast ptosis. Definition and treatment. *Clinics in Plastic Surgery, 3*(2), 193–203.

Rinker, B., Veneracion, M., & Walsh, C. (2010). Breast ptosis: Causes and cure. *Annals of Plastic Surgery, 64,* 579–584. https://doi.org/10.1097/SAP.0b013e3181c39377.

Risius, D., Milligan, A., Berns, J., Brown, N., & Scurr, J. (2017). Understanding key performance indicators for breast support: An analysis of breast support effects on biomechanical, physiological and subjective measures during running. *Journal of Sports Sciences, 35*(9), 842–851. https://doi.org/10.1080/02640414.2016.1194523.

Risius, D., Milligan, A., Mills, C., & Scurr, J. (2015). Multiplanar breast kinematics during different exercise modalities. *European Journal of Sport Science, 15*(2), 111–117. https://doi.org/10.1080/17461391.2014.928914.

Robbins, L., Pender, N., & Kazanis, A. (2003). Barriers to physical activityperceived by adolescent girls. *Journal of Midwifery & Women's Health, 48*(3), 206–212. https://doi.org/10.1016/S1526-9523(03)00054-0.

Ryan, E. L (2000). Pectoral girdle myalgia in women: a 5-year study in a clinical setting. *The Clinical Journal of Pain, 16*(4), 298–303. https://doi.org/10.1097/00002508-200012000-00004.

Sanchez, A., Mills, C., & Scurr, J. (2016). Estimating breast mass-density:a retrospective analysis of radiological data. *The Breast Journal, 23*(2), 237–239. https://doi.org/10.1111/tbj.12725.

Scurr, J., White, J., & Hedger, W. (2009). Breast displacement in three dimensions during the walking and running gait cycles. *Journal of Applied Biomechanics, 25*(4), 322–329. https://doi.org/10.1177/0363546508314791.

Scurr, J., White, J., & Hedger, W. (2010). The effect of breast support on the kinematics of the breast during the running gait cycle. *Journal of Sports Sciences, 28*(10), 1103–1109. https://doi.org/10.1080/02640414.2010.497542.

Scurr, J., White, J., & Hedger, W. (2011). Supported and unsupported breast displacement in three dimensions across treadmill activity levels. *Journal of Sports Sciences, 29*(1), 55–61. https://doi.org/10.1080/02640414.2010.521944.

Shivitz, N. L. (2001). *Adaptation of vertical ground reaction force due to changes in breast support in running.* Oregon State University. Retrieved from http://ir.library.oregonstate.edu/concern/graduate_thesis_or_dissertations/9880vs96k.

Ulger, H., Erdogan, N., Kumanlioglu, S., & Unur, E. (2003). Effect of age, breast size, menopausal and hormonal status on mammographic skin thickness. *Skin Research and Technology, 9*(3), 284–289. https://doi.org/10.1034/j.1600-0846.2003.00027.x.

White, J., Lunt, H., & Scurr, J. (2011). The effect of breast support on ventilation and breast comfort perception at the onset of exercise. In *BASES supplement abstracts* (p. 29). Journal of Sports Sciences.

White, J., Mills, C., Ball, N., & Scurr, J. (2015). The effect of breast support and breast pain on upper-extremity kinematics during running: implications for females with large breasts. *Journal of Sports Sciences, 33*(19), 2043–2050. https://doi.org/10.1080/02640414.2015.1026378.

White, J., Scurr, J., & Smith, N. (2009). The effect of breast support on kinetics during overground running performance. *Ergonomics, 52*(4), 492–498. https://doi.org/10.1080/00140130802707907.

Zhou, J., Yu, W., & Ng, S. (2013). Identifying effective design features of commercial sports bras. *Textile Research Journal, 83*(14), 1500–1513. https://doi.org/10.1177/0040517512464289.

13 The psychology of female sport performance

Claire-Marie Roberts, Leah Ferguson, and Amber Mosewich

Introduction

For those seeking to understand the nuances of gender differences in sport performance, psychology is a discipline that is often overlooked. Rather than having a basis in sex differences, the gender divide in the psychology of sport performance is centred on social-cognitive models and cultural influences (Gill, 2017). That is to say that the social environments of females and males are different from the outset – from physical education to youth sport and all the way through to recreational exercise or elite athletic programmes. Indeed, these environments centred on persistent gender stereotypes in sport, influence perceptions, behaviours, and achievements in sport. Gender differences drive a number of nuanced behaviours that ultimately impact on sport performance. For example, empirical research indicates that there are differences in competitive anxiety responses, confidence, goal orientation, group dynamics, the cohesion-performance relationship, stressors, coping reactions, and preferences of coaching styles in the exercising female. Indeed, gender differences have been reported as being larger in sport than in other domains (Eccles & Harrold, 1991).

Aims of the chapter

The aims of the chapter are as follows:

1   To examine the extant literature focused on the psychology of the exercising female.
2   To examine the likely gender nuances affecting sport performance in this population.

Psychological approaches to sport competition

Competitive anxiety in the exercising female

Competitive state anxiety is a multidimensional construct consisting of both cognitive and somatic anxiety and is one of the most researched constructs in sport psychology (Stadulis, MacCracken, Eidson, & Severance, 2002) due to the potentially negative impact it has on athletic performance. The research examining gender differences in competitive anxiety is sparse (Woodman & Hardy, 2003), although the minimal attention that has been afforded to this area of investigation has resulted in contradictory findings. For example, work in the late 1980s and early 1990s suggested that gender differentiates multidimensional anxiety experiences (e.g., Swain & Jones, 1993), with females supposedly more susceptible to the effects of cognitive anxiety (e.g., Martens, Burton, Vealey, Bump, & Smith, 1990). Yet, in their meta-analysis of studies up to and including January 2002, Woodman and Hardy (2003) concluded 'pre-competitive cognitive anxiety and self-confidence have a greater impact on the performance of men than that of women' (p. 452).

More recent attempts to investigate gender differences in the effects of competitive anxiety on sport performance have further yielded contradictory views. For example, Hagan and associates (2017a) found that elite females were less cognitively anxious, interpreted somatic symptoms as more facilitative, and were more stable seven days before competitive fixtures compared to their male counterparts. In a follow-up study addressing a similar research question in elite table tennis players, Hagan, Pollmann, and Schack (2017b) concluded that their findings contradicted the commonly held belief that gender differentiates multidimensional anxiety experiences, when they found no differences at all. They went on to explain any differences as being attributable to culture, team dynamics, and/or competitive level. Clearly, further research is needed to shed further light on this topic.

Confidence

Confidence is a key skill required for successful athletic performance. Indeed, sport psychology literature delineates between self-confidence, self-efficacy, and sport-confidence as discrete constructs. For example, self-confidence is the belief, as an individual, that you possess the internal resources to achieve success, whereas self-efficacy is a fluctuating state of judgement of one's ability to organise and execute specific actions needed to produce a certain level of performance (Bandura, 1986). Sport-confidence on the other hand is a sport-specific belief in one's ability to succeed in sport (Vealey, 2001).

There are known gender differences in levels and sources of confidence in a sporting context. Males, for example, typically display higher levels of confidence than females (e.g., Vargus-Tonsing & Bartholomew, 2006). In addition, there are gender differences in the antecedents and temporal patterning of self-confidence precompetition (Jones, Swain, & Cale, 1991). To illustrate, personal goals and standards predict confidence in females, whereas males tend to derive theirs from interpersonal comparison and winning (Hays, Maynard, Thomas, & Bawden, 2007). In addition, research has concluded that females may derive confidence from their coach's encouragement, positive feedback/reinforcement, and compliments, akin to the 'social support' source of sport-confidence identified by Vealey (1986). Conversely, no gender differences in self-efficacy in sport have been found (cf. Kocaeksi & Gaziog_u, 2014). Although, when considering sport-confidence, findings from research in the last decade suggest that elite female athletes attribute sources of sport-confidence to: mastering personal skills; reinforcement from significant others; perceptions of their body image; coach's leadership; and feeling comfortable in the competition environment to a greater degree than the male athletes (Kingston, Lane, & Thomas, 2010).

Goal orientation

The achievement goal theory (Nicholls, 1989) provides a social-cognitive approach to understand and study motivation where the main driver is competence. This theory posits that both individuals' achievement goals (the competence-based aim used to guide behaviour) and motivational climate (perception of social environment) can determine the quality of the individuals' affective, cognitive and behavioural experience (Nicholls, 1989). Using this theory as a basis, research has determined that males and females are motivated differently to participate in an action (Duda, 1993). Achievement goals are defined as task- and ego-orientated. With task-orientated goals, competence and satisfaction are derived when a person learns new skills, improves their performance, and does their best – activities all focused on self-referenced standards. Ego-orientated goals on the other hand provide feelings of competence and satisfaction from outperforming others – ability that is normatively or socially referenced (Nicholls, 1989). It is perhaps not surprising that female athletes (both recreational and competitive) often score lower on levels of ego orientation (Li, Harmer, & Acock, 1996) and higher on task-orientation (e.g., Hanrahan, & Cerin, 2009), whereas males place a greater emphasis on competitiveness, winning, and beating others (Duda, 1986). This difference may be driven by parental, school, peer and sociocultural influences, and stereotype threat (Oyer, 2014). An awareness, therefore, of the likely difference in the psychology of female sport performance, will help coaches and athlete-support personnel structure goal setting interventions in an effective manner.

Preferred coaching behaviours

The inability of male coaches to understand how best to engage with female athletes has been determined to be a key barrier to participation, engagement, and progression in this population (Norman & French, 2013). To circumvent these barriers, it is important to understand the exercising female's motivation for participation and competition, their preference in relation to their relationship with their coach, their preferred coaching style, and their coaching needs. With their need for enjoyment (MacKinnon, 2011) and for a good quality personal relationship with the coach, exercising females attribute importance to exploring the rationale behind coaching decisions and will often want to be involved in the decision-making process (Norman, 2016). Coaching style, therefore, is key for the exercising female. Male athletes have been found to favour an autocratic coaching style, whereas female athletes exhibit a greater preference for a democratic coaching style (e.g., Terry, 1984). Indeed, female athletes place more value on being supported as a person as well as a performer, prefer that coaching be a joint endeavour, have a need for positive communication, and finally require that the salience of gender within the coach-athlete dyad is recognised (Norman, 2015). In summary, delivering a more '… democratic, personalised and positive relationship' (Norman, 2015, p. 3) with coaches is an important consideration in improving female athletes' experiences of performance sport (Norman & French, 2013).

Group dynamics and the cohesion-performance relationship in female sport teams

Cohesion represents 'a dynamic process that is reflected in the tendency for a group to stick together and remain united in the pursuit of its instrumental objectives and/or for the satisfaction of member affective needs' (Carron, Brawley, & Widmeyer, 1998, p. 213). In essence, this definition considers the overall unity and individual members' attractions to both task (i.e., performance-related) and social (i.e., relation-orientated) aspects of the group. When examining gender differences in teams, it is important to understand that females tend to be more socially-orientated when it comes to their team (Kidd & Woodman, 1975), defining themselves in terms of relationships.

Although normative data exist (measured by the Group Environment Questionnaire) to suggest that the absolute amount of cohesiveness in female and male teams is similar (Widmeyer, Brawley, & Carron, 1985), female athletes demonstrate significantly higher *perceptions* of cohesion (Wrisberg & Draper, 1988). A posited reason for this is the gender difference in females' greater motivation to create and maintain close relationships with others and the need for belongingness (Cross, Hardin, & Gercek-Swing, 2011). Using this understanding as a baseline, gender has been previously identified as a strong moderator variable in the cohesion-performance relationship (Carron, Colman, Wheeler, & Stevens, 2002).

While on the face of it, a greater perception of cohesion and a stronger orientation towards close relationships and belongingness may appear facilitative to sport team performance, it has been suggested that, 'events that contribute to a loss of cohesiveness might be expected to be more detrimental to team success in female teams' (Carron et al., 2002, p. 183). Likewise, in Eys and colleagues' (2015) recent study exploring perceptions of the cohesion-performance relationship by coaches who have led teams of both genders, one participant noted: 'Group cohesion is harder to achieve in female teams because women handle things more on a personal level' (p. 103). Another participant explained: 'My observations are that for the females, the need for harmony within the training group was stronger than for men' (p. 103). Further observations were made about the ease of formation of subgroups or cliques and the difficulty of handling of personal conflict in female teams, as resentment is often harboured for longer. It is important to emphasise, however, that the existence of psychological differences does not attribute greater significance to one gender's norms over the other. It merely reinforces the need to ensure that coaches and athlete-support personnel fully understand the gender-specific approach to team sport, such that teams can be coached and supported competently to help them achieve optimal performance.

Optimal psychological functioning

In essence, sport and exercise has the potential to promote women's psychological growth, contributing to the likelihood of optimal psychological functioning at one's highest potential. Ryff (1989) provides a framework of striving to reach one's potential, or psychologically flourishing, which has merit in sport and exercise domains. According to Ryff, an individual who is optimally functioning at her highest potential exhibits six core features: (a) autonomy; (b) mastery over one's environment; (c) positive relations with others; (c) personal growth and development; (e) purpose in life; and (f) self-acceptance. Female athletes have indicated that these components are reflective of what it means to reach their potential and flourish in sport (Ferguson, Kowalski, Mack, & Sabiston, 2014).

Although the exercising female may psychologically flourish in sport and exercise contexts, they can also encounter many unpleasant, difficult, and even negative experiences – both competitive and non-competitive in nature – that may hinder psychological growth. For instance, some of the challenges commonly experienced are: body dissatisfaction; injury; bullying; eating disorders; coach conflicts; sexual abuse; performance expectations, evaluations, and slumps; self-criticism; and social comparisons (e.g., Mosewich, Vangool, Kowalski, & McHugh, 2009). Additionally, many women voice the challenge of dealing with an 'appearance-performance' struggle, arising from the conflict of desiring a body that will perform in the physical domain, but also suits non-sport physique expectations and ideals (Mosewich et al., 2009, p. 105). Sport and exercise experiences have the potential to benefit or detrimentally influence female athletes' and exercisers' well-being. Women who have not developed effective coping skills to deal with demands they encounter in sport and exercise contexts may experience negative outcomes such as suboptimal performance, high levels of distress, negative emotional patterns, and dropout (see Hoar, Kowalski, Gaudreau, & Crocker, 2006).

Stressors

The stressors or demands faced by females in sport and exercise can be considered unique from their male counterparts, and warrant acknowledgement, and consideration. Apart from standard sources of performance pressure and competitive anxiety, females may also contend with additional stressors resulting from the perception of unequal or unfair treatment, the often-poor organisation of women's sport, machismo, and the patronising attitudes of male administrators, coaches, and referees. Furthermore, sources of competitive stress may originate from unhelpful gender stereotypes and substandard treatment of women athletes in some elite sports (e.g., Guillén & Sánchez, 2009).

Additionally, there is evidence to suggest that women tend to view and interpret competition settings differently than men (Warner & Dixon, 2015). While the cognitive appraisal of demands and resultant coping strategies and outcomes are individual processes arising from the person-environment interaction, women and girls in sport have acknowledged some unique experiences and demands, as well as differences in resources and approaches that impact how they navigate the sport context (e.g., Mosewich, Crocker, & Kowalski, 2014). Given the many challenges that females may encounter in sport and exercise, which may contribute to stress and thwart their flourishing, it is important to identify resources and tools that may help them navigate their difficult experiences. Managing setbacks through the adoption of a positive approach, with an emphasis on constructive thoughts, has been identified as an effective process by female athletes. Acknowledgement of the positive aspects of a situation, while learning from – as opposed to ruminating on – the negative, positions the exercising female for an optimal focus in the future.

Coping

While there has been some attention to gender differences in coping, the results are largely equivocal and illustrate the complex and individual nature of the coping process (see Hoar et al., 2006). However, in studies that do report differences, female athletes and exercisers tend to use more support-seeking and emotion-focused coping to manage stressors when compared to their male counterparts (e.g., Hammermeister & Burton, 2004). The occasional trend aside, females engaged in sport and exercise adopt a wide array of coping strategies. Of particular importance is the effectiveness of the strategies, and ensuring the exercising female possesses self-awareness and the ability to self-reflect to evaluate – and, if necessary, redirect – their coping efforts, as well as establish external support in addressing deficiencies in coping. Family, friends, significant others, coaches, training partners, psychologists, exercise leaders, and others who have gone through something similar have all been identified as sources of such support (Ingstrup,

Mosewich, & Holt, 2017). While there are diverse coping options and success in many traditional approaches, additional resources should also be considered in an attempt to address the gaps highlighted by women in sport and exercise. Consideration of individual coping efforts, as well as communal coping (see Neely, McHugh, Dunn, & Holt, 2017) has merit.

Self-compassion

One less traditional resource that is beginning to emerge and shows a great deal of potential for women in managing the demands of sport and exercise, while also contributing to positive growth, is self-compassion. Self-compassion is a healthy self-attitude that entails being moved by one's own suffering along with the desire to alleviate that suffering (Neff, 2003a). Self-compassion is compassion turned inward − relating to one's difficult experiences in a self-supporting, rather than self-deprecating, way. Self-compassion has been conceptualised as consisting of three components, each with its own counterpart: self-kindness, common humanity, and mindfulness. Rather than engaging in harsh self-criticism when confronted with suffering, inadequacy, or failure, self-kindness entails offering oneself warmth and non-judgemental understanding. Common humanity involves recognising shared human experiences as opposed to feeling isolated when encountering life's difficulties. Mindfulness represents a balanced awareness of painful feelings and experiences, rather than ruminating on or suppressing one's thoughts. *Self-kindness*, *common humanity*, and *mindfulness* combine and mutually interact to create a self-compassionate frame of mind. Having compassion for oneself is not dependent upon favourable self-evaluations, nor does it require unrealistic positive views of oneself (Neff, 2003a). Extending compassion towards the self is particularly useful during times of difficulty, failure, and struggle (Neff, 2003b), and, as such, can be advantageous for female athletes and exercisers. Self-compassion may be especially useful in helping to manage demands such as excessive self-criticism, rumination, and negative evaluation, which are frequently identified by the exercising female as posing difficulty. Indeed, female athletes and exercisers with higher levels of self-compassion have lower body shame, extrinsic exercise motivations, obligatory exercise, fear of failure and negative evaluation, as well as social physique anxiety (Mosewich, Crocker, Kowalski, & DeLongis, 2013). Moreover, female athletes and exercisers with greater self-compassion have been found to have greater autonomy, body appreciation, intrinsic exercise motivations, positivity, perseverance, self-acceptance, and psychological flourishing (Ferguson et al., 2014).

Practical recommendations

Sport education, whether coaching, management or scientific support-related is currently centred on male performance as the standard (Allen & Shaw,

2009). In essence, the education received by the current workforce is likely to have been gender-blind. Gender-blind education, programmes, policies, and attitudes in sport are unlikely to take into account the different and diverse needs of the exercising female. Clearly, every exercising female is an individual and any coaching, management, or support strategy should be tailored to suit their specific needs. Yet, understanding generalised female tendencies or preferences may help expedite the development of the right strategies for engaging and supporting female athletes individually, and on a team basis (e.g., Norman, 2016). The need for the tailoring of coaching and support to the differing needs of athletes according to gender is supported by research (e.g., Felton & Jowett, 2013; MacKinnon, 2011). It is time now to challenge the status quo in sport, to review the educational provision across disciplines, and to create a diverse workforce that is reflective of gender divide in athletes.

Real-world example

Heidi

The example we have chosen to present features Heidi, a professional football (soccer) player who has played for her current club for 15 years. Her development in football occurred as a result of playing alongside boys throughout her childhood until she was offered the chance to sign for a women's team in her teens. Her career objective is to be the best football player she can be – a mastery-orientated goal that motivates her against all odds to succeed. Although she has had a professional contract for the last five years, her earnings are so small, that she needs to work part-time in a supermarket to be able to afford to live. A combination of the conflict between her work rota and her training and the reactions of her colleagues in her part-time role, who underplay the importance of her athletic career, causes her stress.

Heidi's team is made up of relatively young players. As a group they are high in social cohesion and socialise regularly outside of the sport. In fact, many of the team live together in shared houses, and when conflict inevitably arises between different cliques, the atmosphere at home and in the dressing room is uncomfortable. When this transfers onto the pitch, the team's performance is adversely affected. Meanwhile, the pending contract negotiations with her club mean that Heidi is concerned about her future as a professional footballer as she's one of the oldest players in the team. She has started to reflect on the cost of her football career, since she has focused all her efforts into her training at the expense of everything else. In an attempt to cope, Heidi has contacted a friend who retired from football a few years ago, to seek advice and support. She has also engaged with the sport psychologist at the club in an attempt to start preparing for a life after sport, and identifying new career directions and goals. Early signs suggest that this support is proving to be an effective approach to coping.

Summary

On a macroscale, there are more commonalities in the psychological approach to sport and exercise among males and females than there are differences. However, the nuanced gender-specific psychological approach has the potential to have a significant impact on sport performance. Although the research examining gender differences in competitive anxiety is contradictory, any extant sociocultural gender stereotypes should be taken into consideration when assessing and intervening with competitive anxiety symptoms in female athletes. More compelling are the differences in sources of confidence, goal orientation, and preferred coaching behaviours between male and female athletes. Furthermore, the attainment of cohesion, the need for group harmony, and the difficulty handling personal conflict in all-female teams provide valuable insight into team functioning. Sport and exercise contexts may benefit some females and be of great detriment to others. This difference appears to be driven by the additional stressors associated, in some cases, with sport inequality yet it is moderated by support-seeking and emotion-focused coping – common approaches to coping among females. Finally, self-compassion may be an effective way for females to manage the demands of sport and exercise, at all stages of the lifecycle, to help them reach their potential in this field.

References

Allen, J., & Shaw, S. (2009). Women coaches' perceptions of their sport organizations social environment: Supporting coaches' psychological needs? *The Sport Psychologist, 23*, 346–366. https://doi.org/10.1123/tsp. 23.3.346.

Bandura, A. (1986). *Social foundations of thought and action*. Englewood Cliffs, NJ: Prentice-Hall.

Carron, A. V., Brawley, L. R., & Widmeyer, W. N. (1998). The measurement of cohesiveness in sport groups. In J. L. Duda (Ed.), *Advances in sport and exercise psychology measurement* (pp. 213–226). Morgantown, WV: Fitness Information Technology.

Carron, A. V., Colman, M. M., Wheeler, J., & Stevens, D. (2002). Cohesion and performance in sport: A meta-analysis. *Journal of Sport & Exercise Psychology, 24*, 168–188.

Cross, S. E., Hardin, E. E., & Gercek-Swing, B. (2011). The what, how, why, and where of self-construal. *Personality and Social Psychology Review, 15*, 142–179. https://doi.org/10.1177/1088868310373752.

Duda, J. L. (1986). A cross-cultural analysis of achievement motivation in sport and the classroom. In L. Vander Velden, & J. Humphrey (Eds.), *Psychology and sociology in sport: Current selected research (Vol. I)* (pp. 115–134). New York: AMS Press.

Duda J. L. (1993). Goals: A social cognitive approach to the study of motivation in sport. In: R. N. Singer, M. Murphey, & L. K. Tennant (Eds.), *Handbook of research on sport psychology* (pp. 421–436). New York: Macmillan.

Eccles, J. S., & Harrold, R. D. (1991). Gender differences in sport involvement: Applying the Eccles' expectancy-value model. *Journal of Applied Sport Psychology, 3*, 7–35

Eys, M., Evans, M. B., Martin, L. J., Ohlert, J., Wolf, S. A., Van Bussel, M., & Steins, C. (2015). Cohesion and performance for female and male sport teams. *The Sport Psychologist, 29*, 97–109. https://doi.org/10.1123/tsp. 2014-0027.

Felton, L., & Jowett, S. (2013). The mediating role of social environmental factors in the associations between attachment styles and basic needs satisfaction. *Journal of Sports Sciences, 31*, 618–628. https://doi.org/10.1080/02640414.2012.744078.

Ferguson, L. J., Kowalski, K. C., Mack, D. E., & Sabiston, C. M. (2014). Exploring self-compassion and eudaimonic well-being in young women athletes. *Journal of Sport & Exercise Psychology, 36*, 203–216. https://doi.org/10.1123/jsep.2013-0096.

Ferguson, L. J., Kowalski, K. C., Mack, D. E., & Sabiston, C. M. (2015). Self-compassion and eudaimonic well-being during emotionally difficult times in sport. *Journal of Happiness Studies, 16*, 1263–1280. https://doi.org/10.1007/s10902-014-9558-8.

Gill, D. (2017). Gender and cultural diversity in sport, exercise, and performance psychology. *Oxford Research Encyclopedia of Psychology*. https://doi.org/10.1093/acrefore/9780190236557.013.148.

Guillén, F., & Sánchez, R. (2009). Competitive anxiety in expert female athletes: Sources and intensity of anxiety in national team and first division Spanish basketball players. *Perceptual and Motor Skills, 109*, 407–419. https://doi.org/0.2466/PMS.109.2.407-419.

Hagan, J. E., Pollmann, D., & Schack, T. (2017a). Interaction between gender and skill on competitive state anxiety using the time-to-event paradigm: What roles do intensity, direction, and frequency dimensions play? *Frontiers in Psychology, 8*, 692. https://doi.org/10.3389/fpsyg.2017.00692.

Hagan, J. E., Pollmann, D., & Schack, T. (2017b). Elite athletes' in-event competitive anxiety responses and psychological skills usage under differing conditions. *Frontiers in Psychology, 8*, 2280. https://doi.org/10.3389/fpsyg.2017.02280.

Hammermeister, J., & Burton, D. (2004). Gender differences in coping with endurance sport stress: Are men from Mars and women from Venus? *Journal of Sport Behavior, 27*, 148–164.

Hanrahan, S. J., & Cerin, E. (2009). Gender, level of participation, and type of sport: Differences in achievement goal orientation and attributional style. *Journal of Science and Medicine in Sport, 12*, 508–512. https://doi.org/10.1016/j.jsams.2008 01.005.

Hays, K., Maynard, I., Thomas, O., & Bawden, M. (2007). Sources and types of confidence identified by world class sport performers. *Journal of Applied Sport Psychology, 19*, 434–456. https://doi.org/10.1080/10413200701599173.

Hoar, S. D., Kowalski, K. C., Gaudreau, P., & Crocker, P. R. (2006). A review of coping in sport. In S. Hanton & S. D. Mellalieu (Eds.), *Literature reviews in sport psychology* (pp. 47–90). New York: Nova Science.

Ingstrup, M. S., Mosewich, A. D., & Holt, N. (2017). The development of self-compassion among women varsity athletes. *The Sport Psychologist, 31*(4), 1–32. https://doi.org/10.1123/tsp. 2016-0147.

Jones, G., Swain, A. B. J., & Cale, A. (1991). Gender differences in precompetition temporal patterning and antecedents of anxiety and self-confidence. *Journal of Sport and Exercise Psychology, 13*, 1–15.

Kidd, T. R., & Woodman, W. F. (1975). Sex and orientations toward winning in sport. *Research Quarterly, 46*, 476–483.

Kingston, K., Lane, A., & Thomas, O. (2010). A temporal examination of elite performers sources of sport-confidence. *The Sport Psychologist, 24*(3), 313–332. https://doi.org/10.1123/tsp. 24.3.313.

Kocaeksi, S., & Gazioglu, A. E. (2014). The evaluation of self-efficacy and collective efficacy beliefs in handball in terms of gender. *Procedia Social and Behavioral Science, 159*, 125–127. https://doi.org/10.1016/j.sbspro.2014.12.342.

Li, F., Harmer, P., & Acock, A. (1996). The task and ego orientation in sport questionnaire: construct equivalence and mean differences across gender. *Research Quarterly for Exercise and Sport, 67*, 228–238. https://doi.org/10.1080/02701367.1 996.10607949.

MacKinnon, V. (2011). Techniques for instructing female athletes in traditionally male sports: A case study of LPGA teaching professionals. *The International Journal of Sport and Society, 2*(1), 75–87.

Martens, R., Burton, D., Vealey, R. S., Bump, L. A., & Smith, D. E. (1990). Development and validation of the Competitive State Anxiety Inventory-2. In R. Martens, R. S. Vealey, & D. Burton (Eds.), *Competitive anxiety in sport* (pp. 117–190). Champaign, IL: Human Kinetics.

Mosewich, A. D., Crocker, P. R. E., & Kowalski, K. C. (2014). Managing injury and other setbacks in sport: Experiences of (and resources for) high-performance women athletes. *Qualitative Research in Sport, Exercise, and Health, 6*, 182–204. https://doi.org/10.1080/2159676X.2013.766810.

Mosewich, A. D., Crocker, P. R. E., Kowalski, K. C., & DeLongis, A. (2013). Applying self-compassion in sport: An intervention with women athletes. *Journal of Sport & Exercise Psychology, 35*, 514–524. https://doi.org/10.1123/jsep. 35.5.514.

Mosewich, A. D., Vangool, A. B., Kowalski, K. C., & McHugh, T. F. (2009). Exploring women track and field athletes' meanings of muscularity. *Journal of Applied Sport Psychology, 21*, 99–115. https://doi.org/10.1080/10413200802575742.

Neely, K. C., McHugh, T. L. F., Dunn, J. G., & Holt, N. L. (2017). Athletes and parents coping with deselection in competitive youth sport: A communal coping perspective. *Psychology of Sport and Exercise, 30*, 1–9. https://doi.org/10.1016/j. psychsport.2017.01.004.

Neff, K. (2003a). The development and validation of a scale to measure self-compassion. *Self and Identity, 2*, 223–250. https://doi.org/10.1080/15298860390209035.

Neff, K. (2003b). Self-compassion: An alternative conceptualization of a healthy attitude toward oneself. *Self and Identity, 2*, 85–101. https://doi.org/10.1080/ 15298860390129863.

Nicholls, J. G. (1989). *The competitive ethos and democratic education.* Cambridge, MA: Harvard University Press.

Norman, L. (2015). The coaching needs of high performance female athletes within the coach-athlete dyad. *International Sport Coaching Journal, 2*, 15–28. https://doi. org/10.1123/iscj.2013-0037.

Norman, L. (2016). Is there a need for coaches to be more gender responsive? A review of the evidence. *International Sport Coaching Journal, 3*, 192–196. https:// doi.org/10.1123/iscj.2016-0032.

Norman, L., & French, J. (2013). Understanding how high performance women athletes experience the coach-athlete relationship. *International Journal of Coaching Science, 7*, 3–24.

Oyer, M. H. (2014). *Investigating gender differences in achievement goal orientation in example-based algebra learning.* Philadelphia, PA: Temple University.

Ryff, C. D. (1989). Happiness is everything, or is it? Explorations on the meaning of psychological well-being. *Journal of Personality and Social Psychology, 57*, 1069–1081. https://doi.org/10.1037/0022-3514.57.6.1069.

Stadulis, R. E., MacCracken, M. J., Eidson, T. A., & Severance. C. (2002). The children's form of the CSAI: The CSAI–2C. *Measurement in Physical Education and Exercise Science, 6,* 147–165. https://doi.org/10.1207/S15327841MPEE0603_1.

Swain, A. B. J., & Jones, G. (1993). Intensity and frequency dimensions of competitive state anxiety. *Journal of Sport Sciences, 11,* 533–542. https://doi.org/0.1080/02640419308730024.

Terry, P. (1984). The coaching preferences of elite athletes competing at Universiade '83. *Canadian Journal of Applied Sport Sciences, 9,* 201–208.

Vargas-Tonsing, T. M., & Bartholomew, J. B. (2006). An exploratory study of the effects of pregame speeches on team on team efficacy beliefs. *Journal of Applied Sport Psychology, 36,* 918–933. https://doi.org/10.1111/j.0021-9029.2006.00049.x.

Vealey, R. (1986). Conceptualization of sport-confidence and competitive orientation: Preliminary investigation and instrument development. *Journal of Sport Psychology, 8,* 221–246. https://doi.org/10.1123/jsp. 8.3.221.

Vealey, R. (2001). Understanding and enhancing self-confidence in athletes. In R. Singer, H. Hausenblas, & C. Janelle (Eds.), *Handbook of sport psychology* (pp. 550–565). New York: Wiley.

Warner, S., & Dixon, M. A. (2015). Competition, gender and the sport experience: An exploration among college athletes. *Sport, Education and Society, 20,* 527–545. https://doi.org/10.1080/13573322.2013.774273.

White, S. A., & Duda, J. L. (1994). The relationship of gender, level of sport involvement, and participation motivation to task and ego orientation. *International Journal of Sport Psychology, 25,* 4–18.

Widmeyer, N., Brawley, L., & Carron, A. (1985). *The measurement of cohesion in sport teams. The Group Environment Questionnaire.* London, Ontario.

Woodman T., & Hardy L. (2003). The relative impact of cognitive anxiety and self-confidence upon sport performance. A meta-analysis. *Journal of Sports Science, 21,* 443–457. https://doi.org/10.1080/0264041031000101809.

Wrisberg, C. A., & Draper, M. V. (1988). Sex, sex role orientation, and the cohesion of intercollegiate basketball teams. *Journal of Sport Behavior, 11,* 45–54.

14 The changing nature of lesbian athletes coming out in competitive organised team sports

Rachael Bullingham

Introduction

The stories of athletes 'coming out' as lesbian, gay, or bisexual differ significantly throughout research depending on the cultural epoch in which the research was conducted (Anderson & Bullingham, 2015; Anderson, Magrath, & Bullingham, 2016; Griffin, 1998). Using Griffin's taxonomy of climates, this chapter tracks the transition from the hostile climates of the 1980s, through conditional tolerance, to the open and inclusive zeitgeist of today in many Western contexts. Previously, only athletes who were integral to their team's success had been able to come out in climates of conditional tolerance (Anderson, 2002; Anderson & Bullingham, 2015). Athletes (both male and female) at a recreational level are increasingly able to come out regardless of their place on the team (Anderson et al., 2016). In fact, it could be argued now that it is psychologically beneficial to come out rather than remaining closeted (Anderson et al., 2016). The potential reason for this change is that the lesbian label is being negated in today's more inclusive sporting environment.

Lesbian athletes were significantly researched in the 1990s (Cahn, 1994; Griffin, 1998; Hekma, 1998; Lenskyj, 1991). Griffin (1998) acknowledged that three climates exist for lesbian athletes: hostile, conditionally tolerant, and open and inclusive – with hostility being evident in the 1980s and 1990s. A product of their culture, the authors of these investigations may have used their research as a warning to other athletes thinking of coming out of the closet. As a result, lesbian athletes frequently use silence as a form of protection in hostile sporting environments. Silence regarding their sexual orientation serves as a means of surviving constant hostility (Elling, De Knop, & Knoppers, 2003; Griffin, 1998; Krane & Barber, 2005). Yet, silence carries social-emotional implications as well. Silence is a form of oppression that is faced by lesbian women and its impact can be exceptionally damaging (Cahn, 1994). Nonetheless, lesbian athletes, participating within the male-dominated world of sport, often maintain that it is safer to stay silent than to disclose their sexual identity (Lenskyj, 2003).

Aim of the chapter

The aim of the chapter is as follows:

1   To examine the coming out process of lesbian athletes through different climates of homophobia. By exploring the taxonomy of Griffin's climates (1998), it is possible to note the positive changes for lesbian athletes and their ability to come out.

Climates within a sporting environment

Griffin's (1998) taxonomy of climates for lesbian athletes (from hostile, through conditionally tolerant, to open and inclusive) can help analyse not only if lesbian athletes are able to come out, but also how they do so. Griffin (1998) denotes the hostile climate as one in which lesbian participation in sport is not just disapproved of, but completely forbidden. However, the hostility goes beyond simple secrecy surrounding lesbianism, but one where lesbians are actually blamed for issues within sport (Griffin, 1998), which creates problems for all women, as both homophobic and sexist attitudes are left unchallenged (Drury, 2011). Within a hostile environment in sport, lesbian women may fear coming out and, therefore, lesbian athletes keep their identity secret, ensuring that they 'maintain deep cover at all times' (Griffin, 1998, p. 253). It is in hostile environments that lesbian women use silence as a survival strategy (Elling et al., 2003; Lenskyj, 2003).

A hostile environment can be defined as any climate where athletes must resort to survival strategies such as silence, denial, or the projection of a feminised image in order to dismiss or minimise the lesbian label (Griffin, 1998). Research on specific sports shows particularly hostile individual environments. For example, some football (soccer) environments have been found to be highly homophobic where lesbians have experienced challenges with expressing their sexuality (Mennesson & Clément, 2003). Additionally, the Australian cricket environment in the 1990s has also been described as hostile to lesbians (Burroughs, Ashburn, & SeeBohm, 1995). Likewise, in the American collegiate sport system, two of 12 athletes interviewed by Anderson and Bullingham (2015) in their recent research reported homophobic language being used by players on their team.

While lesbian athletes are expected to remain in the closet in hostile climates, in conditionally tolerant climates, the closet becomes transparent (Griffin, 1998). Within a conditionally tolerant climate, the closet still exists but is made of glass instead, where lesbians 'keep their identities "secret" but everyone knows who they are' (Griffin, 1998, p. 100). Plymire and Forman (2001) acknowledge that in order to ensure media coverage and continued spectatorship, those involved in women's sport need to maintain clear boundaries confined within heterosexuality. Additionally, within sporting organisations, employees demonstrate conformity towards the norm of heterosexuality, therefore silencing the lesbian issue (Melton & Cunning-ham, 2014).

Within a conditionally tolerant climate, the issue is not lesbian participa-tion but rather their visibility within sport; lesbians are allowed to parti-cipate providing they subscribe to a set of rules (Griffin, 1998). This environment has more recently been described as 'don't ask, don't tell' (Anderson, 2002; Anderson & Bullingham, 2015), a policy implemented until recently within the US military. Within a 'don't ask, don't tell' policy, athletes may temporarily emerge from the closet to reveal their sexual iden-tity, but after the revelation, normal play is resumed, with teammates ignor-ing the incident. Krane and Barber (2005) have also discovered this climate within US sports coaching environments.

In Anderson's (2002) first study of openly gay male athletes, he found that teams readily implemented 'don't ask, don't tell' policies. Of note within his study, gay male athletes remained oblivious to this environment, even defending its existence. Anderson (2002) discovered that this policy of 'don't ask, don't tell' was practised between homosexual and heterosexual players, but also *between* two homosexual athletes. Homosexual athletes themselves helped to reinforce this climate, also having to remain within the glass closet, as nobody would talk about their sexuality post revelation. Similar findings are outlined in Anderson and Bullingham's (2015) study of openly lesbian athletes. Again, athletes defended a 'don't ask, don't tell' policy, claiming that sport was not the right forum for a discussion on sexu-ality. Within a conditionally tolerant environment, lesbian athletes have to conform to a set of rules, which include silence surrounding their sexuality (Anderson & Bullingham, 2015).

Interestingly, Anderson (2002) found that gay male athletes were only con-doned by the team if they conformed to a winning mentality and if the team were successful. Anderson (2005, p. 23) describes how 'masculine capital' aids the reception of the athletes who come out. He defines the masculine capital dynamic as: '... the more a male adheres to these traits the more he raises his masculine capital – his worth among other boys and men'. Anderson dis-covered in both his research of 2002 and 2005 that the more valuable the gay male player is to the team's success, the more likely it is that he will be accepted. Indeed, there was a distinct pattern between the athlete's importance to the team and how well they were received when they came out as gay (Anderson, 2002). Athletic ranking – otherwise known as athletic capital – relates to how integral a player is to the success of the team. Anderson (2002) found that 22 of the 26 openly gay male athletes he interviewed had high ath-letic capital. Thus, athletic capital may influence the decision to come out, especially within conditionally tolerant climates. Anderson (2002) also found in his initial study that athletes expected to face homophobia when they came out, either in the form of abuse or deselection from the team.

Since 2002, Anderson has updated his research on athletic capital. In 2011, Anderson found that athletes who came out did *not* expect to face any homophobia from teammates. Perhaps most interestingly, in his follow-up study Anderson (2011b) found that athletic capital had been nullified, when it was no longer only the top athletes coming out, but fringe members of the team were also disclosing their sexuality. Research on female athletes' capital is limited, but Anderson and Bullingham (2015) found that all of the lesbians they interviewed were valuable to the team, with seven even labelling themselves the most valuable player. This research demonstrates that the possession of predisclosure, high athletic capital influences the decision to come out. Therefore, high athletic capital is also a currency and coping mechanism adopted by lesbian athletes to gain acceptance within a team.

Griffin's final category is an environment described as open and inclusive. This environment was viewed by Hargreaves (2000) as a distant dream for lesbian athletes in the 1990s. Where an open environment has been achieved, lesbian women have been able to express their identity freely, with some even using the sporting environment as a safe zone. Because of the high representation of lesbians within sport (Lenskyj, 2003), athletes have found mutually supportive lesbian communities within teams (Cahn, 1994; Griffin, 1998). However, this support mechanism only exists where athletes are 'out'. Griffin (1998) shows how high-profile lesbian athletes influence values and help educate others. Likewise, Melton and Cunningham (2014) note that when sportsmen and women come out, they create an opportunity to challenge preconceived ideas concerning human sexuality.

Some inclusive environments were uncovered by Fink, Burton, Farrell, and Parker (2012) in their study of the US collegiate system. Likewise, Hardy (2015) found a positive environment for female rugby players in Canada. Anderson, Magrath, and Bullingham (2016) showed that open and inclusive environments have also been found in women's recreational sport in the UK. Additionally, some improvements have been demonstrated within elite sport in general, but there is a need for further research in this area (Anderson, Magrath, & Bullingham, 2016).

Changing nature of coming out

Previous literature on athletes coming out has shown athletic capital to be important, not only in the athlete's initial decision to come out, but also on their acceptance within the team and sport (Anderson, 2002; Anderson & Bullingham, 2015). Essentially, the research demonstrates that the ethos of winning enables high quality and important homosexual players to gain acceptance, as they are essential to the success of the team, whereas those who are fringe players are rarely tolerated, as they lack importance to the team's success (Anderson, 2002, 2011; Anderson & Bullingham, 2015). Anderson's results show that, as cultural homophobia continues to decrease, the correlation between athletes' abilities and their acceptance has diminished in men's sport (Anderson, 2011a). However, lesbian athletes have historically shared different experiences to those of gay athletes; lesbian athletes often find a supportive community among other closeted athletes within their sport (Griffin, 1998).

A 'coming out' story, male or female, used to be a significant event; athletes came out by wearing gay pride jewellery or making statements, like shouting out in the middle of a movie (Anderson, 2002; Anderson & Bullingham, 2015). Regardless of the circumstances, it was clearly an event that athletes could vividly recall. However, since the 1990s, there has been a significant cultural shift in terms of decreasing homophobia (Clements & Field, 2014). This decline has been linked to increased access to the internet, increased visibility of gay athletes and celebrities, and more athletes choosing to come out, which have led to a more open and inclusive environment (Anderson, 2011a).

In Anderson's initial study on gay male athletes (2002), he found that some athletes remained closeted owing to the homophobia demonstrated by their teammates. Women, in the meantime, faced the 'lesbian' label. Such fears not only secured the closet doors, they also saw female athletes idealise and assume feminine characteristics, in order to distance themselves from lesbian suspicion (Blinde & Taub, 1992; Griffin, 1998; Lenskyj, 2003; Wright & Clarke, 1999). In this way, labels have historically been used as a political tool for controlling female athletes (Griffin, 1998). Cahn (1994) describes how numerous participants refused to subscribe to either the 'gay' or 'lesbian' label. Instead, they hid their relationships by suggesting they had a 'roommate' – a process described as survival strategy (Cahn, 1994). However, the more recent dismissal of binary labels has changed matters. As Better (2014, p. 32) explains, 'Sexuality for women today is fluid and evolving'. Correspondingly, athletes may define their sexuality in a number of different ways, not necessarily ascribing to the lesbian label.

Griffin notes that open female athletes are 'out and proud' (1998, p. 152), wearing symbols of their sexual identity, while at the same time actively advocating their position in teams and society. However, with more people publicly owning their sexual identity, combined with decreasing cultural homophobia, it may be that coming out has become a non-event – perhaps even normalised. Athletes can now come out quietly, without the need to make a big political statement (Anderson, Magrath, & Bullingham, 2016). In fact, research has shown that some lesbian athletes did not even know when, or indeed how, their teammates found out they were gay, as their coming out was deemed insignificant, with no party or preplanning required (Anderson, Magrath, & Bullingham, 2016).

Research on lesbian athletes competing in team sports has previously shown high levels of homophobia from teammates, coaches, and administration (Anderson & Bullingham, 2015; Fink et al., 2012; Griffin, 1998). More recent research in this domain has mirrored findings from men's team sports, indicating decreasing levels of homophobia (Anderson, Magrath, & Bullingham, 2016); this has, in turn, resulted in increasing numbers of female athletes coming out of the closet. In addition, the value of athletic capital in acceptance of lesbian athletes has also diminished. Previously, athletes who came out were shown to be more accepted where they had a tangible benefit on the team's success (Anderson, 2002; Anderson & Bullingham, 2015). However, research in recreational sport has found that athletic capital has ceased to be a factor in coming out among both gay and lesbian athletes (Anderson, Magrath, & Bullingham, 2016).

Athletic capital had previously been shown to be important for both gay and lesbian athletes coming out within a sporting environment (Anderson, 2002; Anderson & Bullingham, 2015). Although Anderson's (2011a) updated study demonstrates a significant decline in the importance of athletic capital for men, it was nevertheless still evident. It could be argued that athletic capital will always remain essential for those competing at the highest level of sport; within elite sport, performance is ascribed a higher value, since sporting success is the most important outcome. But, this does not mean that high athletic capital is required to come out in highly-supportive environments within recreational environments (Anderson, Magrath, & Bullingham, 2016). However, it should be noted that 17 openly lesbian women competed in the semi-finals of the 2015 FIFA Women's World Cup. Additionally, Outsports has noted that, while there were 23 out athletes (both men and women) at London 2012, there were 56 at the Rio Olympics in 2016, showing continued improvement in the climates of both male and female athletes.

Research has shown that athletes are no longer afraid to come out; therefore, it can be proposed that the lesbian label has lost its damaging and pejorative association (Anderson, Magrath, & Bullingham, 2016). This change could be due to women's increasing sexual fluidity (as identified by Better, 2014). It could also be argued that the negative impact of the lesbian label has dissipated. For example, if athletes no longer conceptualise sexuality in its binary form of heterosexuality and homosexuality, supporting recent research findings (e.g., Better, 2014), then sexuality can be considered more fluid. The fluidity of sexuality expressed and presented by the women in this study mirrors findings from the more abundant research on male athletes (Anderson & Adams, 2011) and their increasing willingness to describe themselves as something beyond the hetero-/homosexual binary.

Practical recommendations

In 1998 Griffin wrote about the 'unplayable lies' needed to be overcome to allow women to compete in sport. She also provided strategies to support sport changing. She outlined the key factors that needed to be implemented: education, information, legislation, institutionalisation, connection, agitation, and visibility. A number of Griffin's suggestions were evident in a recent British government report (Culture, Media and Sport Committee, 2017). This report noted the importance of the visibility of the lesbian, gay, bisexual, and transsexual (LGBT) community through initiatives such as the *Rainbow Lace Campaign* – a way for everyone involved in sport to show their support for LGBT equality and inclusivity. Additionally, the significance of education is acknowledged as essential in terms of training, advice, and support from grassroots to national level sport (Culture, Media and Sport Committee, 2017). Finally, there is an urgent need for more research at all levels of competitive team sport as well as for the individual exercising female to ensure we continue to understand how best to support this population in the sporting environment.

Real-world examples

Although research has shown significant improvements within male sporting culture, women's sport is more complex, since women who play sport challenge gender norms and, therefore, often face both sexism and homosexual suspicion through participation (Griffin, 1998; Lenskyj, 1995). The number of high-profile men coming out has not impacted on the level of homophobia in women's sport at any point (Griffin, 2012). In the 1980s, both Martina Navratilova and Billie Jean King (both retired professional tennis players) were outed (the sexuality was revealed by someone else). As a result, they promptly lost sponsorship and gained negative media coverage (Forman & Plymire, 2005; Hargreaves, 2000). Since coming out in 1999, Amélie Mauresmo (retired professional tennis player) received negative coverage from her fellow players and came under intense scrutiny from all sections of society (Forman & Plymire, 2005; Tredway, 2014). Prior to coming out, the situation was no better; Hargreaves (2000) describes how Mauresmo regularly faced derogatory remarks with constant inferences that she was a lesbian. Indeed, a media analysis by Forman and Plymire (2005) showed evidence of her muscular body causing alarm and even panic. They concluded that, rather than being portrayed as a 'lesbian hero', Mauresmo appears to be more of an 'underdog hero' (Forman & Plymire, 2005, p. 121). The underdog hero is described as 'someone to root for' who might achieve against all the odds (Forman & Plymire, 2005, p. 130).

Despite negative media coverage and disparaging remarks from fellow professionals, such as Martina Hingis (who attracted negative crowd reactions as a result; see Krane & Barber, 2003), Mauresmo continued to be sponsored by Nike, Inc., amassing career earnings of around US$7,000,000 (Forman & Plymire, 2005). In fact, rather than covering up Mauresmo's body, her clothing sponsors, Nike, Inc., actively encouraged her to reveal her muscular physique and designed clothing specifically to expose her athletic build (Forman & Plymire, 2005). This change in approach caused Tredway (2014) to re-examine the heterosexual matrix with its failure to acknowledge openly lesbian athletes. However, her adaptation fails to account for openly lesbian athletes who do not acknowledge their muscularity. As Tredway (2014, p. 175) explains: 'Once we know that a woman is a lesbian, we are prepared, even eager, to reread her physique in masculine terms, presumably because lesbians are socially coded as masculine'. However, athletes who have come out in more recent times do not always fit this notion of masculine social coding.

Sheryl Swoopes, who was the first player to be signed to the Women's National Basketball Association (WNBA) in America, can be considered one of the most prominent female athletes, having won the most valuable player award on three occasions and featuring in the Hall of Fame. She came out in a magazine article in 2005 while at the height of her career in the WNBA (Chawansky & Francombe, 2011). In order to prevent any potential damage to her career earnings, Swoopes signed a sponsorship deal with a holiday company aimed at the lesbian travel market (Chawansky & Francombe, 2011). The timing of her coming out demonstrates awareness of previous negative experiences faced by lesbian athletes. As Anderson (2002) discusses, the most valuable player status on a team helps with acceptance of (homo) sexuality. Swoopes was not only the most important person on the team, but the most valuable player in the entire league. This high athletic capital guaranteed her place on the team, and she also had the foresight to organise additional endorsements prior to coming out. In fact, she cited this contract with the lesbian travel firm as an influential factor in facilitating her coming out of the closet (Chawansky & Francombe, 2011). Swoopes' career hit a low in 2009 when she was not offered a new WNBA contract. After a short break from the sport, she returned in 2011 (Ogden & Rose, 2013). In the two years out of the sport, she has seemingly split with her female partner and become engaged to a man (Ogden & Rose, 2013). This was a significant development, since she had originally come out as a lesbian and not bisexual. This example could link to the argument of Better (2014), who acknowledges the complexity of the categories of sexuality, particularly in its binary form, and notes changing sexual fluidity of women.

In England in 2013, field hockey players, Kate Walsh and Helen Richardson announced they were getting married to very little press coverage, despite both players competing for the same domestic and international team – a unique media angle, which has yet to be analysed by an academic peer-reviewed journal. An article on the BBC Sport website noted how understated the event: '... sparked little coverage beyond congratulations. There was no discussion – the players said none was needed' (Williams, 2014). This was despite Kate Walsh previously having been in a relationship with Brett Garrard (England and Team GB's most capped male hockey player), with their relationship being described as 'The Posh and Becks' of hockey (Harris, 2013). Walsh and Richardson received an overwhelming positive reaction to their civil partnership, but still found it difficult initially to make the relationship public (Harris, 2013). Interestingly, Helen Richardson-Walsh's exclusion from the World Cup and Commonwealth Games in 2014 and then subsequent inclusion for the World League semi-final appeared to spark more media interest then the Richardson–Walsh civil partnership (Archer, 2015; Wilson, 2014).

Casey Stoney, a retired footballer who represented England, Team GB, and played league football, came out in 2014, announcing that she was in a relationship with another footballer. Since coming out, her partner has given birth to their three children – events that attracted significant media coverage. Stoney has openly acknowledged the positive reception she received as a result of coming out, but has also made public the anonymous abuse she received on Twitter (Steinberg, 2014). Interestingly, this invisibility is also indicative of an inclusive society, since so-called Twitter trolls tweet behind a cloak of anonymity, enabling them to challenge culturally declining homophobia without fear of personal repercussions. Her decision to come out was aided by the reception that British diver, Tom Daley, received when he came out. Indeed, Stoney was quick to acknowledge that Daley's experience helped her make the decision (McCloskey, 2014). Since coming out she continued to play for England before retiring and recently being appointed as the manager of Manchester United's women's team.

Summary

This chapter has examined the climates of homophobia that women engaged in competitive organised team sports have faced from the 1980s onwards. Using Griffin's (1998) climates as a framework, it has been possible to show the changes in climate from the hostility of the 1980s through to the more inclusive climate of today. Additionally, the changing nature of the process of coming out has been analysed. Previously, athletes needed high athletic capital to ensure acceptance in sporting contexts and, in many cases, coming out was making a statement. More recently, gay and lesbian athletes of all abilities have been able to safely come out in a climate that is open and inclusive. However, there is clearly a need for research and further work to be conducted with lesbian women competing at the elite level as well as those exercising females outside the competitive, organised, team sport arena.

References

Anderson, E. (2002). Openly gay athletes. Contesting hegemonic masculinity in a homophobic environment. *Gender & Society, 16,* 860–877. https://doi.org/10.1177/0891243202237892.

Anderson, E. (2005). *In the game: Gay athletes and the cult of masculinity*. Albany, NY: State University of New York Press.

Anderson, E. (2009). *Inclusive masculinity the changing nature of masculinities*. London: Routledge.

Anderson, E. (2011a). Updating the outcome: Gay athletes, straight teams and coming out at the end of the decade. *Gender & Society, 25,* 250–268. https://doi.org/10.1177/0891243210396872.

Anderson, E. (2011b). Masculinities and sexualities in sport and physical cultures: Three decades of evolving research. *Journal of Homosexuality, 58,* 565–578. https://doi.org/10.1080/00918369.2011.563652.

Anderson, E., & Adams, A. (2011). 'Aren't we all a little bisexual?': The recognition of bisexuality in an unlikely place. *Journal of Bisexuality, 11,* 3–22. https://doi.org/10.1080/15299716.2011.545283.

Anderson, E., & Bullingham, R. (2015). Openly lesbian team sport athletes in an era of decreasing homohysteria. *International Review for the Sociology of Sport, 50*, 647–660. https://doi.org/10.1177/1012690213490520.

Anderson, E., Magrath, R., & Bullingham, R. (2016). *Out in sport.* London: Routledge.

Archer, B. (2015, 9 June). Olympic dream masks the back pain for Helen Richardson-Walsh as GB head to Valencia. *Express* [Online] Retrieved from www.express.co.uk/sport/othersport/583248/Helen-Richardson-Walsh-interview-Great-Britain-women-s-hockey-team.

Better, A. (2014). Redefining queer: Women's relationships and identity in an age of sexual fluidity. *Sexuality & Culture, 18*, 16–38. https://doi.org/10.1007/s12119-013-9171-8.

Blinde, E. M., & Taub, D. E. (1992). Homophobia and women's sport: The disempowerment of athletes. *Sociological Focus, 25*, 151–166. https://doi.org/10.1080/00380237.1992.10570613.

Burroughs, A., Ashburn, L., & SeeBohm, L. (1995). 'Add sex and stir'. Homophobic coverage of women's cricket in Australia. *Journal of Sport and Social Issues, 19*, 266–286. https://doi.org/10.1177/019372395019003004.

Cahn, S. (1994). *Coming on strong: Gender and sexuality in Twentieth-Century women's sport.* Cambridge, Massachusetts: Harvard University Press.

Chawansky, M., & Francombe, J. M. (2011). Cruising for Olivia: Lesbian celebrity and the cultural politics and coming out in sport. *Sociology of Sport Journal, 28*, 461–477. https://doi.org/10.1123/ssj.28.4.461.

Clements, B., & Fields, C. D. (2014). Public opinion toward homosexuality and gay rights in Britain. *Public Opinion Quarterly, 78*, 523–547. https://doi.org/10.1093/poq/nfu018.

Culture, Media and Sport Committee. (2017, 7 February). *Homophobia in sport.* Retrieved from https://publications.parliament.uk/pa/cm201617/cmselect/cmcumeds/113/113.pdf.

Drury, S. (2011). 'It seems really inclusive in some ways, but … inclusive just for people who identify as lesbian': Discourses of gender and sexuality in a lesbian-identified football club. *Soccer & Society, 12*, 421–442. https://doi.org/10.1080/14660970.2011.568108.

Elling, A., De Knop, P., & Knoppers, K. (2003). Gay/lesbian sport clubs and events. Places of homo-social bonding and cultural resistance? *International Review for the Sociology of Sport, 38*, 441–456. https://doi.org/10.1177/1012690203384005.

Fink, J. S., Burton, L. J., Farrell, A. O., & Parker, H. M. (2012). Playing it out: Female intercollegiate athletes' experiences in revealing their sexual identities. *Journal for the Study of Sports and Athletes in Education, 6*, 83–106. https://doi.org/10.1179/ssa.2012.6.1.83.

Forman, P. J., & Plymire, D. C. (2005). Amélie Mauresmo's muscles: The lesbian heroic and women's professional tennis. *Women's Studies Quarterly, 33*, 120–133.

Griffin, P. (1998). *Strong women, deep closets.* Leeds: Human Kinetics.

Griffin, P. (2012). LGBT equality in sports: Celebrating our successes and facing our challenges. In G. B. Cunningham (Ed.), *Sexual orientation and gender identity in sport: Essays from activists, coaches, and scholars* (pp. 1–13). Texas: The Center for Sport Management Research and Education.

Hardy, E. (2014) The female 'apologetic' behaviour within Canadian women's rugby: Athlete perceptions and media influences. *Sport in Society, 18*, 155–167. https://doi.org/10.1080/17430437.2013.854515.

Hargreaves, J. A. (2000). *Heroines of sport*. London: Routledge.

Harris, C. (2013, Dec 4). Partners make name for themselves. *The Times*. Retrieved from www.thetimes.co.uk/article/hockey-partners-make-name-for-themselves-bqmgs 3025x8.

Hekma, G. (1998). 'As long as they don't make an issue of it…': Gay men and lesbians in organized sports in the Netherlands. *Journal of Homosexuality, 35*, 1–23. https://doi.org/10.1300/J082v35n01_01.

Krane, V., & Barber, H. (2005). Identity tensions in lesbian intercollegiate coaches. *Research Quarterly for Exercise and Sport, 76*, 67–81. https://doi.org/10.1080/02701 367.2005 10599263.

Lenskyj, H. J. (1991). Combating homophobia in sport and physical education. *Sociology of Sport Journal, 8*, 61–69. https://doi.org/10.1123/ssj.8.1.61.

Lenskyj, H. J. (1995). Sport and the threat to gender boundaries. *Sporting Traditions, 12*, 47–60.

Lenskyj, H. J. (2003). *Out on the field*. Toronto: Women's Press.

McCloskey, J. (2014, 11 February). England women's football player Casey Stoney comes out as lesbian. *Daily Star* [Online] Retrieved from www.dailystar.co.uk/news/latest-news/364907/England-women-s-football-player-Casey-Stoney-comes-out-as-lesbian.

Melton, N. E., & Cunningham, G. B. (2014). Examining the workplace experiences of sport employees who are LGBT: A social categorization theory perspective. *Journal of Sport Management, 28*, 21–33. https://doi.org/10.1123/jsm.2011-0157.

Mennesson, C., & Clément, J-P. (2003). Homosociability and homosexuality: The case of soccer played by women. *International Review for the Sociology of Sport, 38*, 311–330. https://doi.org/10.1177/10126902030383004.

Ogden, D. C., & Rose, J. N. (2013). *A locker room of her own: Celebrity, sexuality and female athletes*. Jackson: University Press of Mississippi.

Outsports. (2016, 11 July). *A record 56 out LGBT athletes compete at Rio Olympics*. Retrieved from www.outsports.com/2016/7/11/12133594/rio-olympics-teams-2016-gay-lgbt-athletes-record.

Plymire, D. C., & Forman, P. J. (2001). Speaking of Cheryl Miller: Interrogating the lesbian taboo on a women's basketball newsgroup. *NWSA Journal, 12*, 1–21. https://doi.org/10.1353/nwsa.2001.0020.

Steinberg, J. (2014, Oct 11). Football: Saturday interview: Casey Stoney: 'The positives far outweigh the negatives. Being gay isn't a choice … I'm still the same person': The Arsenal player believes revealing her sexuality has helped to change lives. *Guardian (London, England)*. Retrieved from www.theguardian.com/football/2014/oct/10/casey-stoney-positives-gay-arsenal-england.

Tredway, K. (2014). Judith Butler redux – the heterosexual matrix and the out lesbian athlete: Amélie Mauresmo, gender performance, and women's professional tennis. *Journal of the Philosophy of Sport, 41*, 163–176. https://doi.org/10.1080/009 48705.2013.785420.

Williams, O. (2014, 21 May). England's Kate Richardson-Walsh on marrying her team-mate. Retrieved from www.bbc.co.uk/sport/hockey/27491319.

Wilson, G (2014, 19 May). Helen Richardson-Walsh breaks silence over world cup snub. *Express* [Online]. Retrieved from www.express.co.uk/sport/other-sport/475881/Helen-Richardson-Walsh-breaks-silence-over-World-Cup-snub.

Wright, J., & Clarke, G. (1999). Sport, the media and construction of compulsory heterosexuality. *International Review for the Sociology of Sport, 34*, 227–248. https://doi.org/10.1177/101269099034003001.

15 Pregnancy and the exercising female

Robin Pickering

Introduction

Until somewhat recently, pregnancy has been perceived by many professionals and laypeople as a time of 'rest'. Indeed, prenatal exercise was seen as a danger to both the mother and the unborn foetus. Many myths exist regarding the impact of exercise on maternal and foetal outcomes. As more data regarding exercise efficacy in pregnancy emerges, most find that if used appropriately and occasionally with accommodation, maternal exercise during the prenatal and postnatal period can be a very important key to lifelong health and fitness in women. Although there are global differences in recommendations for physical activity, sport, and exercise during the prenatal period, several helpful guidelines exist to aid health professionals. In order to appropriately facilitate ideal levels of health and fitness during the prenatal period, it is important to understand the anatomical and physiological changes of pregnancy, exercise guidelines and contraindications for sport and exercise, and prenatal weight management recommendations. This chapter outlines those areas to assist in the facilitation supporting improved health in mothers and infants.

Aims of the chapter

The aims of the chapter are as follows:

1 To discuss the anatomical and physiological changes that occur during pregnancy.
2 To describe the risks and contraindications of sport and exercise during the prenatal period.
3 To describe appropriate guidelines for weight gain during pregnancy relative to pre-pregnancy body mass index (BMI).
4 To describe evidence-based recommendations for exercise and sport during the prenatal and postnatal periods.

A consideration of the current evidence base

Anatomy and physiology of pregnancy

Pregnancy has a profound impact on many body systems, which can impact a woman's ability to perform physical exercise at the same level as before pregnancy. Some of the key system changes are described in the following sections.

Endocrine system

Several hormones are necessary to create ideal circumstances for both implantation of the fertilised egg and pregnancy maintenance. Levels of these hormones vary throughout the prenatal and postnatal periods. The increased production of the hormones can cause profound body changes that can impact a woman's approach to exercise. The roles of key hormones produced during pregnancy are described on pp. 199–200.

Oestrogen

Oestrogen is released from the corpus luteum in the first trimester, and then from the placenta. One of the important functions of oestrogen during pregnancy is to stimulate breast growth and the growth of duct cells within the breast. Additionally, the hormone stimulates the secretion of prolactin, which promotes breast growth and milk production. Oestrogen prepares the body for the delivery of the infant by stimulating the growth of the myometrium, which allows for the forceful contractions necessary for delivery of the foetus as well as the placenta. Oestrogen also increases the body's responsiveness to oxytocin during labour – the hormone that stimulates contractions. Also, during this birthing preparation, oestrogen helps prostaglandin synthesis, which is responsible for the ripening of the cervix, allowing it to soften and dilate, and aids in the myometrial contractions.

Progesterone

Progesterone is released from the corpus luteum in the first trimester, and then from the placenta. One of the important roles of this hormone is to prevent contractions by promoting relaxation of the myometrium. Along with oestrogen, progesterone suppresses the release of the follicle-stimulating hormone and the luteinising hormone. Progesterone aids in the formation of the maternal portion of the placenta. In preparation for lactation, it also stimulates breast growth and milk-producing cells in the glands of the breast.

Relaxin

Though additionally synthesised by other reproductive organs, the hormone relaxin is primarily produced by the corpus luteum during pregnancy. Relaxin works to promote the anatomical changes necessary to prepare the body for pregnancy and the birthing process. During pregnancy, the hormone stimulates uterine growth and vascularisation. Relaxin also aids in pregnancy and delivery by relaxing the pelvic girdle, increasing the mobility of joints, and facilitating the cervical ripening in preparation for labour.

Cardiovascular system

Cardiovascular changes during pregnancy occur as the metabolic demands of the mother and foetus increase. Some of these changes include changes in blood volume, blood composition, cardiac output, cardiac size and position, and venous distension. Blood volume increases throughout pregnancy and includes a plasma volume increase by about 40–50 per cent at its maximum (Rodger, Sheppard, Gándara, & Tinmouth, 2015). The plasma volume increases because there is a need for additional blood circulation between the mother and foetus as well as fluid for the placenta. There is also a smaller increase in red blood cells (RBCs), resulting in a decrease in haemoglobin concentration when measuring haematocrit – a test used to identify anaemia. The increase in RBCs is independent of the increased plasma volume. The increase is needed because more oxygen is required as the metabolic rate increases due to the work of the pregnancy.

Pregnancy necessitates a two- to three-fold increase in iron consumption (Soma-Pillay et al., 2016). Iron-deficiency anaemia happens when the mother does not have enough iron to make new RBCs to carry the iron on the haemoglobin. Poor diet, not enough iron sources, vomiting from morning sickness, or deficiencies of either folate or $B_{12,}$ both of which are needed to form the RBCs, are all possible causes. This decrease necessitates an increase in supplemental iron and folic acid, which are commonly prescribed during this period. Pregnant women are also at higher risk for being incorrectly diagnosed with iron-deficiency anaemia due to the changes in blood volume. The increase in the plasma volume can mask the increase in RBCs just as it does in sports anaemia – this is not a true diagnosis of the anaemia – rather a pseudo-anaemia. The third trimester of pregnancy poses the greatest risk for true anaemia because of the rapid growth of the foetus and the expanded blood volume and RBCs in the foetus. Up to one-third of pregnant women are anaemic, with the most common causes being iron and folate deficiency (Friel, n.d.).

The work of pregnancy – increased body weight, the growth process of the foetus, and the increased demand on the mother to supply everything to the foetus – causes adaptations in the circulatory system. Cardiac output is a measure of the work of the circulatory system and is measured by stroke volume multiplied by heart rate. The vascular system builds blood vessels for the foetus and the placenta. To support the blood volume needed to supply the necessary oxygen and fuel, and to remove metabolic by-products through this vascular system, the vessels must grow. Cardiac output increases slowly throughout the pregnancy by up to about 40 per cent in total (Soma-Pillay et al., 2016). Cardiac output is most influenced during pregnancy by the increase in stroke volume, and through minimal increases in heart rate.

The demand is gradual during the first trimester and increases more rapidly through the last two trimesters. This larger volume of blood and increased work of the heart to deliver it also results in increased left ventricular volume and a thicker muscular wall. These changes are similar to aerobic training in an athlete except that heart rate normally decreases with increased training. In pregnancy the changes are too great and too rapid to allow heart rate to decline. These conditions mean that the increased cardiac output is not solely a marker of training as it is in an athlete. Additionally, concentrations of blood-clotting factors change throughout pregnancy and for some time following, increasing the risk of venous thrombosis (Soma-Pillay et al., 2016).

During the second and third trimesters, the foetus and placenta are growing rapidly, and their weight can decrease venous return if the mother is lying supine (on her back) for any length of time. Venous return is decreased as pressure is exerted on the inferior vena cava, which will lead to decreased cardiac output. The decrease in blood pressure can be severe enough to cause the mother to lose consciousness. At the same time, blood flow to the placenta and foetus comes through the abdominal aorta, which can also be compressed when the mother is lying supine. Both of these conditions, caused by aortocaval compression, can negatively affect the foetus; thus, pregnant women in their second and third trimesters are discouraged from lying in the supine position during sleep or during exercise.

Respiratory system

The respiratory system is affected during pregnancy by both mechanical and hormonal factors. Mechanical changes occur due to the increasing size of the uterus, which results in upward displacement of the diaphragm. These changes result in a reduction of overall lung capacity and residual volume. Because of these changes, women may notice shortness of breath during exercise and exertion that was not noticed before pregnancy. Hormonal effects of pregnancy also contribute to changes in the respiratory system, largely due to the presence of progesterone and prostaglandin. Some of these changes include increased minute ventilation, lowering of the carbon dioxide threshold of the respiratory centre, and decreasing airway resistance, which facilitate a greater airflow during pregnancy.

Hormonal changes can cause swelling in the lining of the nose, oropharynx, larynx, and trachea. The results are noticed as nasal congestion and changes in the voice; some women may have a greater risk of upper respiratory tract infections throughout their pregnancy. In the second and third trimesters, the hormone relaxin is released to allow the pubic joint to open for the eventual delivery. The hormone is not specific to that area, so, as the uterus is growing and pushing up on the diaphragm, the ribs are expanded, and relaxin can relax the ligaments between the ribs as well. This means greater muscular work for breathing to compress the ribs.

Other notable changes

A number of other changes occur during pregnancy that can impact sport and exercise. Postural changes occur during pregnancy as a result of the compensatory adjustment due to the changing weight distribution. These changes are typically marked by exaggerated lordosis of the lower back, forward flexion of the neck, downward movement of the shoulders, and sacral posterior inclination (Soma-Pillay et al., 2016). Prolonged postural changes may lead to elongation and decreased tone of the abdominal muscles as well as back pain. Additionally, as body weight redistributes as a result of pregnancy, the forces on the joints change. When combined with the effects of joint laxity from relaxin, weight gain, and postural change, balance may be affected. It is important to keep this in mind when engaging in activity that requires rapid acceleration or sudden directional changes. Changes in the centre of mass, weight, and joint laxity can also contribute to difficulty with balance in the pregnant sport and exercise participant.

Weight management during pregnancy

Perhaps one of the most important impacts of exercise and sport participation throughout pregnancy is the facilitation of weight management. Excess maternal weight gain is associated with increased birth weight and foetal growth, and postpartum (postnatal) weight retention (Siega-Riz et al., 2009). Generally speaking, the placenta, amniotic fluid, and the foetus account for about a third of the weight gain acquired during pregnancy. Many confounders exist when attempting to define 'normal' foetal growth (Zhang, Merialdi, Platt, & Kramer, 2010). Generally speaking growth generally begins slowly in the first trimester, rapidly in the second, and slowly and steadily in the third. The other two-thirds is weight gain in the mother. The gain includes fluids that will go away after the baby is born, plus a proportion of body fat. Besides the amniotic fluid, the larger fluid volume includes the increased plasma volume in the mother.

Throughout pregnancy, maternal changes, insulin sensitivity, maternal hyperplasia, and hyperlipidaemia impact lipid metabolism, which result in greater lipogenesis. These stimulate increased maternal subcutaneous fat deposition that is necessary for a healthy pregnancy. Changes in lipid metabolism are necessary to ensure an adequate glucose supply for the developing foetus and increased triglyceride levels to assist with maternal energy requirements (Soma-Pillay et al., 2016). Fat also is deposited in the breast tissue in preparation for lactation. Maternal fat stores can typically return to pre-pregnancy levels with committed effort. An additional component impacting prenatal weight gain is change in lean body mass (LBM). The growing uterus and the increase in RBCs contribute to increased LBM. The rest of the increase in LBM is, in part, due to the weight increase and the work of the mother to carry increased body weight. Muscles can hypertrophy, and bones can become denser as a result of the increased workload requirements, which may contribute to postnatal weight retention.

Historically, guidelines for weight gain during pregnancy, and adherence to them, have varied considerably. In the first half of the 20th century, published studies started citing recommended weight gain in pregnancy. Early recommendations suggested gaining no more than 6.8 kg (15 pounds) during pregnancy (Gilmore, Klempel-Donchenko, & Redman, 2015). A variety of factors influence the more individualised, gestational weight gain recommendations as put forward by the American College of Obstetricians and Gynecologists (2013), including greater knowledge of the health impacts of weight gain during pregnancy, as well as specific recommendations for underweight, normal weight, overweight, and obese women. Generally speaking, the number of women who are overweight or obese when they get pregnant has increased, and the number of multiple births of twins or more, has also increased. All these conditions have to be considered when weight gain recommendations are made.

A second concern is associated with research that indicates that weight gain during pregnancy is a predictor of weight retention following pregnancy (S ega-Riz et al., 2009). Data suggest that the presence of obesity and excess weight gain increases a person's risk of developing certain cancers, diabetes, and other diseases (Garg, Maurer, Reed, & Selagamsetty, 2014). Maternal weight gain recommendations consider not only health outcomes during pregnancy, but also the long-term impact that may be associated with pregnancy weight gain. In addition, gestational diabetes is a precursor for developing type 2 diabetes later in life. With these health risks in mind, current guidelines set forth by the Institute of Medicine (2009) recommend that women gain between 5 and 18 kg (11 and 40 pounds) during pregnancy based on their BMI prior to the pregnancy; underweight women should gain weight on the upper end of the range (13–18 kg), normal weight women, 11–16 kg, overweight women, 7–11 kg, and obese women should gain weight on the lower end of the range (5–9 kg). There is lack of consensus regarding universal guidelines for weight gain during pregnancy (Scott et al., 2014). Additional global confounders impacting universal recommendations include the differences in maternal anthropometry that exist cross-culturally. For example, according to Ota and colleagues (2011), Asian women have statistically lower pre-pregnancy BMIs and less weight gain compared to other ethnicities, which may impact recommendations when compared with Western populations. It is also important to note that steady weight gain is important and should mostly take place during the second and third trimesters.

Obesity during pregnancy is unfortunately a common condition that can cause various complications for the mother and the baby, as well as contributing to increased health care costs. Research out of the United States indicates that obesity during pregnancy is associated with a change in the use of health care services, including an increase in use of inpatient and outpatient services, increased length of hospital stays for delivery, greater use of physician services, and decreased use of services by nurse practitioners and physician assistants during prenatal visits (Chu et al., 2008).

One of the key issues with excess weight gain during pregnancy is the increased risk of developing gestational diabetes. Gestational diabetes occurs during pregnancy and is marked by an inability of the body to process carbohydrates effectively, which increases glucose in the bloodstream. The mother is supposed to transition to fat metabolism, leaving the glucose for the foetus, but maternal glucose is used in the storage of fat joining with free-fatty acids to create triglycerides (TG). When the mother becomes insulin resistant she does not use the glucose for TG effectively, and the foetus is overwhelmed with extra glucose. The foetus secretes more insulin to handle the excess glucose, part of which becomes TG and excess fat storage in the foetus. The second concern is postdelivery when glucose is provided in the milk or formula in normal amounts, but there is still too much insulin, which can result in postdelivery hypoglycaemia in the infant.

Individuals with gestational diabetes are unable to produce enough insulin to accommodate the demands of the pregnancy or become insulin resistant. Women with the condition are more likely to deliver infants that are large for gestational age when the foetus creates TG from the excess glucose. Although gestational diabetes goes away upon delivery, women with gestational diabetes are at a significantly increased risk of developing type 2 diabetes later in life (Herath, Herath, & Wickremasinghe, 2017). Lifestyle modification, including a healthy diet, exercise, and weight management, can be effective in reducing the risk of developing gestational diabetes. Postnatal diabetes' testing is recommended for all women who are diagnosed with gestational diabetes.

Calorific management during pregnancy

Proper nutritional intake during pregnancy is one important component of proper foetal development and maternal health. The energy demand required for maintaining a pregnancy varies throughout each trimester. Calorific demands also increase if activity levels increase. Many misconceptions exist regarding calorific need during pregnancy, with many believing that it is important to literally 'eat for two'. More recent recommendations set forth in 2009 by the Institute of Medicine indicates that no additional calories are to be consumed during the first trimester, followed by an increase calorific intake by 340 kcal/day during the second trimester and 450 kcal/day during the third for a singleton pregnancy. Current Institute of Medicine (2009) guidelines suggest that women should also consider pre-pregnancy BMI when determining calorific consumption along with their suggested weight gain, with underweight women consuming more and overweight women consuming less. Women who move into a higher BMI category as a result of postpartum weight retention are at increased risk of complications during subsequent pregnancies, especially gestational diabetes, in addition to long-term maternal health complications.

Practical recommendations

Exercise guidelines during pregnancy

Though the health benefits of physical activity and exercise during pregnancy are well documented, there is some variance in global recommendations in terms of recommended type, frequency, duration, and intensity. A meta-analysis (Evenson et al., 2014) of research examining guidelines for physical activity during pregnancy throughout the world indicated the presence of the following justified contraindication to exercise during pregnancy: 'anaemia, persistent bleeding, cardiovascular disease, cerclage or incompetent cervix, multiple gestation, preeclampsia or pregnancy-induced hypertension, premature contractions or labour, premature rupture of membranes, and thyroid disease'. Other guidelines included the presence of diabetes mellitus, eating disorder, morbid obesity, and placenta previa as cause to avoid exercise during pregnancy.

The review of the literature additionally supports the recommendations that specific sport activities should be avoided during pregnancy, because they can compromise both maternal and foetal safety. One example of these contraindicated activities includes downhill snow skiing (and one might also assume other alpine activities like snowboarding). Maternal change in centre of mass can increase the risk of falling. Altitude sickness may also be a concern. Contact sports (e.g., hockey, basketball, handball, rugby, and football [soccer]) with high risk of falls can result in increased risk of foetal trauma. Scuba diving is contraindicated due to the risk of foetal decompression sickness, which results from changes in pressure surrounding the body.

Based on the previously discussed anatomical and physiological changes that occur during pregnancy, additional considerations should also be taken into account when exercising during pregnancy. Consistent recommendations include avoiding exercises in the supine position after the first trimester. Additionally, several recommendations include variances in guidelines for exercising at altitude. Most guidelines ranged from moderate exercise at altitudes up to 1800–2500 m as considered safe during pregnancy, with the caution that women should be aware of the signs of altitude sickness (Evenson et al., 2014). Current United Kingdom (UK) guidelines include risks associated with sedentary lifestyle. Other guidelines include advising against prolonged periods of motionless standing during pregnancy. Many guidelines specifically state that it is appropriate to avoid exercise in hot, humid weather or when a fever is present (Evenson et al., 2014). Other recommendations included in the literature suggest it is reasonable to suggest wearing comfortable clothing that will help maintain thermoregulation and wearing a bra during exercise that supports the breasts (see Chapter 12, for a review of breast health) and gives adequate protection. Another important recommendation for sport and exercise is to maintain adequate fluid balance and to consume adequate calorific intake consistent with activity levels (Evenson et al., 2014).

Mode of exercise

In addition to understanding when not to exercise, it is important to understand appropriate mode, duration, frequency, and progression of prenatal exercise in order to make appropriate prenatal recommendations. Recommendations surrounding engaging in vigorous exercise vary, and range from the Spanish guidelines stating that women should have no more than 15 min of vigorous activity and should decrease intensity by 20–30 per cent, to guidelines stating that women could continue to exercise vigorously throughout pregnancy as long it was tolerated well (Evenson et al., 2014).

Most international guidelines support participation in aerobic activities as an acceptable exercise modality. Weight training can also be an effective way to improve fitness during pregnancy, which is supported by guidelines from Australia, Canada, Denmark, Norway, and the UK. Though little research has been conducted examining weight training during pregnancy, a key concern that exists involves breath control during lifting heavy weights. Risk of performing the Valsalva manoeuvre increases while participating in heavy lifting. The manoeuvre occurs with moderately forceful attempted exhalation against a closed airway, which can result in rapid and unfavourable changes in heart and blood pressure. Holding one's breath is contraindicated during pregnancy. It is also important to consider balance and coordination changes that occur during pregnancy when selecting exercises to be performed. Consistent guidelines (either stated or implied) described in the literature review by Evenson and colleagues (2014) include the following as 'examples of exercises to do' during the prenatal period: cross-country skiing, Nordic walking, pelvic floor exercises, strengthening, stretching, swimming, running, stationary cycling, aerobic activities, walking, and water exercise such as swimming and yoga.

Intensity of exercise

Recommendations regarding intensity of exercise can vary considerably based on pre-pregnancy fitness levels. Some recommendations include maximum heart rate recommendations (both Japan's and Spain's guidelines include maximums of 150 and 140 beats/min, respectively) (Evenson et al., 2014). Guidelines from the UK advocate moderate-intensity exercise for women attempting to maintain pre-pregnancy fitness (Smith et al., 2018). In the United Sates, the American College of Sports Medicine (2009) guidelines for competitive athletes are consistent with those for maintaining and improving fitness of the non-pregnant population (60–90 per cent of maximal heart rate, or 50–85 per cent of either maximal oxygen uptake or heart rate reserve). The upper level may be appropriate for well-conditioned pregnant women. However, using heart rate to monitor exertion levels in pregnant women may be misleading. Resting heart rate tends to increase during pregnancy, which may make that method of monitoring exertion unreliable. In that case, according to the American College of Obstetrics and Gynecology (2002), using ratings of perceived exertion may be appropriate, with a 'moderate to hard' rating being acceptable.

Duration of exercise

Current guidelines in Canada indicate a minimum of 15-min sessions 3 times per week, progressing to 30 min, 4 times per week if intensity was reduced (Evenson et al., 2014). New guidelines in the UK suggest 150 min of exercise per week throughout pregnancy (Smith et al., 2018). Japanese recommendations include aerobic exercise up to 60 min, 2–3 times per week. The American College of Sports Medicine (ACSM) (2002) recommends that pregnant women who fall in the low-risk category are recommended to participate in physical activity for 30 min or more on most, if not all, days of the week. According to the ACSM, an athlete already doing more than 30 min prior to becoming pregnant does not need to reduce activity duration unless contraindications develop.

Exercise progression

According to the meta-analysis conducted by Evenson and colleagues (2014), most recommendations encourage women who were not exercisers prior to pregnancy to begin an exercise programme during pregnancy as long as they are healthy enough to exercise. Progression can begin with as little as 5 min of exercise per day, adding 5 min each week until the participant can maintain 30 consecutive minutes per day. Fitness levels and activity volume will likely gradually decline as the pregnancy progresses. Because of the weight gain, some fitness increase happens in all pregnant women with or without being active. The demands of the pregnancy prevent the woman from training at an ever-increasing intensity, especially in the third trimester. This means that someone already extremely fit prior to the pregnancy will probably not gain fitness, but any loss will be minimal and can be easily regained following the birth. A woman who had a very low fitness level, especially if overweight prior to becoming pregnant, and is starting a fitness programme might make some effective changes in body composition – gaining LBM and losing or not gaining additional fat mass – which might result in an increased fitness level at the end of the pregnancy, which may also make recovering from the pregnancy easier (Moyer, Reoyo, & May, 2016).

Real-world example

Stacy, an American college professor and first-time mother, reflects on the physical and emotional challenges of maintaining exercise during the final trimester of pregnancy.

> Pregnancy has been a very difficult experience. I feel more unfit now than I have in my entire life. With my growing belly, a lot of the high intensity activities I used to enjoy (running, calisthenics) are off of the table. It is also becoming increasingly difficult to do even low-impact activities like cycling, since I cannot bend over to reach the handle bars or move my legs fast enough to get my heart rate up on the elliptical. I have been using greater resistance, but I prefer to just walk around my neighbourhood or on hills if I am going that slow.
>
> The greatest challenge with all of these activities, however, is my body's response. In addition to finding clothes that allow me to move without being constricting, I am never really comfortable during my workouts. I have difficulty catching my breath, even with simple exercises like walking. I can get light headed when using light free weights, and I easily overheat during exercise (so much so, that I have had to step out of the shower or refrained from using the hair dryer because I couldn't get my body back to normal temperature).
>
> It is emotionally exhausting to put so much effort into wanting to be healthy and feeling your body making it more and more difficult to keep up the pace, to feel strong, and to feel comfortable in my own skin. I have left the gym after 10 min of working out because my motivation for being there plummeted after not feeling comfortable in my clothes. I have cried to my spin instructor that I have to modify everything she asks of us. I have laid on my back on the running trail after a run, coming to grips with that fact that I was probably done with running after a slow mile and a half jog. The only thing that keeps me motivated to maintain an active lifestyle at this point is to make my labour and postpartum recovery easier and faster.
>
> (S. Keogh-George, personal communication, 4 December 2017)

Summary

Exercise during the prenatal period is essential to maintaining ideal levels of health for both the mother and the unborn foetus. In order to appropriately facilitate this behaviour, it is important to understand the anatomy and physiology of pregnancy, as it can clarify the need for specific adaptations. Understanding weight management and exercise and sport guidelines for that period are essential for optimising safety and effectiveness of prenatal sport and exercise.

References

American College of Obstetricians and Gynecologists. (2013). ACOG Committee Opinion No. 548: Weight gain during pregnancy. *Obstetrics and Gynecology, 121*, 210–212. https://doi.org/10.1097/01.AOG.0000425668.87506.4c.

Chu, S. Y., Bachman, D. J., Callaghan, W. M., Whitlock, E. P., Dietz, P. M., Berg, C. J., ... Hornbrook, M. C. (2008). Association between obesity during pregnancy and increased use of health care. *The New England Journal of Medicine, 58*, 1444–1453. https://doi.org/10.1056/NEJMoa0706786.

Evenson, K. R., Barakat R., Brown W. J., Dargent-Molina, P., Haruna, M., Mikkelsen, E. M., ... Yeo, S. (2014). Guidelines for physical activity during pregnancy: Comparisons from around the world. *American Journal of Lifestyle Medicine, 8*, 102–121. https://doi.org/10.1177/1559827613498204.

Friel, L. A. (n.d.) Anemia in pregnancy [Merck Manual]. Retrieved from www.merckmanuals.com/professional/gynecology-and-obstetrics/pregnancy-complicated-by-disease/anemia-in-pregnancy.

Garg, S. K., Maurer, H., Reed, K., & Selagamsetty, R. (2014). Diabetes and cancer: Two diseases with obesity as a common risk factor. *Diabetes, Obesity & Metabolism, 16*, 97–110. https://doi.org/10.1111/dom.12124.

Gilmore, L. A., Klempel-Donchenko, M., & Redman, L. M. (2015). Pregnancy as a window to future health: Excessive gestational weight gain and obesity. *Seminars in Perinatology, 39*, 296–303. https://doi.org/10.1053/j.semperi.2015.05.009.

Herath, H., Herath, R., & Wickremasinghe, R. (2017). Gestational diabetes mellitus and risk of type 2 diabetes 10 years after the index pregnancy in Sri Lankan women – A community based retrospective cohort study. *PLoS ONE, 12*(6), e0179647. https://doi.org/10.1371/journal.pone.0179647.

Institute of Medicine. (2009). *Weight gain during pregnancy: Re-examining the guidelines*. Washington, DC: National Academies Press.

Moyer, C., Reoyo, O. R., & May, L. (2016). The influence of prenatal exercise on offspring health: A review. *Clinical Medicine Insights. Women's Health, 9*, 37–42. https://doi.org/10.4137/CMWH.S34670.

Ota, E., Haruna, M., Suzuki, M., Anh, D. D., Tho le, H., Tam, N. T., ... Yanai. H. (2011). Maternal body mass index and gestational weight gain and their association with perinatal outcomes in Vietnam. *Bulletin of the World Health Organization, 89*, 127–136. https://doi.org/10.2471/BLT.10.077982.

Rodger, M., Sheppard, D., Gándara, E., & Tinmouth, A. (2015). Haematological problems in obstetrics. Best Practice in Research. *Clinical Obstetrics & Gynecology, 29*, 671–684. https://doi.org/10.1016/j.bpobgyn.2015.02.004.

Scott, C., Andersen, C. T., Valdez, N., Mardones, F., Nohr, E. A., Poston, L., & Abrams, B. (2014). No global consensus: A cross-sectional survey of maternal weight policies. *BMC Pregnancy and Childbirth, 14*, 167. https://doi.org/10.1186/1471-2393-14-167.

Siega-Riz, A. M., Viswanathan, M., Moos, M.-K., Deierlein, A., Mumford, S., Knaack, J., … Lohr, K. N. (2009). A systematic review of outcomes of maternal weight gain according to the Institute of Medicine recommendations: Birth-weight, fetal growth, and postpartum weight retention. *American Journal of Obstetrics & Gynecology, 201*, 339.e1–339.e14. https://doi.org/10.1016/j.ajog.2009. 07.002.

Soma-Pillay, P., Catherine, N. -P., Tolppanen, H., Mebazaa, A., Tolppanen, H., & Mebazaa, A. (2016). Physiological changes in pregnancy. *Cardiovascular Journal of Africa, 27*, 89–94. https://doi.org/10.5830/CVJA-2016-021.

Smith, R., Reid, H., Matthews, A., Calderwood, C., Knight, M., & Foster, C. (2018). Infographic: Physical activity for pregnant women. *British Journal of Sports Medicine, 52*, 532–533. https://doi.org/10.1136/bjsports-2017-098037.

Zhang, J., Merialdi, M., Platt, L. D., & Kramer, M. S. (2010). Defining normal and abnormal fetal growth: Promises and challenges. *American Journal of Obstetrics & Gynecology, 202*, 522–528. http://doi.org/10.1016/j.ajog.2009.10.889.

16 Postnatal depression and the exercising female

Amanda J. Daley and Ruth V. Pritchett

Introduction

Many women experience depression after having a baby, which can have adverse consequences for the mother and detrimental effects on the well-being and development of the baby. In this chapter, we aim to summarise the evidence regarding the effectiveness of exercise as an intervention for postnatal (postpartum) depression (PND), and whether health professions can recommend exercise as a treatment. The chapter draws on evidence from both quantitative and qualitative research, although the focus is on findings from systematic reviews and meta-analyses of randomised controlled trials (RCTs), since these studies provide the best evidence on which to draw conclusions regarding effectiveness. The potential mechanisms of action for exercise on symptoms of PND are discussed, as are the practical implications for promoting exercise with this population of women.

Aims of the chapter

The aims of the chapter are as follows:

1   To describe the prevalence and symptoms of PND.
2   To provide a case for the role of exercise as a treatment for PND.
3   To summarise the evidence for the effects of exercise on the symptoms of PND.
4   To provide a summary of the potential mechanisms of action for exercise on the symptoms of PND.
5   To describe what women think and feel about exercise as a treatment for PND.
6   To debate the implications for health professionals promoting exercise with women experiencing PND.

Postnatal depression

PND (also known as postpartum depression), is a highly prevalent, global health concern, affecting 13 million women annually (World Health

Organization, 2005). Depression can affect mothers at any point in the post-natal period, with a peak incidence at six weeks after childbirth (Horowitz & Goodman, 2004); however the Diagnostic and Statistical Manual, 5th edition (DSM-5) does not differentiate PND from prenatal depression, providing the broader diagnosis of 'depressive disorder' with 'peripartum onset' (American Psychiatric Association, 2013). The psychological and psychomotor symptoms of PND vary in severity from mild to severe and are those of a major depressive episode, including continuous depressed mood, fatigue, diminished pleasure in activities, significant changes in weight and sleeping patterns, psychomotor agitation or retardation, feeling of worthlessness and excessive guilt, indecisiveness, and suicidal ideation, plans, or attempts (American Psychiatric Association, 2013). Some mothers will also experience thoughts of harming their child (Jennings, Ross, Popper, & Elmore, 1999), though in the vast majority of cases, no action is taken. Many mothers gradually recover; however, they are at an increased risk of depression later in life, particularly following subsequent pregnancies (Alasoom & Koura, 2014).

For many women, including the exercising female, the postnatal period brings substantial physical and psychological changes (Highet, Stevenson, Purtell, & Coo, 2014). Women have described feeling an altered or lost sense of personal identity (Pritchett et al., 2017). The contrast between a woman's expectations of motherhood and the reality of caring for an infant, breastfeeding, sleep deprivation, and changes in the relationship with a partner can cause frustration and self-doubt (Highet et al., 2014). PND can also affect the interaction between a mother and her baby, with some mothers responding less sensitively to their infant (Field, 2010). This altered interaction between depressed mothers and their children, as well as reported physiological differences in children's neurological development, may have a long-term impact on children's social and cognitive development (National Institute of Child Health and Human Development Early Child Care Research Network, 1999).

The aetiology of PND

The aetiology of PND is multifaceted. Among the strongest predictors of PND are depressive or anxiety symptoms during pregnancy (Abdollahi et al., 2014; Katon, Russo, & Gavin, 2014), a family history of depression, or a personal history of anxiety, depression or PND (Alasoom & Koura, 2014; Alfayumi-Zeadna, Kaufman-Shriqui, Zeadna, Lauden, & Shoham-Vardi, 2014). Researchers have revealed a range of psychosocial stressors associated with an increased risk of PND, such as: delayed perinatal care, poor infant health, and unwanted pregnancy (Abdollahi et al., 2014; Alasoom & Koura, 2014); marital or family conflict (Parsons, Young, Rochat, Kringelbach, & Stein, 2012); perceived social isolation (Parsons et al., 2012; Robertson, Grace, Wallington, & Stewart, 2004); and bereavement, abuse, addiction, work, and financial concerns (Katon et al., 2014).

A further facet of PND is thought to be the influence of chemical pathways in the body. A connection has been suggested between the substantial fluctuations in postnatal oestrogen and progesterone and the development of PND; however, a recent systematic review has concluded that empirical evidence does not support this association (Yim, Tanner Stapleton, Guardino, Hahn-Holbrook, & Dunkel Schetter, 2015). There is evidence to suggest that dysregulation in many of the body's chemical pathways, including thyroid hormone production, reactivity to stress, production of neurones, the immune system, and lower perinatal oxytocin levels may be related to depression (Yim et al., 2015).

Treatment

Guidelines from the National Institute for Health and Care Excellence (NICE, a clinical guideline body in England) for the treatment of depression in the postnatal period recommend a combination of facilitated self-help, psychological interventions such as cognitive behavioural therapy (CBT), and antidepressants (National Collaborating Centre for Mental Health, 2014). If a mother chooses to breastfeed, the neurodevelopmental risk associated with some antidepressants must be weighed up with the risks of untreated depression for both mother and child (National Collaborating Centre for Mental Health, 2014).

The case for exercise as a treatment for PND

There has been considerable interest in the effectiveness of exercise as a treatment for depression. While in England exercise is not explicitly recommended for the treatment of PND, NICE recommend that adults with persistent subthreshold depressive symptoms or mild-moderate depression should be advised of the benefits of participating in a structured group physical activity programme (National Institute for Health and Care Excellence, 2009). This chapter provides an up-to-date overview of systematic reviews on the question of whether exercise is an effective treatment for PND.

The first systematic review and meta-analysis of exercise as an intervention for PND was published in 2009 (Daley, Jolly, & MacArthur, 2009). This review of RCTs and quasi-RCTs reported that exercise significantly reduced symptoms of depression compared with no exercise comparator groups; however, the authors noted that there was significant heterogeneity and the analysis was based on five small trials that had randomised a total of only 221 women. The review also noted a number of methodological issues in the trials, the most concerning being that women who did not have a confirmed diagnosis of depression had been recruited.

Since the first systematic review by Daley and colleagues (2009), several more systematic reviews on this topic have been published, but space does not allow detailed discussion of these here (McCurdy, Boulé, Sivak, & Davenport, 2017; Poyatos-León et al., 2017; Saligheh, Hackett, Boyce, &

Cobley, 2017). The systematic review with the latest search dates (up to September 2016) was conducted by Pritchett, Daley, and Jolly (2017). The review included 13 RCTs that had evaluated aerobic exercise-based interventions in women who had given birth within 1 year of randomisation. Both general populations of postnatal women and depressed postnatal women were included in the trials. From this meta-analysis, it was shown that aerobic exercise significantly reduced depression scores. There were high levels of heterogeneity, however, and the authors stated that these results should, therefore, be interpreted cautiously. Subgroup analyses to compare the effects of aerobic exercise on depression scores in general populations of postnatal women (prevention) versus depressed postnatal women (treatment), different intervention types and exercise context were also conducted. Results for these analyses are listed in Table 16.1. In summary, exercise appeared to be equally effective for both the prevention and treatment of PND, and group-based exercise was also particularly effective, relative to non-group-based interventions, although these analyses were based on small sample sizes.

In terms of future research, relatively little is known about the ideal exercise type and context for this population of women, and research on these questions would be welcome (Pritchett et al., 2017). Studies that compare exercise 'head to head' with other treatments for PND are also important. Trials that recruit and offer an exercise intervention during pregnancy with follow-up prenatally and postnatally would also be worthwhile, as this would help to provide evidence about whether exercise could alleviate prenatal depression and prevent PND from occurring.

Table 16.1 Subgroup meta-analysis by population, intervention type, and exercise context

Category	SMD[1]	CI[2]	I[2][3] (%)	Number of trials	Number of participants
Depressed postnatal populations	−0.32	−0.63 to −0.00	55	7	416
General postnatal populations	−0.57	−1.12 to −0.02	92	6	891
Exercise-only interventions	−0.56	−1.13 to 0.01	89	8	528
Exercise co-interventions	−0.35	−0.66 to −0.04	72	5	779
Group exercise interventions	−1.10	−1.99 to −0.21	9	6	406
Participant choice exercise	−0.20	−0.33 to −0.06	0	7	901

Source: Pritchett, Daley, and Jolly, 2017.

Notes
1 SMD: standard mean difference.
2 CI: confidence intervals.
3 I^2: heterogeneity.

Postnatal depression and physical health

Depressive illness is strongly associated with physical health status; therefore the rationale for exercise may extend beyond the mental health benefits it provides for women experiencing PND (Bica, Castelló, Toussaint, & Monteso-Curtó, 2017). Moreover, exercise can provide benefits in terms of weight loss, which is a particular concern for many women after having a baby, and cardiovascular benefits, which may be beneficial given many women engage in more sedentary behaviour towards the end of pregnancy and postnatally (Albright, Maddock, & Nigg, 2005).

Mechanisms of action

Exercise may reduce depressive symptoms through biochemical, physiological, psychological, and psychosocial mechanisms, or pathways. Despite extensive research regarding the exercise and depression relationship, the mechanisms of action are not well understood. A brief overview of some of the more prominent explanations is provided here; it is possible that different mechanisms interact, and/or that more than one explanation is responsible for the effects of exercise on depression.

Biochemical and physiological explanations

Arguably the most well-known explanation for the effect of exercise on depression is the endorphin hypothesis (Steinberg & Sykes, 1985). This hypothesis proposes that participation in exercise is associated with the release of endogenous opiates, such as beta-endorphins, that consequently result in lower feelings of depression. Several researchers have reported increases in plasma endorphins after exercise (Bortz et al., 1981; Farrell, Gates, Maksud, & Morgan, 1982), but it remains unclear whether such changes reflect brain chemistry and are directly linked to reductions in depression. Similarly, the monoamine hypothesis (Pierce, Kupprat, & Harry, 1976) has suggested that exercise results in an increase in the availability of brain neurotransmitters (dopamine, serotonin, and noradrenaline) that are typically found to be reduced with depression. While studies involving animals have indicated that exercise increases levels of serotonin and noradrenaline in the brain (Dunn, Reigle, Youngstedt, Armstrong, & Dishman, 1996), this relationship remains unclear in humans.

Psychological hypothesis and explanations

Exercise can provide a different focus to life, whether through the activity itself or the surroundings in which it is undertaken (Pritchett et al., 2017). It has been suggested that exercise can serve as a type of distraction or a 'time out' strategy from every day worries and depressive feelings (Bahrke &

Morgan, 1978; Gleser & Mendelberg, 1990). Researchers have reported that exercise is associated with self-esteem and self-efficacy enhancement in a range of clinical and non-clinical populations (Fox, 2000; Taylor & Fox, 2005). It is possible, therefore, that exercise influences symptoms of depression via enhancement of self-esteem. People who are depressed often feel they lack control and feelings of mastery in and over their lives, and correspondingly, do not feel they have skills or resources to bring about change in their lives or how they are feeling (Denis & Luminet, 2017). Exercise may provide individuals with a sense of achievement, efficacy and self-determination in their recovery process. Exercise may be a form of behavioural activation, which is typically an important component of effective psychotherapy interventions for depression (Brosse, Sheets, Lett, & Blumenthal, 2002).

Social hypotheses and explanations

Evidence has demonstrated that social support is, in itself, an effective intervention for depression (Paykel & Cooper, 1992). Many types of exercise involve groups and interaction with others, and the connections experienced with others in such contexts may have benefits for mental health (Bailey & McLaren, 2005). This element of exercise could provide women with an opportunity for social integration and expansion of social networks (Stathi, Fox, & McKenna, 2002), rather than isolation (which can be common in people with depression). More specifically, exercise can provide valuable social interaction with other mothers who share experiences and thought processes (Doran & Hornibrook, 2013; Pritchett et al., 2017). In a small qualitative study, postnatal women in Australia (with and without PND) were interviewed about their experiences of participating in pram (stroller) walking groups (Watson, Milat, Thomas, & Currie, 2005). The main reasons women gave for enjoying pram walks were socialising, 'getting out the house' and developing new friendships for social support.

Real-world example

What do women think about exercise as treatment for postnatal depression?

Much of the information presented in this chapter so far has been generated by quantitative research studies; however, much can also be learned from qualitative research. A few researchers have explored the views and experiences of women, who are expecting a baby, or have young children, regarding exercise (Currie & Develin, 2002; Doran & Hornibrook, 2013). More specifically, a recent qualitative study, nested within an RCT of an exercise intervention for PND, explored women's experiences of the practicalities of postnatal exercise and their beliefs about exercise as a treatment for PND (Daley et al., 2015; Pritchett et al., 2017).

Research has found that many mothers have a positive view of exercise as a treatment for PND (Pritchett et al., 2017). In particular, depressed mothers have described their experiences of exercise as reducing the severity of their depression and improving the rapidity of their recovery (Pritchett et al., 2017): '… that's what kept me sane really, putting the children into the pushchair and just going, walking and walking' (female, 37 years, intervention).

In relation to other treatments for PND, a reluctance has been reported among postnatal women to taking antidepressants due to possible side effects, fears of dependency, previous negative personal or family experiences with their use, and the stigma attached to them (Turner, Sharp, Folkes, & Chew-Graham, 2008). In contrast, exercise, and the endorphins released, are often seen as natural and preferable to traditional pharmaceutical treatments (Battle, Salisbury, Schofield, & Ortiz-Hernandez, 2013; Pritchett et al., 2017). As reflected in research with depressed adults, however, postnatal women have also described exercise as a first step, providing short-term alleviation of low mood, while medication can provide 'constant cover' for the more severely depressed (Pritchett et al., 2017; Searle et al., 2011). Postnatal women have also reported a view that the optimum treatment for their depression involved a combination of exercise with medication or counselling (Pritchett et al., 2017).

One of the principal benefits reported by depressed exercising mothers is a feeling of increased energy (Cramp & Bray, 2010; Pritchett et al., 2017). Body image can also be of great importance to postnatal women, with weight loss and the accompanying improvements in self-esteem being reported to reduce low mood (Pritchett et al., 2017). Psychologically, exercise has been reported to provide a sense of temporary freedom from the mothering role, allowing mothers to focus on themselves and regain a sense of personal achievement:

> I run out the front door and I could almost do that [hands in the air] because it's like 'yes, I'm away'. There's no-one tugging on my trousers, 'mummy can I have a drink'. It is that real sense of freedom and I think that's so important when you've got little kids because you just don't have that (female, 37 years, intervention).
>
> (Pritchett et al., 2017)

It is noteworthy that for many mothers, the desire to prioritise their child can lead to a struggle not to view exercise as selfish (Barkin & Wisner, 2013; Pritchett et al., 2017). Women taking part in yoga sessions for pregnant and postnatal women have described their experience of a safe, nurturing, space where they can receive support, empathy, and advice (Doran & Hornibrook, 2013). Group exercise within a peer group was felt to reduce isolation and provide reassurance when new mothers were struggling with the psychological challenges of sleep deprivation and crying infants (Doran & Hornibrook, 2013).

It is important to acknowledge that many mothers report barriers to postnatal exercise, some of which are common to all postnatal women such as recovery from giving birth, the practicalities of childcare, time limitations, poor weather, and financial pressures (Currie & Develin, 2002; Pritchett et al., 2017). Some barriers, however, are unique to depressed mothers. Postnatal depression and anxiety are often comorbid (Farr, Dietz, O'Hara, Burley, & Ko, 2014) and can prove a serious impediment to certain types of exercise (Pritchett et al., 2017; Rogerson, Murphy, Bird, & Morris, 2012). Depression can result in very low motivation, and anxiety can cause self-isolation, with the prospect of new environments such as group exercise classes becoming overwhelming (Pritchett et al., 2017): 'When I'm feeling low you won't get me out of the house … I lock myself in my bedroom and just stay there' (female, 23 years old, intervention) (Pritchett et al., 2017). A self-critical, self-doubting attitude in some mothers with PND can occur, which can inhibit public exercise through insecurities about one's appearance or negative comparisons to previous fitness levels: 'Knowing what I used to be able to do to then only be able to manage 10 min or something like that would be just too much for me to bear' (female, 34 years, intervention) (Pritchett et al., 2017).

Women have reported success in incorporating exercise into daily life. Several practical factors have been found to be conducive to postnatal exercise, such as informal childcare from family and friends, walking to school, home exercise, and exercising once a partner returned from work (Pritchett et al., 2017). In summary, despite the substantial practical, physical, and psychological barriers to exercise faced by depressed mothers, successful incorporation of certain types of activity is possible, and physical and psychological benefits can be gained (Pritchett et al., 2017).

Helping women with PND to exercise

Taken together, current evidence indicates that exercise can be an effective treatment for PND, with minimal side effects, although women will only experience the benefits that exercise can provide if they participate regularly. We will now discuss the ways in which women with PND can be supported to be active, or recommence activity (if they were active prior to pregnancy).

First, as discussed earlier, there can be barriers to exercise for women with PND, in addition to the practical difficulties of recovery from childbirth, childcare, breastfeeding, and limited free time (Pritchett et al., 2017). Anxiety, depression, low motivation, self-critical thoughts, and maladaptive coping strategies appear to form significant obstacles, specifically to the initiation, but also to the maintenance, of exercise (Pritchett et al., 2017). Making psychological therapies such as CBT accessible to women with PND may prove beneficial for those struggling to initiate exercise. It is also important that exercise programmes are targeted and designed to address these challenges. Postnatal walking groups have the potential to create an exercise environment based on an empathetic peer group that may provide valuable social support (Armstrong & Edwards, 2003, 2004; Currie & Develin, 2002).

Mental health benefits have been reported from even walking at a slow pace (Hanson & Jones, 2015), so it is important to highlight to women that even low-intensity exercise might be beneficial and that exercise does not have to be performed at a high intensity. Short bouts of exercise have also been shown to have health benefits (Patel et al., 2018). Encouraging short bouts of exercise may, therefore, be a useful step in getting women to at least initiate, or re-initiate exercise (if already active prior to pregnancy). Women can then work towards gradually increasing the time engaged in exercise.

Many women experience a change or loss of identity through motherhood (Nelson, 2003). Exercise can provide mothers with a period of time away from the mothering role to focus on themselves. Health professionals need to recognise that mothers may need to overcome a sense of guilt, both innate and societal, at focusing on themselves rather than their child for a time. Health professionals can encourage women to exercise regularly by emphasising the importance of their physical and psychological health, and the impact this can have on the health and development of their child.

There must be recognition that returning to exercise may not be suitable for all women, such as those recovering from a difficult childbirth or for women experiencing very severe mental health difficulties. Furthermore, people experiencing poor mental health may be lacking in the motivation to engage with tasks in their everyday lives and may feel socially isolated. Consequently, it may be difficult for women with PND to feel they have the energy and confidence to be proactive in finding opportunities to exercise, whether that be on their own, or with others in their community.

Summary

In several meta-analyses of the effects of exercise on PND, it has been reported that exercise can reduce the symptoms of PND. There are also many other reasons why exercise should be encouraged with this population of women, such as opportunities for social integration and connections and physical health benefits. Unlike medication, exercise has minimal side effects and does not necessarily require equipment or specialist clothing, nor does it have to be costly. For these reasons, women who are experiencing PND should be encouraged to exercise regularly as part of their recovery process, and clinical guidance for postnatal mental health should reflect this evidence.

References

Abdollahi, F., Rohani, S., Sazlina, G. S., Zarghami, M., Azhar, M. Z., Lye, M. S., … Mozafari, S. (2014). Bio-psycho-socio-demographic and obstetric predictors of postpartum depression in pregnancy: A prospective cohort study. *Irazian Journal of Psychiatry and Behavioural Sciences, 8*(2), 11–21.

Alasoom, L. I., & Koura, M. R. (2014). Predictors of postpartum depre;sion in the eastern province capital of saudi arabia. *Journal of Family Medicine and Primary Care, 3*(2), 146–150. https://doi.org/10.4103/2249-4863.137654.

Albright, C., Maddock, J. E., & Nigg, C. R. (2005). Physical activity before pregnancy and following childbirth in a multiethnic sample of heal-hy women in Hawaii. *Women & Health, 42*(3), 95–110. https://doi.org/10.1300/J013 v42n03_06.

Alfayumi-Zeadna, S., Kaufman-Shriqui, V., Zeadna, A., Lauden, A., & Shoham-Vardi, I. (2014). The association between sociodemographic characteristics and postpartum depression symptoms among arab-bedouin women in southern israel. *Depression and Anxiety, 32*(2). https://doi.org/10.1002/da.22290.

American Psychiatric Association. (2013). *Diagnostic and statistical manual of mental disorders* (5th ed.). Arlington VA, USA: American Psychiatric Associatþn. https://doi.org/10.1176/appi.books.9780890425596.

Armstrong, K., & Edwards, H. (2003). The effects of exercise and social support on mothers reporting depressive symptoms: A pilot randomized controlled trial. *International Journal of Mental Health Nursing, 12*, 130–138. https://doi.org/10.1046/j.1440-0979.2003.00229.x.

Armstrong, K., & Edwards, H. (2004). The effectiveness of a pram-walking exercise programme in reducing depressive symptomatology for postnatal women. *International Journal of Nursing Practice, 10*, 177–194. https://doi.org/10.1111/j.1440-172X.2004.00478.x.

Bahrke, M. S., & Morgan, W. P. (1978). Anxiety reducation following exercise and meditation. *Cognitive Therapy and Research, 2*(4), 323–333. https://doi.org/10.1007/BF01172650.

Bailey, M., & McLaren, S. (2005). Physical activity alone and with other; as predictors of sense of belonging and mental health in retirees. *Aging & Mental Health, 9*(1), 82–90. https://doi.org/10.1080/13607860512331334031.

Barkin, J. L., & Wisner, K. L. (2013). The role of maternal self-care in new motherhood. *Midwifery, 29*, 1050–1055. https://doi.org/10.1016/j.midw.2012.10.001.

Battle, C. L., Salisbury, A. L., Schofield, C. A., & Ortiz-Hernandez, S. (2013). Perinatal antidepressant use: Understanding women's preferences and concerns. *Journal of Psychiatrric Practice, 19*(6), 443–453. https://doi.org/10.1097/01.pra.0000438183.74359.46.

Bica, T., Castelló, R., Toussaint, L. L., & Monteso-Curtó, P. (2017). Depression as a risk factor of organic diseases: An international integrative review. *Journal of Nursing Scholarship, 49*(4), 389–399. https://doi.org/10.1111/jnu.12303.

Bortz, W. M., 2nd, Angwin, P., Mefford, I. N., Boarder, M. R., Noyce, N., & Barchas, J. D. (1981). Catecholamines, dopamine, and endorphin levels during extreme exercise. *New England Journal of Medicine, 305*(8), 466–467.

Brosse, A. L., Sheets, E. S., Lett, H. S., & Blumenthal, J. A. (2002). Exercse and the treatment of clinical depression in adults: Recent findings and future directions. *Sports Medicine, 32*(12), 741–760. https://doi.org/10.2165/00007256-200232120-00001.

Cramp, A. G., & Bray, S. R. (2010). Postnatal women's feeling state responses to exercise with and without baby. *Maternal and Child Health Journal, 14*, 343–349. https://doi.org/10.1007/s10995-009-0462-5.

Currie, J. L., & Develin, E. (2002). Stroll your way to well-being: A survey of the perceived benefits, barriers, community support, and stigma associated with pram walking groups designed for new mothers, Sydney, Australia. *Health Care for Women International,* 23(8), 882–893. https://doi.org/10.1080/073993302 90112380

Daley, A. J., Blamey, R. V., Jolly, K., Roalfe, A. K., Turner, K. M., Coleman, S., … MacArthur, C. (2015). A pragmatic randomized controlled trial to evaluate the effectiveness of a facilitated exercise intervention as a treatment for postnatal depression: The PAM-PeRS trial. *Psychological Medicine,* 45(11), 2413–2425. https://doi.org/10.1017/S0033291715000409.

Daley, A., Jolly, K., & MacArthur, C. (2009). The effectiveness of exercise in the management of post-natal depression: Systematic review and meta-analysis. *Family Practice, 26,* 154–162. https://doi.org/10.1093/fampra/cmn101.

Denis, A., & Luminet, O. (2017). Cognitive factors and post-partum depression: What is the influence of general personality traits, rumination, maternal self-esteem, and alexithymia? *Clinical Psychology & Psychotherapy.* https://doi.org/10.1002/cpp. 2168.

Doran, F., & Hornibrook, J. (2013). Women's experiences of participation in a pregnancy and postnatal group incorporating yoga and facilitated group discussion: A qualitative evaluation. *Women and Birth, 26,* 82–86. https://doi.org/10.1016/j.wombi.2012.06.001.

Dunn, A. L., Reigle, T. G., Youngstedt, S. D., Armstrong, R. B., & Dishman, R. K. (1996). Brain norepinephrine and metabolites after treadmill training and wheel running in rats. *Medicine & Science in Sports & Exercise, 28*(2), 204–209. https://doi.org/10.1097/00005768-199602000-00008.

Farr, S. L., Dietz, P. M., O'Hara, M. W., Burley, K., & Ko, J. Y. (2014). Postpartum anxiety and comorbid depression in a population-based sample of women. *Journal of Women's Health, 23*(2), 120–128. https://doi.org/10.1089/jwh.2013.4438.

Farrell, P. A., Gates, W. K., Maksud, M. G., & Morgan, W. P. (1982). Increases in plasma beta-endorphin/beta-lipotropin immunoreactivity after treadmill running in humans. *Journal of Applied Physiology, 52*(5), 1245–1249. https://doi.org/10.1152/jappl.1982.52.5.1245.

Field, T. (2010). Postpartum depression effects on early interactions, parenting, and safety practices: A review. *Infant Behavior and Development, 33*(1), 1–6. https://doi.org/10.1016/j.infbeh.2009.10.005.

Fox, K. (2000). The effects of exercise on self-perceptions and self-esteem. In S. Biddle, K. Fox, & S. Boutcher (Eds.), *Physical activity and psychological well-being* (p. 88). London: Routledge.

Gleser, J., & Mendelberg, H. (1990). Exercise and sport in mental health: A review of the literature. *Israel Journal of Psychiatry and Related Sciences, 27*(2), 99–112.

Hanson, S., & Jones, A. (2015). Is there evidence that walking groups have health benefits? A systematic review and meta-analysis. *British Journal of Sports Medicine, 49*(11), 710–715. https://doi.org/10.1136/bjsports-2014-094157.

Highet, N. S., Stevenson, A. L., Purtell, C., & Coo, S. (2014). Qualitative insights into women's personal experiences of perinatal depression and anxiety. *Women and Birth, 27*(3), 179–184. https://doi.org/10.1016/j.wombi.2014.05.003.

Horowitz, J. A., & Goodman, J. (2004). A longitudinal study of maternal postpartum depression symptoms. *Research and Theory for Nursing Practice, 18,* 149–163.

Jennings, K. D., Ross, S., Popper, S., & Elmore, M. (1999). Thoughts of harming infants in depressed and nondepressed mothers. *Journal of Affective Disorders*, *54*(1–2), 21–28. https://doi.org/10.1016/S0165-0327(98)00185-2.

Katon, W., Russo, J., & Gavin, A. (2014). Predictors of postpartum depression. *Journal of Women's Health*, *23*(9), 753–759. https://doi.org/10.1089/jwh.2014.4824.

McCurdy, A. P., Boulé, N. G., Sivak, A., & Davenport, M. H. (2017). Effects of exercise on mild-to-moderate depressive symptoms in the postpartum period: A meta-analysis. *Obstetrics & Gynecology*, *129*(6), 1087–1097. https://doi.org/10.1097/aog.0000000000002053.

National Collaborating Centre for Mental Health. (2014). *Clinical guideline 192. Antenatal and postnatal mental health: Clinical management and service guidance.* Retrieved from www.nice.org.uk/guidance/cg192.

National Institute for Health and Care Excellence. (2009). *Clinical guideline 90. Depression in adults: The treatment and management of depression in adults (update).* Retrieved from www.nice.org.uk/guidance/CG90.

National Institute of Child Health and Human Development, Early Child Care Research Network. (1999). Chronicity of maternal depressive symptoms, maternal sensitivity, and child functioning at 36 months. *Developmental Psychology*, *35*, 1297–1310. https://doi.org/10.1037/0012-1649.35.5.1297.

Nelson, A. M. (2003). Transition to motherhood. *Journal of Obstetric, Gynecologic, & Neonatal Nursing*, *32*(4), 465–477. https://doi.org/10.1177/0884217503255199.

Parsons, C. E., Young, K. S., Rochat, T. J., Kringelbach, M. L., & Stein, A. (2012). Postnatal depression and its effects on child development: A review of evidence from low- and middle-income countries. *British Medical Bulletin*, *101*, 57–79. https://doi.org/10.1093/bmb/ldr047.

Patel, A. V., Hildebrand, J. S., Leach, C. R., Campbell, P. T., Doyle, C., Shuval, K., … Gapstur, S. M. (2018). Walking in relation to mortality in a large prospective cohort of older U.S. adults. *American Journal of Preventive Medicine*, *54*(1), 10–19. https://doi.org/10.1016/j.amepre.2017.08.019.

Paykel, E., & Cooper, Z. (1992). Life events and social stress. In E. S. Paykel (Ed.), *Handbook of affective disorders* (pp. 149–170). New York: Guilford Press.

Pierce, D., Kupprat, I., & Harry, D. (1976). Urinary epinephrine and norepinephrine levels in women athletes during training and competition. *European Journal of Applied Physiology and Occupational Physiology*, *36*(1), 1–6. https://doi.org/10.1007/BF00421628.

Poyatos-León, R., García-Hermoso, A., Sanabria-Martínez, G., Álvarez-Bueno, C., Cavero-Redondo, I., & Martínez-Vizcaíno, V. (2017). Effects of exercise-based interventions on postpartum depression: A meta-analysis of randomized controlled trials. *Birth*, *44*(3), 200–208. https://doi.org/10.1111/birt.12294.

Pritchett, R., Daley, A., & Jolly, K. (2017). Does aerobic exercise reduce postpartum depressive symptoms? A systematic review and meta-analysis. *British Journal of General Practice*, *67*(663), e684–e691. https://doi.org/10.3399/bjgp17X692525.

Pritchett, R., Jolly, K., Daley, A., Turner, K., Bradbury-Jones, C., & PAM-PeRS Study Team. (2017). Women's experiences of exercise as a treatment for their postnatal depression: A nested qualitative study. *Journal of Health Psychology, Epub ahead of print*. https://doi.org/10.1177/1359105317726590.

Robertson, E., Grace, S., Wallington, T., & Stewart, D. E. (2004). Antenatal risk factors for postpartum depression: A synthesis of recent literature. *General Hospital Psychiatry*, *26*(4), 289–295. https://doi.org/10.1016/j.genhosppsych.2004.02.006.

Rogerson, M. C., Murphy, B. M., Bird, S., & Morris, T. (2012). 'I don't have the heart': A qualitative study of barriers to and facilitators of physical activity for people with coronary heart disease and depressive symptoms. *International Journanl of Behavioral Nutrition and Physical Activity, 9*, 140–148. https://doi.org/10.1186/1479-5868-9-140.

Saligheh, M., Hackett, D., Boyce, P., & Cobley, S. (2017). Can exercise or physical activity help improve postnatal depression and weight loss? A systematic review. *Archives of Women's Mental Health, 20*(5), 595–611. https://doi.org/10.1007/s00737-017-0750-9.

Searle, A., Calnan, M., Lewis, G., Campbell, J., Taylor, A., & Turner, K. (2011). Patients' views of physical activity as treatment for depression: A qualitative study. *British Journal of General Practice, 61*(585), 149–156. https://doi.org/10.3399/bjgp11X567054.

Stathi, A., Fox, K., & McKenna, J. (2002). Physical activity and dimensions of subjective well-being in older adults. *Journal of Aging and Physical Activity, 10*(1), 76–92. https://doi.org/10.1123/japa.10.1.76.

Steinberg, H., & Sykes, E. A. (1985). Introduction to symposium on endorphins and behavioural processes; review of literature on endorphins and exercise. *Pharmacology, Biochemistry and Behavior, 23*(5), 857–862. https://doi.org/10.1016/0091-3057(85)90083-8.

Taylor, A. H., & Fox, K. R. (2005). Effectiveness of a primary care exercise referral intervention for changing physical self-perceptions over 9 months. *Health Psychology, 24*(1), 11–21. https://doi.org/10.1037/0278-6133.24.1.11.

Turner, K. M., Sharp, D., Folkes, L., & Chew-Graham, C. (2008). Women's views and experiences of antidepressants as a treatment for postnatal depression: A qualitative study. *Family Practice, 25*, 450–455. https://doi.org/10.1093/fampra/cmn056.

Watson, N., Milat, A. J., Thomas, M., & Currie, J. (2005). The feasibility and effectiveness of pram walking groups for postpartum women in western sydney. *Health Promotion Journal of Australia, 16*(2), 93–99. https://doi.org/10.1071/HE05093.

World Health Organization. (2005). *World health report 2005: Make every mother and child count*. Retrieved from www.who.int/whr/2005/en/.

Yim, I. S., Tanner Stapleton, L. R., Guardino, C. M., Hahn-Holbrook, J., & Dunkel Schetter, C. (2015). Biological and psychosocial predictors of postpartum depression: Systematic review and call for integration. *Annual Review of Clinical Psychology, 11* 99–137. https://doi.org/10.1146/annurev-clinpsy-101414-020426.

17 Motherhood in the exercising female

Claire-Marie Roberts and Göran Kenttä

Introduction

Up to this point, *The Exercising Female: Science and Its Application* has examined both the biological idiosyncrasies of women in the context of sport and exercise, and in addition, some of the gender-based considerations in society's expectations of behaviour and attitudes of the exercising female. Indeed, one of the primary biological distinctions between females and males relate to the fact that only females can become pregnant. Although the biological topic of pregnancy is discussed at length in Chapter 15, the present chapter aims to provide a more gender-based examination of the social and psychological implications of motherhood in the exercising female. These social and psychological implications are driven by gender ideology – the cultural norms and attitudes regarding the appropriate roles, rights, and responsibilities of women and men in society. Traditionally, gender ideologies emphasise the value of distinctive roles for females and males in society. In the case of motherhood in athletes, gender ideology would assert that the true role and natural suitability of the female is to have children due to their biology (Johnston & Swanson, 2003; Weedon, 1997). Males, on the other hand, are the providers for their family, working outside of the home and leaving all homemaking duties to the woman (Dixon & Wetherell, 2004). Furthermore, a fundamental component of a female's moral development is that of the ethic of care (Gilligan, 1982), where they sacrifice their own needs to take care of others (O'Brien, Lloyd & Ringuet-Riot, 2014). Such expectations are incongruent with the pursuit of a career in sport, and in some cases, engagement in exercise.

This ideal and somewhat mythological world of mothering does not translate into practice in most Westernised nations. When cultural norms prevail, and females work, or perhaps make time for their own leisure, those who have children are often criticised for being selfish or bad mothers, which often results in negative and distressing psychological reactions (Batey & Owton, 2014). Athlete mothers may be particularly susceptible to potentially distressing psychological reactions arising from the gender ideology-led attitudes, expectations, and behaviour. For example, the job of an elite athlete often involves intense training loads, a high degree of time spent away travelling, attending training camps and competitions (Freeman, 2008; Pedersen, 2001). Moreover, there is an unrealistic expectation that athlete mothers can 'do it all' (Douglas & Carless, 2009), which may, in turn, lead to further distress when that fails to be achieved.

Aims of the chapter

The aims of the chapter are as follows:

1   To present a gender-based examination of the social and psychological implications of motherhood in the exercising female.
2   To provide practical recommendations for governing bodies of sport for the purposes of enhancing support to elite athlete mothers.

Pregnancy and motherhood in the exercising female

Historically, elite female athletes would end their careers to have children, or at least were encouraged to do so (Palmer & Leberman, 2009; Pedersen, 2001), for the reason that motherhood and sport were seen to be incompatible due to reproductive concerns (Jette, 2011; Kardel, 2005; Vertinsky, 1994). As a result, pregnancy and motherhood have been singled out as reasons why female athletes may end their sport careers or fail to reach their full potential in sport (Palmer & Leberman, 2009; Pedersen, 2001). Certainly, the cultural norms in sport have previously been to delay childbearing until athletic retirement, not least because negotiating time for high-level training and competing may leave little time for motherhood (Appleby & Fisher, 2009; Freeman, 2008).

Although research suggests that 69.8 per cent of athletes report a history of hormonal contraception use (Martin, Sale, Cooper, & Elliott-Sale, 2017; see Chapter 4), anecdotal evidence points to a reluctance in some athlete circles to use this form of birth control for fear of common side effects such as fluid retention and weight gain (Brown, 2017). In addition, athletes report a lack of education in relation to the interaction between training load and the reproductive cycle with misconceptions associated with high levels of fitness driving shorter menstrual cycles and impaired fertility (Brown, 2017). As a result, unplanned pregnancies may occur during an athletic career, which, if unwanted, may result in termination due to a combination of competitive anxieties and a lack of understanding about how pregnancy may affect elite sport performance (Brown, 2017).

Conversely, there are an increasing number of elite female athletes competing well into their 30s, some of whom may wish to become pregnant during their athletic career, and to continue to compete after childbirth (Bø et al., 2016). For these individuals, having a child and becoming a parent brings with it vast changes in life circumstances and accompanying psychological changes. Anecdotally, however, many female athletes are put off having children, because in most sports the general consensus suggests that there is never a good time to have a baby.

Motherhood in elite athletes

Despite the historical, cultural norms associated with childbearing and an athletic career, research examining the media's coverage of athlete mothers demonstrates that there is a growing number in elite sport (McGannon, Curtin, Schinke, & Schweinbenz, 2012). In the elite athletic population, motherhood is more often than not meticulously planned (Kenttä, 2014). For those planning motherhood, there are two clear choices to consider when deciding the timing of pregnancy: (1) to cause as little disruption as possible to the athletic career with a view to returning to sport after the birth; and/or (2) to coincide with the cessation of an athletic career. The consequences of both choices for the exercising female are now examined in the chapter.

Planned pregnancy and return to sport

In female Olympians and Paralympians, any contemplation of planned pregnancies is often considered against the backdrop of the 4-year Olympic and Paralympic cycles. Under these circumstances, athletes will often opt to become pregnant immediately after the cessation of one Olympic or Paralympic Games in order that peak physical fitness and preparedness is attainable for the next Games in 4 years' time. Similarly, elite female athletes representing non-Olympic/Paralympic sports often make planned pregnancy decisions in the context of major sports competitions and tournaments with a view to continuing with their athletic career after the birth (e.g., Nash, 2011). That said, there is a different category of athlete mothers emerging – those who opt for a career break after failing to achieve their sporting goals, during which time they start a family. Although research in this area is sparse, there is one empirical account of an elite female fencer experiencing 'sport saturation' after fighting for and failing to secure Olympic selection for 14 to 15 months (Debois, Ledon, Argiolas, & Rosnet, 2012, p. 665). At this point in her career she planned a break away from sport and started a family, which she reported as adding a new dimension to her identity and a different perspective on life. After this period of renewal, she was able to resume her elite fencing career and continue to work towards her athletic goals.

If female athletes do decide to become mothers during their athletic career, they, like their non-athletic counterparts, are faced with the prospect of leaving the 'job market' at a critical time, resulting in a significant interruption in their career trajectory. This significant career interruption may mean that the pinnacle of one's career is now unattainable. As an individual athlete, this is often a challenging period of time, none more so for team athletes, as their stepping away from the team is likely to have wide-ranging consequences for all team members.

Despite planning on returning to an athletic career post pregnancy, first-time mothers do not necessarily know to what extent the continuation is going to be possible. Certainly in exercising females, as in the general population, one rule does not apply to all when returning to sport after having a baby. Some individuals appear to make a quick return, while for others the journey back to training and competition is more complex and prolonged.

To further compound the issue, most sports offer no financial protection for pregnant athletes. Typically, when a pregnant athlete takes maternity leave, they more often than not fall into the 'not competing' category, and, therefore, any funding (e.g., athlete performance awards) is withheld. This situation places added pressure on athletes to return quickly postpartum at a time when balancing the demands of new motherhood, a change in family dynamics and a return to a physically demanding job is all playing out.

Breastfeeding

A further social expectation associated with the ethic of care on athlete mothers includes breastfeeding, which creates strain for those looking to return to training and competition postpartum (Giles, Phillipps, Darroch, & McGettigan-Dumas, 2016). As societal expectations dominate, the impact of breastfeeding on training, both from an energy perspective and from potentially running around with a full bust, is rarely discussed. When returning to training and competition, it is important to note that exercise intensity can elevate lactic acid concentration in breast milk for up to 1 hr post-exercise (Wright, Carey, & Quinn, 2002), which may affect the taste. Nevertheless, for athletes choosing to breastfeed and return to training and competition, the logistical scheduling of breastfeeding may present a barrier to a return to a normal training routine. Many athletes choose to pump breast milk in order to manage feeding schedules (Giles et al., 2016).

There are further implications that need to be considered when determining whether to start or continue breastfeeding in the context of returning to training and competition. For example, breastfeeding can have an impact on training and recovery, driven by an energy deficit, which leads to depleted energy levels. Thus, athlete mothers often, against the ethic of care, make an informed decision about breastfeeding and a consideration of their ability to train and compete and decide to discontinue (e.g., Giles et al., 2016).

One of the most concerning findings of Giles and colleagues' (2016) study was the lack of relevant information and inconsistencies in recommendations from health care professionals for female athletes wishing to breastfeed and train at high levels. The athletes in Giles and colleagues' study (2016) were keen to breastfeed for prolonged periods yet did not want to negatively influence their own health or the health of their babies.

Sleep

A general lack of energy, fatigue, and irregular sleep patterns are common issues during the postpartum period and may hamper the exercising female's efforts to engage in physical activity and exercise (Beilock, Feltz, & Pivarnik, 2001; Evenson, Aytur, & Borodulin, 2009). Postpartum sleep disturbances arise predominantly from night-time newborn care – specifically sleep management and feeding patterns – along with a combination of changes in the new mother's levels of progesterone and melatonin (e.g., Hunter, Rychnovsky, & Yount, 2009). As before, the ethic of care and the social stereotypes of motherhood lead to the expectation that females are the sole provider of nutrition for their baby and hence must bear the responsibility of night-time newborn care. This expectation is often described as 'overwhelming' by new mothers (e.g., Spencer, Greatrex-White, & Fraser, 2014, p. 87). If babies are breastfed, expressing milk so that the mother's partner may become involved in night-time feeds has the potential to relieve this onus of responsibility and to reduce sleep disturbances.

The deficit accumulated from weeks of disrupted sleep reduces the exercising female's ability to return to competition-level fitness and to recover in between training. Specifically, the detrimental consequences of sleep deprivation on cognitive, motor functioning, and psychomotor performance is well documented (Fullagar, Skorski, Duffield, Hammes, Coutts, & Meyer, 2015; Thun, Bjorvatn, Flo, Harris, & Pallesen, 2015). Psychomotor performance skills typically involve the production of motor actions and an awareness of the environmental conditions that trigger those actions (Fadde, 2010). These include vigilance, sustained attention, concentration, visual pursuit, and decisive tasks such as simple and choice reaction time (e.g., Monleon, Afif, Mahdavi, & Rezayi, 2018). Psychomotor performance is a vital determinant of successful performance in athletic events and therefore, any impairment in this area puts the individual at a disadvantage. A sleep deficit may require the exercising female to reduce their training load to accommodate the fatigue and reduction in recovery capacity.

Identity

Traditionally, the role of mother and of athlete were, and perhaps in some circles still are, considered polarised, insinuating that women should have to choose between an athletic career and motherhood (McGannon et al., 2015). Indeed, McGannon and colleagues found that the polarity of these identities was often promoted by the media, where the care of children is considered as solely women's responsibility and a true calling (Miller & Brown, 2005; Vertinsky, 1994), and that a transformative journey back to an athletic career following the birth of a child is only in fact worth it when 'good mother ideals are attained' (Miller & Brown, 2005, p. 56).

An additional portrayal of identity in McGannon and colleague's (2015) study was one of the 'athlete and mother as superwoman' (p. 56), meaning one who performs in both sport and domestic duties. This status, in reality, is an unattainable cultural illusion (Appleby & Fisher, 2009; Freeman, 2008); moreover, striving for it causes psychological distress and burnout (Choi, Henshaw, Baker, & Tree, 2005; Douglas & Michaels, 2004; McGannon & Schinke, 2013). Other identities attributed to athlete mothers like British long-distance runner Paula Radcliffe were based around redemption, where, after having children, she was labelled as a 'better athlete and more complete person' (McGannon, Curtin, Schinke, & Schweinbenz, 2012, p. 823).

In spite of these challenges, it is the process of adding a motherhood identity to an existing athletic identity that may bring about improvements in sport performance in the exercising female. This identity dimensionality allows pressure in high-performance sport to be reframed, bringing about a greater sense of perspective and an enhanced level of confidence due to the need to negotiate multiple identities (Appleby & Fisher, 2009; Debois et al., 2012). Consequently, it is clear that sociocultural norms and narratives surrounding athlete mothers are both facilitative and constraining for athletic careers, which may lead to guilt and distress in some instances and identity dimensionality and life satisfaction in others (Freeman, 2008; McGannon et al., 2015). However, from an identity perspective, the negotiation of motherhood and an athletic career is not straightforward.

Advantages of being an athlete mother

Research supports the compatibility of the dual roles of elite athlete and motherhood. For example, motherhood has been shown to decrease performance pressure and provide an additional and alternative perspective on life (Palmer & Leberman, 2009; Pedersen, 2001; Spowart, Burrows, & Shaw, 2010). Elite athletes who are also mothers successfully continue to strive for and achieve performance excellence (Pedersen, 2001) and see themselves as positive role models for others (Leberman & Palmer, 2009; Spowart et al., 2010). As mentioned above, an enhanced focus, a better life balance, and greater resilience may all result. However, there are also a number of disadvantages to consider.

Consequences of being an athlete mother

Despite the clear benefits of combining an athletic career and motherhood, research has addressed the complexities of negotiating both roles. For example Appleby and Fisher (2009) recruited elite runners with young children who provided accounts of their guilt associated with the time their sport took them away from their children, despite the clear psychological gains of time away. In support of these findings, an unpublished doctoral dissertation featured reports of psychological distress associated with athlete mothers travelling to training camps and competitions without families. In addition, despite having support for their athletic training, the support for the athletes' roles as mothers was often lacking causing a high degree of psychological discomfort (Freeman, 2008). It is also clear that the high-performance standards attained by elite athletes (Douglas & Carless, 2009) may generate an added pressure to strive for the cultural expectation that women 'do it all' (both motherhood and an athletic career) perfectly. This often unattainable and unrealistic standard leads to psychological distress due to the inability to meet that expectation (Choi et al., 2005).

In addition to the psychological struggles of balancing the two roles, the athletic patriarchy creates a sporting environment that may prevent many exercising females from excelling once they have had children. Sub-standard maternity structures driven by an outdated gender ideology was highlighted by Victoria Azarenka, former world number 1, Belarusian professional tennis player in 2017. She publicly expressed her dissatisfaction with the way the scheduling was organised at Wimbledon 2017, claiming that she spent hours away from her then 6-month-old baby son while waiting to hear of the timing of her first-round match (Sabur & Sawer, 2017). In addition, due to a dispute with her former partner and a resulting custody battle, she was not able to leave her home in California to resume her competitive career. Such examples shine a light on the structures of sport, and, in some cases, society in general that internalise gender ideologies requiring females to place childcare above athletic pursuits, making high-performance goals more stressful (Cosh & Crabb, 2012; Douglas & Carless, 2009) or masking the difficulties of trying to do it all as a super mum (Choi et al., 2005; McGannon et al., 2015).

Planned pregnancies and athletic career termination

Sport is not a mother-friendly industry. This incompatibility (e.g., Jette, 2011; Kardel, 2005; Vertinsky, 1994) drives many exercising females to wait to have children until the termination of their athletic career. Anecdotally, many athletes feel that they cannot have a baby during their athletic career due to the competitive nature of selection and end up delaying the process against their better judgement. However, these plans do not guarantee fertility. The Female Athlete Triad – a state of inadequate energy status leading to functional hypothalamic amenorrhoea and low bone mineral density (see Chapter 6), which is common in endurance athletes – can cause infertility. On the other hand, those athletes who do manage to start families after retirement often experience an expedited adaptation to life after sport (Stambulova, 2001).

Motherhood in the recreational exercising female

An examination of motherhood in the recreational exercising female is almost more significant due to the inverse relationship between motherhood and exercise participation (Bellows-Riecken & Rhodes, 2008; McIntyre & Rhodes, 2009). One of the reasons for this may relate, in part, to the socio-cultural gender ideologies and practices that are less likely to emphasise the importance of mothers' engagement in physical activity and exercise (Miller & Brown, 2005; Thomsson, 1999). Specifically, the outdated expectation that, women are the primary caregivers and sacrifice their own needs to look after others, constrain engagement in exercise and physical activity (McGannon & Schinke, 2013). Furthermore, the likelihood of women negotiating motherhood and a career make them more likely to suffer guilt when taking time to engage in exercise and physical activity, (Miller & Brown, 2005; Thomsson, 1999). Nevertheless, by reconfiguring time for exercise and physical activity as time for themselves to benefit the family, the exercising female may be able to stay active (Lewis & Ridge, 2005; Miller & Brown, 2005).

Practical recommendations

Both the recreational and elite sporting environment remain inherently patriarchal, and as a result there are few guidelines to help new mothers understand how best to return to their sport or exercise regime. At the elite end of the continuum, organisational policies and procedures often make little to no reference of how to support pregnant or nursing athletes on a day-to-day basis, or even at competitive events. It is recommended that urgent steps are taken by governing bodies of sport worldwide to consider how they can assist their female athletes to balance work (i.e., their sport) and parenthood, if chosen.

Anecdotally, the issue of maternity rights in the context of the sporting environment has been referred to as an 'omnishambles' (Bona, 2017, p. 1), which may contribute to the already numerous barriers preventing females from excelling professionally once they have had children. Sports should be expected to promote and support their athlete mothers by providing them with the right advice to help them train safely during pregnancy, and to transition back into their sport at a time of their choosing.

Real-world example

Perhaps one of the most inspirational female athletes to mention in the context of combining motherhood and an athletic career is Dame Jessica Ennis-Hill. A British double Olympic medallist, three-time World Champion, and 2010 European Champion in the Heptathlon, she had her first child, Reggie, during her athletic career. In his book, *How to Support a Champion:*

The Art of Applying Science to the Elite Athlete, Ingham (2016), Jessica's performance scientist, explains how her life perspective changed once she had given birth to Reggie. He recalls how she changed the timing of her training, so that it could all be completed in the morning, to enable her to spend the rest of the day with her son. By prioritising Reggie, the expectation was that her training had to fit around his needs.

In an account of her return to training after giving birth, Jessica's Coach, Tony Minichiello, noted the beneficial impact of her increased blood volume and in the range of movement in her joints as a result of the hormone relaxin (see Chapter 15), which stays in the body for up to a year post childbirth. Yet, Jessica had lost her speed, which was reported as having a significant negative impact on her confidence (Oxley & Aloia, 2018). By introducing post pregnancy personal best goals, and, in effect, starting from scratch with her training, her coaches, and athlete-support personnel helped create an environment that allowed her to thrive. In her first World Championships 15 months after giving birth, she won gold in the Heptathlon and went on to claim silver in the same event at the 2016 Olympic Games in Rio de Janeiro.

Summary

Gender ideology views females as suited to caregiving roles as a result of their biology. Furthermore, this ideology would suggest that having children is deemed a natural rite of passage that all females must achieve to realise happiness (Choi et al., 2005; Douglas & Michaels, 2004). Clearly, many females have no such desires, including many of those who participate and compete in sport. However, for those female athletes that do desire to have a family, the timing of their decision to become pregnant is a critical consideration within the context of their athletic career. By aspiring to have a baby *during* their athletic career, they remove themselves from the job market temporarily. That time away from sport impacts ranking, preparation and competition, and results in the risk of not being able to reach the pinnacle of their career when they attempt to return. Furthermore, a return to previous levels of performance postpartum is not guaranteed. If a successful return to an athletic career is possible, female athlete mothers face a myriad of barriers to success including gender ideology and the athletic patriarchy, which must be overcome in order to continue to attain their athletic goals.

References

Appleby, K. M., & Fisher, L. A. (2009). Running in and out of motherhood: Elite distance Runners' experiences of returning to competition after pregnancy. *Women in Sport and Physical Activity Journal, 18*, 3–17. https:/doi.org/10.1123/wspaj.18.1.3.

Batey, J., & Owton, H. (2014). Team mums: Team sport experiences of athlete mothers. *Women in Sport and Physical Activity Journal, 22*, 20–36. https://doi.org/0.1122/wspaj.2014-0010.

Bellows-Riecken, K., & Rhodes, R. E. (2008). The birth of inactivity? A review of physical activity and parenthood. *Preventive Medicine, 46*, 99–110. https://doi.org/10.1016/j.ypmed.2007.08.003.

Beilock, S. L., Feltz, D. L., & Pivarnik, J. M. (2001). Training patterns of athletes during pregnancy and postpartum. *Research Quarterly for Exercise and Sport, 72*, 39–46. https://doi.org/10.1080/02701367.2001.10608930.

Bø, K., Artal, R., Barakat, R., Brown, W., Davies, G. A. L., Dooley, M., … Khan, K. M. (2016). Exercise and pregnancy in recreational and elite athletes: 2016 evidence summary from the IOC expert group meeting, Lausanne. Part 1 – exercise in women planning pregnancy and those who are pregnant. *British Journal of Sports Medicine, 50*, 571–589. https://doi.org/10.1136/bjsports-2016-096218.

Bona, N. (2017). From birth to rebirth: How athletes get back in the game after pregnancy. *Vice Sports*. Retrieved from: https://sports.vice.com/en_ca/article/mgzpa8/from-birth-to-rebirth-how-athletes-get-back-in-the-game-after-pregnancy.

Brown, O. (2017, 8 June). Sanya Richards-Ross breaks silence on sport's last taboo with incendiary claim about prevalence of abortions. *Telegraph*. Retrieved from www.telegraph.co.uk/athletics/2017/06/08/sanya-richards-ross-breaks-silence-sports-last-taboo-incendiary/.

Carless, D., & Douglas, K. (2009). 'We haven't got a seat on the bus for you' or 'All the seats are mine': Narratives and career transition in professional golf. *Qualitative Research in Sport and Exercise, 1*, 51–66. https://doi.org/10.1080/19398440802567949.

Choi, P., Henshaw, C., Baker, S., & Tree, J. (2005). Supermum, superwife, super-everything: Performing femininity in the transition to motherhood. *Journal of Reproductive and Infant Psychology, 23*, 167–180. https://doi.org/10.1080/02646830500129437.

Cosh, S., & Crabb, S. (2012). Motherhood within elite sport discourse: The case of Keli Lane. *Psychology of Women Section Review, 14*, 41–49.

Debois, N. Ledon, A., Argiolas, C., & Rosnet, E. (2012). A lifespan perspective on transitions during a top sports career: A case of an elite female fencer. *Psychology of Sport & Exercise, 13*, 660–668. https://doi.org/10.1016/j.psychsport.2012.04.010.

Dixon, J., & Wetherell, M. (2004). On discourse and dirty nappies: Gender, the division of household labour and the social psychology of distributive justice. *Theory & Psychology, 14*, 167–189. https://doi.org/10.1177/0959354304042015.

Douglas, S., & Michaels, M. (2004). *The mommy myth: The idealization of motherhood and how it has undermined women.* New York: Free Press.

Evenson, K. R., Aytur, S. A., & Borodulin, K. (2009). Physical activity beliefs, barriers, and enablers among postpartum women. *Journal of Women's Health, 18*, 1925–1934 https://doi.org/10.1089/jwh.2008.1309. http://doi.org/10.1089/jwh.2003.1309.

Fadde, P. J. (2010). Training complex psychomotor performance skills: A part-task approach In K. H. Silber & R. Foshay (Eds.), *Handbook of training and improving workplace performance. Volume 1: Instructional design and training delivery.* New York: Wiley & Sons.

Freeman, H. V. (2008). *A qualitative exploration of the experiences of mother-athletes training for and competing in the Olympic Games* (Doctoral dissertation). Philadelphia: Temple University.

Fullagar, H. H., Skorski, S., Duffield, R., Hammes, D., Coutts, A. J., & Meyer, T. (2015). Sleep and athletic performance: The effects of sleep loss on exercise performance, and physiological and cognitive responses to exercise. *Sports Medicine, 45*, 161–186. https://doi.org/10.1007/s40279-014-0260-0.

Giles, A. R., Phillipps, B., Darroch, F. E., & McGettigan-Dumas, R. (2016). Elite distance runners and breastfeeding: A qualitative study. *Journal of Human Lactation, 32*, 627–632. https://doi.org/10.1177/0890334416661507.

Gilligan, C. (1982). *In a different voice.* Cambridge, MA: Harvard University Press.

Hunter, L. P., Rychnovsky, J. D., & Yount, S. M. (2009). A selective review of maternal sleep characteristics in the postpartum period. *Journal of Obstetric, Gynaecologic and Neonatal Nursing, 38*, 60–68. https://doi.org/10.1111/j.1552-6909.2008.00309.x.

Ingham, S. (2016). *How to support a champion: The art of applying science to the elite athlete.* London: Simply Said.

Jette, S. (2011). Exercising caution: the production of medical knowledge about physical exertion during pregnancy. *Canadian Bulletin of Medical History, 28*, 293–313.

Johnston, D., & Swanson, D. (2003). Invisible mothers: A content analysis of motherhood ideologies and myths in magazines. *Sex Roles, 49*, 21–33. https://doi.org/10.1023/A:1023905518500.

Kardel, K. R. (2005). Effects of intense training during and after pregnancy in top level athletes. *Scandinavian Journal of Medicine and Science in Sports, 15*, 79–86. https://doi.org/0.1111/j.1600-0838.2004.00426.x.

Kenttä, G. (2014). *Being an elite female athlete: A psychological perspective.* Stockholm: SISU sport Books.

Lewis, B., & Ridge, D. (2005). Mothers reframing physical activity: Family oriented politicism, transgression and contested expertise in Australia. *Social Science and Medicine, 60*, 2295–2306. https://doi.org/10.1016/j.socscimed.2004.10.011.

Martin, D., Sale, C., Cooper, S. B., & Elliott-Sale, K. J. (2017). Period prevalence and perceived side effects of hormonal contraceptive use and the menstrual cycle in elite athletes. *International Journal of Sports Physiology & Performance, 28*, 1–22. https://doi.org/10.1123/ijspp. 2017–0330.

McGannon, K. R., Curtin, K., Schinke, R. J., & Schweinbenz, A. N. (2012). (De) Constructing Paula Radcliffe: Exploring media representations of elite running, pregnancy and motherhood through cultural sport psychology. *Psychology of Sport and Exercise, 13*, 820–829. https://doi.org/10.1016/j.psychsport.2012.06.005.

McGannon, K. R., Gonsalves, C. A., Schinke, R. J., & Busanich, R. (2015). Negotiating motherhood and athletic identity: A qualitative analysis of Olympic athlete mother representations in media narratives. *Psychology of Sport and Exercise, 20*, 51–59. https://doi.org/10.1016/j.psychsport.2015.04.010.

McGannon, K. R., & Schinke, R. J. (2013). 'My first choice is to work out at work; then i don't feel bad about my kids': A discursive psychological analysis of motherhood and physical activity participation. *Psychology of Sport & Exercise, 14*, 179–188. https://doi.org/10.1016/j.psychsport.2012.10.001.

McIntyre, C. A., & Rhodes, R. E. (2009). Correlates of leisure-time physical activity during transitions to motherhood. *Women and Health, 49*, 66–83. https://doi.org/10.1080/03630240802690853.

Miller, Y. D., & Brown, W. J. (2005). Determinants of active leisure for women with young children – an 'ethic of care' prevails. *Leisure Sciences, 27*, 405–420. https://doi.org/10.1080/01490400500227308.

Monleon, C. Afif, A. H., Mahdavi, S., & Rezayi, M. (2018). The acute effect of low intensity aerobic exercise on psychomotor performance of athletes with nocturnal sleep deprivation. *International Journal of Sport Studies for Health, 1*, e66783. https://doi.org/10.5812/intjssh.66783.

Nash, M. (2011). 'You don't train for a marathon sitting on the couch': Performances of pregnancy 'fitness' and 'good' motherhood in Melbourne, Australia. *Women's Studies International Forum, 34*, 50–65. https://doi.org/10.1016/j.wsif.2010.10.004.

O'Brien, W., Lloyd, K., & Ringuet-Riot, C. (2014). Mothers governing family health: From an 'ethic of care' to a 'burden of care'. *Women's Studies International Forum, 47* 317–325. https://doi.org/0.1016/j.wsif.2013.11.001.

Oxley S., & Aloia, A. (2018, 11 July) Bumps, boobs and bouncing back: An athlete's path through pregnancy. *BBC News*. Retrieved from www.bbc.co.uk/news/resources/dt-sh/bumps_boobs_and_bouncing_back.

Palmer, F. E., & Leberman, S. I. (2009). Elite athletes as mothers: managing multiple sport identities. *Sport Management Review, 12*, 241–254. https://doi.org/10.1016/j.smr.2009.03.001.

Pedersen, I. K. (2001). Athletic career: 'Elite sports mothers' as a social phenomenon. *International Review for the Sociology of Sport, 36*, 259–274. https://doi.org/10.1177/101269001036003001.

Sabur, P., & Sawer. R. (2017, 4 July). Wimbledon: 'Sexist' scheduling leaves new mum Azarenka away from baby all day. *Telegraph*. Retrieved from www.telegraph.co.uk/news/2017/07/04/wimbledon-sexist-scheduling-leaves-new-mum-azarenka-away-baby/.

Spencer, R. Greatrex-White, S., Fraser, D. M. (2014) 'I was meant to be able to do this': A phenomenological study of women's experiences of breastfeeding. *Evidence Based Midwifery, 12*, 83–88.

Spowart, L. Burrows, L., & Shaw, S. (2010). I just eat, sleep and dream of surfing: When surfing meets motherhood. *Sport in Society, 13*, 1186–1203. https://doi.org/10.1080/17430431003780179.

Stambulova, N. B. (2001). Sport career termination of Russian athletes: Readiness for the transition. Paper presented at the *10th World Congress of Sport Psychology, Skiathos, Hellas, Greece*.

Thomsson, H. (1999). Yes, I used to exercise, but … a feminist study of exercise in the life of Swedish women. *Journal of Leisure Research, 31*, 35–56. https://doi.org/10.1080/00222216.1999.11949850.

Thun, E., Bjorvatn, B., Flo, E., Harris, A., & Pallesen, S. (2015). Sleep, circadian rhythms, and athletic performance. *Sleep Medicine Reviews, 23*, 1–9. https://doi.org/10.1016/j.smrv.2014.11.003.

Vertinsky, P. A. (1994). *The eternally wounded woman: Women, doctors and exercise in the late nineteenth century*. Manchester, UK: Manchester University Press.

Weedon, C. (1997). *Feminist practice and poststructuralist theory* (2nd ed.). Oxford: Blackwell.

Wright, K. S., Carey, G. B., & Quinn, T. J. (2002). Infant acceptance of breast milk after maternal exercise. *Pediatrics, 109*, 585–589. https://doi.org/0.1097/00005768-199905001-00164.

18 Athletic career termination in females

Claire-Marie Roberts

Introduction

Placing the well-being of athletes at the centre of research has helped develop knowledge and understanding of a number of features of an athletic career, starting with the development of talent in sport (for a review see: Coutinho, Mesquita, & Fonseca, 2016), negotiating within-career transitions throughout the lifecycle of an athletic career, and finishing at the endpoint (Stambulova & Ryba, 2013). This endpoint is referred to as athletic career termination (e.g., Wylleman, Alfermann, & Lavallee, 2004). Athletes facing career termination approach a notoriously difficult transition to a life after sport, which brings with it a set of demands that require adequate coping processes (Stambulova & Wylleman, 2014).

The reasons for athletic career termination are understood to be multi-faceted (Stambulova, Alfermann, Statler, & Côté, 2009). That is to say that there are often a number of factors that either drive or influence the end of an athlete's sport career, which include: freely choosing to retire; career-ending injuries; deselection; age; and problems with coaching staff, to name a few (Park, Tod, & Lavallee, 2012). The reasons for athletic career termination are often referred to as antecedents or preconditions of retirement (e.g., Taylor & Ogilvie, 1994). These antecedents or preconditions are understood to hold significant influence over the way in which the individual reacts to their retirement from sport, and ultimately their adaptation to a post sport life (Roberts & Davis, 2017). Indeed, there is a large body of research that supports the benefits of a planned and voluntary retirement from sport as opposed to an unplanned or involuntary career transition (e.g., Young, Pearce, Kane, & Pain, 2006). However, recent attempts to clarify this dichotomy have found no support for it at all (e.g., Roberts, Mullen, Evans, & Hall, 2015). Instead, it is suggested that the fluctuating nature of life satisfaction (indicative of adaptation) after athletic career termination, driven by different barriers and resources at different times in individuals' lives, does not support the conceptual and theoretical perspectives of a linear, dichotomous healthy- versus crisis-transition outcome.

The diversity in athletic career termination experiences can be attributed to cultural- and national-specific factors (Seiler, Anders, & Irlinger, 1998; Wylleman et al., 2004), and in addition, the sport environment and its associated cultural traditions and norms may account for differences in the experiences of athletic career termination (Roberts, 2010). With this in mind and given the gender roles that still exist in society (see Chapter 17), gender is likely to influence athletes' status within their respective sports and, therefore, their experiences of athletic career termination (e.g., Moesch, 2012).

Aims of the chapter

The aims of the chapter are as follows:

1 To explore the female-specific experiences of athletic career termination.
2 To provide associated practical recommendations for female athletes facing retirement from sport.

Gender equality

One may assume that experiences of athletic career termination between genders are equal, since there has been progress towards gender equity in sport in Westernised nations in the past 50 years (Salinas & Bagni, 2017). Any progress made, however, has been slow and inconsistent, certainly in the sport domain (Scraton & Flintoff, 2002). Recent stories of inappropriate behaviour displayed by the former England football manager, Mark Sampson, towards female athletes, the failure of the England Rugby Football Union to offer full-time professional contracts to the England's Women Rugby World Cup final-reaching side, and stories of bullying of female members of British Cycling by (now former) coach, Shane Sutton, suggest gender equality in sport is still a long way off. The media perpetuates this stance with female athletes such as Anna Kournikova, Maria Sharapova, and the Williams' sisters, who are identified and valued for how they look rather than their exceptional sporting abilities. It is clear, therefore, that women and men are unlikely to experience similarities in the way their sport is governed, the manner in which they are coached (see Chapter 13), and the training and competition support available to them. Therefore, it is safe to assume that these differences drive divergent experiences during the athletic career lifecycle.

Gender differences

Dropout and athletic career termination are closely related concepts, with no clear delineation. The general difference relates to, but is limited to, the confines of age. For example, in elite sport, dropout relates to a *premature* termination of a sport career before one reaches peak performance. Athletic career termination, however, tends to relate to retirement, inferring that athletes have reached peak performance before leaving their sport, although this, in reality, is not always the case. In research, the two concepts are studied separately. The available statistics suggest that females drop out from sport at a much higher level than do male athletes, and at the peak age of 17 (Enoksen, 2011). Perhaps, as a marker of gender ideology, those females that drop out of sport report negative personal experience, a lack of support, and a negative social environment as key factors in their decision-making (Enoksen, 2011). Certainly, cultural expectations and influence from parents are key determinants of what young girls choose to prioritise (Higginson, 1985; Fasting, 1996), which may, in part, be responsible for the high dropout rates among females.

If young girls are able to successfully negotiate dropout from sport, progression in this domain leads them to an often male-dominated structure, where their training and competitions are most likely to be managed and coached by males. As a result, some scholars have suggested that the needs and values of women are not understood, appreciated, or even acknowledged (Douglas & Carlees, 2009).

Age of athletic career termination

The length of the athletic lifecycle is sport-specific. For example, distinct differences exist between early specialisation sports such as gymnastics, and late specialisation sports such as long-distance running (see Chapter 2). There is, however, a variation in athletic lifespans between males and females, where females reach peak performance at younger ages than do men, especially for long-distance swimming events (i.e., 800 m and 1500 m) and gymnastics, and subsequently retire earlier (Schulz & Curnow, 1988). In the past, far more female athletes terminated their athletic career prematurely because of a variety of reasons, including family commitments, loss of motivation, injury, and financial motives. There is, however, an emerging trend of women's peak-performance age increasing in the six Olympic disciplines of 100-m and 400-m running, 100-m and 400-m swimming events, single sculls (rowing), and 500-m speed skating at least (Elmenshawy, Machin, & Tanaka, 2015). A slow change in societal expectations towards women in the past 50 years may have allowed female athletes to continue to compete at older ages when, in the past, athletes would have retired upon marriage and/or childbirth. This increase in age of peak performance in women is bringing them in line with the peak performance ages of male athletes. Knowledge of this trend may be important for female athletes and their coaches, if a premature termination of their athletic career is being considered.

Body image

Females, in general, are more susceptible to problems with body image (see Chapter 8), and although some sports such as swimming (e.g., Howells & Grogan, 2012) provide a focus on bodily experiences and functionality (e.g., Alleva, Tylka, & Kroon Van Diest, 2017), engaging in lean (e.g., distance running) and aesthetic (e.g., gymnastics) sports, may intensify pressures to be thin (Martinsen & Sundgot-Borgen, 2013). For those athletes with body image problems during their sport career, there may be an expectation that those problems dissipate on retirement (Papathomas, Smith, & Lavallee, 2015); however, evidence exists to suggest that weight and body image concerns continue to evolve.

For female athletes, who put on weight when they retire from sport as a direct result of a reduced or non-existent training load, negative emotional consequences may result, since a discrepancy emerges between their current and former bodies (Papathomas, Petrie, & Plateau, 2018). Furthermore, after an athletic career focused on extensive body monitoring, retired female athletes in particular, may develop a heightened sensitivity to even small body-related changes (Kerr et al., 2006; McMahon & Penney, 2013). Retired female athletes, who subscribe to both an athletic ideal and a feminine thin ideal, labelled the 'retired female athlete paradox' by Papathomas and colleagues (2018, p. 40), are likely to struggle with prolonged body dissatisfaction as these two body ideals are completely incompatible. Where body dissatisfaction was present, it is suggested that the broadening of identity into domains outside of sport (e.g., career and romantic relationships) can help bring about a different perspective and increased worth (Papathomas et al., 2018).

'Family reasons'

The broadening of identity on retirement from sport is easily brought about by a switch in focus from the sport career to relationships and/or family. Although research, investigating the impact of 'family reasons' on females' retirement from sport, how it is defined, and how it is brought about, is sparse, there are a few studies that offer an insight. In 2012, Moesch, Mayer, and Elbe investigated gender differences as potential correlates, as reasons for career termination in Danish athletes. They found that female athletes reported ending their career for family-related reasons significantly more frequently than did males. This finding supports Reints' (2011) study, where female athletes reported having or wanting children as the second most important reason for athletic retirement; support also comes from Stambulova, Stephan, and Jäphag's (2007) research, in which family reasons were positioned as the third most popular factor for career termination among Swedish female athletes. Additionally, Alfermann (2000) suggested that female athletes were more likely to terminate their athletic career to start a family or due to family obligations.

Pregnancy and motherhood

Of course, family-related reasons are most often reduced to the topic of pregnancy and motherhood, both of which, more often than not, lead to a dropout from competitive sport (Roberts & Kenttä, 2018). In Chapter 17, this topic is examined in greater detail, but in summary, the female athlete may perceive an incompatibility between motherhood and an athletic career and opt to invest her energies into the former at the expense of her sport career. In fact, this perceived incompatibility is often a reality, where the athletic patriarchy is both intolerant of and unprepared for motherhood in the athletic population (Roberts & Kenttä, 2018). When female athlete mothers experience problems in the sporting environment, Crosset (1995) suggests that sport culture places the blame for underperformance with the character or the talent of the athlete.

Adaptation to life after sport

There is a body of evidence emerging that suggests that former female athletes adapt quicker following retirement from sport than do men (e.g., Stambulova, 2001). Certainly, in their recent study into motherhood as a career transition in Olympic athletes, Roberts and Kenttä (2018) found that athletes retiring for the purpose of having a child were protected against any negative outcomes of career termination. However, career termination is multifaceted, and the athletes at the centre of the research had all enjoyed long careers in their respective sports, which may have contributed to their positive responses to sport retirement. It is not particularly clear as to why females appear, in general, to be less affected than males by athletic career termination. For those female athletes who are mothers, or go on to become mothers following their sports career, a new perspective, a different focus and a broader identity help ameliorate negative reactions to retirement (Roberts & Kenttä, 2018). Furthermore, it has been proposed that a greater resilience results from the need to negotiate multiple identities (e.g., Debois, Ledon, Argiolas, & Rosnet, 2012) and retiring on your own terms. The other construct to highlight in the context of athletic career termination is flourishing – a state in which an individual experiences positive emotions towards life and functions well psychologically and socially (Keyes, 2003). There are suggestions that females may experience higher levels of flourishing post athletic retirement than do males, which may explain the greater capacity for adaptation after retirement among females (e.g., Knights, Sherry, & Ruddock-Hudson, 2015).

Practical recommendations

As a coach or a member of athlete-support personnel, being mindful of the high levels of dropout in adolescent female athletes and at the same time demonstrating that the needs and values of females are acknowledged, understood, and appreciated in sport may help reduce the numbers of females leaving competitive sport. For those coming to the end of their career, the encouragement of planning, and open and frank conversations between coach, athlete, and athlete-support personnel, is key. In the case of female athletes, however, the desire to start a family may coincide with plans for career termination on the basis of the perception that an elite athletic career and motherhood are incompatible. As a coach or member of athlete-support personnel, knowledge of the increasing age of peak performance in female athletes may help with discussing the options of a return to sport postpartum with the athlete in question. Motherhood should not automatically signal the end of an athletic career.

For female athletes, who do decide to retire from sport, a careful management of expectations and the provision of advice regarding post career nutrition and training may help prevent the evolution of body image problems into retirement. Finally, for those athletes wishing to end their career to have children, an anticipation of a more positive reaction to retirement may help facilitate this response and encourage flourishing in a post sport life.

Real-world example

Eni

Eni retired from lightweight rowing two years ago, when she found that she was unable to return to her previous levels of performance after rehabilitating from shoulder surgery. During her career, Eni found it difficult to stay on top of the weight requirements of her sport, and the intense focus on her diet led her to develop disordered eating that was evident throughout her career. Her retirement was unanticipated, and, as such, she had no plans regarding a second career to work towards, when she retired from sport. After a period of indecision regarding her future, she decided to pursue a Master's degree while planning on her next career move.

As Eni was left with a restricted range of movement in her shoulder as a result of surgery, she felt that this prevented her from engaging in regular exercise. Additionally, since her calorific intake was restricted when she was training and competing, the release from such a controlled existence meant that she was now able to eat anything she liked – nothing was off limits anymore. In an extension of the disordered eating from her sport career, her retirement drove her to develop a binge-eating disorder. A combination of much reduced activity levels and a large increase in calorific intake meant that Eni put on weight rapidly following her retirement. This weight gain led her to suffer from extreme body dissatisfaction, which led to a depressive episode during which she sought help from a psychologist. The psychologist used cognitive behavioural therapy to help Eni overcome her body image problems and referred her to a nutritionist who advised her on her diet post athletic retirement. Eni also started working with a personal trainer, who helped introduce her to exercises she could do without aggravating her weak shoulder. As a result, Eni has a maintenance exercise regime, a better understanding of a healthy diet, and a more compassionate view of herself and her body image. With her Master's degree and a new sense of well-being, she was prepared to tackle the next phase of her life.

Summary

Cultural expectations sustained by significant influencers in children's lives mean that significantly more adolescent females than males dropout of sport prematurely. If females do persist with competitive sport and develop in to an athletic career, their sport is almost certainly going to be structured and governed by males. While on the face of it, this situation seems innocuous, the gender inequality present in most sports means that females may experience their athletic careers in a different way to males, up to and including retirement. The reasons for retirement from sport are multifaceted, but in females there are a significant number of athletes who cite family reasons as their main driver for athletic career termination. Family reasons most often reflect the desire to have children, and in many cases this maternal drive means a premature ending of a sport career. For others, the desire to start or add to a family may coincide with the natural end of their sporting career. In both cases, the new focus and responsibility that a child brings allows athletes to adopt a new perspective on life, where the relative importance of their athletic career is reduced. This renewed focus means that, for retiring athletes, the adaptation to a life after sport is facilitated. Although female athletes are more at risk of problems with their body image on retirement from sport, there are suggestions that females may experience higher levels of flourishing post athletic retirement than do males, which may explain the greater capacity for adaptation after retirement among females.

References

Alfermann, D., & Stambulova, N. B. (2012). Career transitions and career termination. In G. Tenenbaum, & R. C. Eklund (Eds.), *Handbook of sport psychology* (4th ed., pp. 712–736). New York: Wiley.

Alleva, J. M., Tylka, T. L., & Kroon Van Diest, A. M. (2017). The functionality appreciation scale (FAS): Development and psychometric evaluation in U.S. community women and men. *Body Image, 23*, 28–44. https://doi.org/10.1016/j.bodyim.2017.07.008.

Coutinho, P., Mesquita, I., & Fonseca, A. M. (2016). Talent development in sport: A critical review of pathways to expert performance. *International Journal of Sports Science & Coaching, 11*, 279–293. https://doi.org/10.1177/1747954116637499.

Crosset, T. W. (1995). *Outsiders in the clubhouse: The world of women's professional golf.* New York: The State University of New York.

Debois, N., Ledon, A., Argiolas, C., & Rosnet, E. (2012). A lifespan perspective on transitions during a top sports career: A case of an elite female fencer. *Psychology of Sport and Exercise, 13*, 660–668. http://doi.org/10.1016/j.psychsport.2012.04.010.

Douglas, K., & Carless, D. (2009). Abandoning the performance narrative: Two women's stories of transition from professional sport. *Journal of Applied Psychology, 21*, 213–230. https://doi.org/10.1080/10413200902795109.

Elmenshaw, A. R., Machin, D. R., & Tanaka, H. (2015). A rise in peak performance age in female athletes. *Age, 37*, 57. https://doi.org/10.1007/s11357-015-9795-8.

Enoksen, E. (2011). Dropout rate and dropout reasons among promising Norwegian track and field athletes. *Scandinavian Sport Studies Forum, 2*, 19–43.

Fasting, K. (1996). *Hvor går kvinneidretten?* [What is the direction of women's sport?]. Oslo: Norges idrettsforbund.

Higginson, D. C. (1985). The influence of social agents in the female sport-participation process. *Adolescence, 20*, 73–82.

Howells, K., & Grogan, S. (2012). Body image and the female swimmer: muscularity but in moderation. *Qualitative Research in Sport, Exercise and Health, 4*, 98–116. https://doi.org/10.1080/2159676X.2011.653502.

Kerr, G., Berman, E., & De Souza, M. J. (2006). Disordered eating in women's gymnastics: Perspectives of athletes, coaches, parents, and judges. *Journal of Applied Sport Psychology, 18*, 28–43. https://doi.org/10.1080/10413200500 471301.

Keyes, C. L. M. (2003). Complete mental health: An agenda for the 21st century. In C. L. M. Keyes & J. Haidt (Eds.), *Flourishing: Positive psychology and the life well-lived* (pp. 293–312). Washington, DC, US: American Psychological Association. http://do.org/10.1037/10594-013.

Knights, S., Sherry, E., & Ruddock-Hudson, M. (2015). Investigating elite end-of-athletic-career transition: A systematic review. *Journal of Applied Sport Psychology, 28*, 291–308. https://doi.org/10.1080/10413200.2015.1128992.

Martinsen, M., & Sundgot-Borgen, J. (2013). Higher prevalence of eating disorders among adolescent elite athletes than controls. *Medicine and Science in Sports and Exercise, 45*, 1188–1197. http://doi.org/10.1249/MSS.0b013e318281a939.

McMahon, J. A., & Penney, D. (2013). (Self-) surveillance and (self-)regulation: Living by fat numbers within and beyond a sporting culture. *Qualitative Research in Sport, Exercise and Health, 5*, 157–178. http://doi.org/10.1080/2159676X.2012. 712998.

Moesch, K., Mayer, C., & Elbe, A. -M. (2012). Reasons for career termination in Danish elite athletes: Investigating gender differences and the time-point as potential correlates. *Sport Science Review, 21*, 49–68. https://doi.org/10.2478/ v10237-012-0018-2.

Papathomas, A., Petrie, T. A., & Plateau, C. R. (2018). Changes in body image perceptions upon leaving elite sport: The retired female athlete paradox. *Sport, Exercise, and Performance Psychology, 7*, 30–45. https://doi.org/10.1037/spy0000111.

Papathomas, A., Smith, B., & Lavallee, D. (2015). Family experiences of living with an eating disorder: A narrative analysis. *Journal of Health Psychology, 20*, 313–325. https://doi.org/10.1177/1359105314566608.

Park, S., Tod, D., & Lavallee, D. (2012). Exploring the retirement from sport decision-making process based on the transtheoretical model. *Psychology of Sport and Exercise, 13*, 444–453. https://doi.org/10.1016/j.psychsport.2012.02.003.

Reints, A. (2011). *Validation of the holistic athletic career model and the identification of variables related to athletic retirement.* Brussels: VUB Press.

Roberts, C. -M. (2010). A cross-cultural evaluation of rugby union transitions. *Paper presented at the 26th Annual Conference of the Association of Applied Sport Psychology*, Providence, Rhode Island.

Roberts, C. -M., & Davies, M. O. (2017). Career transition: Current issues in assessment. In J. Taylor (Ed.), *Assessment in sport psychology consulting.* Champaign, IL: Human Kinetics.

Roberts, C. -M., & Kenttä, G. (2018). Motherhood as an athletic career transition. *Paper presented at the Inaugural Women in Sport & Exercise Conference*, Stoke-on-Trent, Staffordshire.

Roberts, C. -M., Mullen, R., Evans, L., & Hall, R. J. (2015). An in-depth appraisal of career termination experiences in elite cricket. *Journal of Sport Science, 33*, 935–944. https://doi.org/10.1080/02640414.2014.977936.

Salinas, P. C., & Bagni, C. (2017). Gender equality from a European perspective: Myth and reality. *Neuron, 96*, 721–729. https://doi.org/10.1016/j.neuron.2017.10.002.

Schulz, R., & Curnow, C. (1988). Peak performance and age among superathletes: Track and field, swimming, baseball, tennis, and golf. *Journal of Gerontology, 43*, 113–120. https://doi.org/10.1093/geronj/43.5.P113.

Scraton, S., & Flintoff, A. (2002). *Gender and sport: A reader.* London: Routledge.

Seiler, R., Anders, G., & Irlinger, P. (Eds.). (1998). *Das Leben nach dem Spitzensport. La vie après le sport de haut niveau* [Life after elite level sport]. Paris: INSEP.

Stambulova, N. B. (2001). Sport career termination of Russian athletes: Readiness for the transition. *Paper presented at the 10th World Congress of Sport Psychology*, Skiathos, Hellas, Greece.

Stambulova, N. B. (2009). Talent development in sport: The perspective of career transitions. In E. Tsung-Min Hung, R. Lidor, & D. Hackfort (Eds.), *Psychology of sport excellence* (pp. 63–74). Morgantown, WV: Fitness Information Technology.

Stambulova, N. B., Alfermann, D., Statler, T., & Côté, J. (2009). ISSP Position stand: Career development and transitions of athletes. *International Journal of Sport and Exercise Psychology, 7*, 395–412. https://doi.org/10.1080/1612197X.2009.9671916.

Stambulova, N. B., & Ryba, T. V. (2013). *Athletes' careers across cultures.* New York: Routledge.

Stambulova, N., Stephan, Y., & Jäphag, U. (2007). Athletic retirement: A crossnational comparison of elite French and Swedish athletes. *Psychology of Sport and Exercise, 8*, 101–118. https://doi.org/10.1016/j.psychsport.2006.05.002.

Stambulova, N. B., & Wylleman, P. (2014). Athletes' career development and transitions. In A. G. Papaioannou & D. Hackfort (Eds.), *Routledge companion to sport and exercise psychology.* London: Routledge.

Taylor, J., & Ogilvie, B. (1994). A conceptual model of adaptation to retirement among athletes. *Journal of Applied Sport Psychology, 6*, 1–20. https://doi.org/10.1080/10413209408406462.

Wylleman, P., Alfermann, D., & Lavallee, D. (2004). Career transitions in sport: European perspectives. *Psychology of Sport & Exercise, 5*, 7–20. https://doi.org/10.1016/S1469-0292(02)00049-3.

Young, J. A., Pearce, A. J., Kane, R., & Pain, M. (2006). Leaving the professional tennis circuit: exploratory study of experiences and reactions from elite female athletes. *British Journal of Sports Medicine, 40*, 477–483. https://doi.org/10.1136/bjsm.2005.023341.

19 Cardiovascular health and the exercising female

Karen Birch and Gemma Lyall

Introduction

Cardiovascular disease (CVD) remains a leading cause of morbidity and mortality accounting for 31 per cent of worldwide deaths (Hajar, 2016). Moreover, the World Health Organization (WHO) estimates that the burden of CVD will increase further.

Females typically present with fewer CVD risk factors compared to age-matched males, while the development of CVD has been reported to occur 7–10 years later in women than in men (Maas et al., 2011). Increasing CVD risk in females coincides with the onset of menopause and resultant loss of oestrogen, with CVD risk becoming equivalent to risk in age-matched males. Specific CVD risk factors appear to have a greater impact upon females: the relative risk of myocardial infarction in female smokers was 50 per cent higher than risk in male smokers (Prescott, Hippe, Schnohr, Hein, & Vestbo, 1998); hypertension is more prevalent in older females, attributed to a steeper rise in systolic blood pressure (Staessen et al., 2001); type 2 diabetes in females results in higher cardiovascular-related mortality than in male counterparts (Maas & Appelman, 2010); and prevalence of hypercholesterolaemia is lower in younger females compared with aged-matched males, but above 55 years of age low-density lipoprotein cholesterol (LDL-C) is higher in females (Maas & Appelman, 2010). Cardiovascular disease risk factors of this nature account for 60 per cent of CVD risk, with the remaining 40 per cent thought to be directly related to changes in the vascular environment. As circulating oestrogens are capable of conveying direct effects upon the vasculature, the role of oestrogen deficiency in enhancing CVD risk may be via alterations in both traditional risk factors and/or alterations in vascular integrity. The potential impact of oestrogen loss is summarised in Figure 19.1.

A number of CVD risk factors in women have been targeted with menopausal hormone treatment; however, following the original results of the Women's Health Initiative (WHI) indicating a potential increase in risk of breast cancer and risk of coronary heart disease, prescriptions have significantly fallen. Later analysis of the WHI data revealed a protective

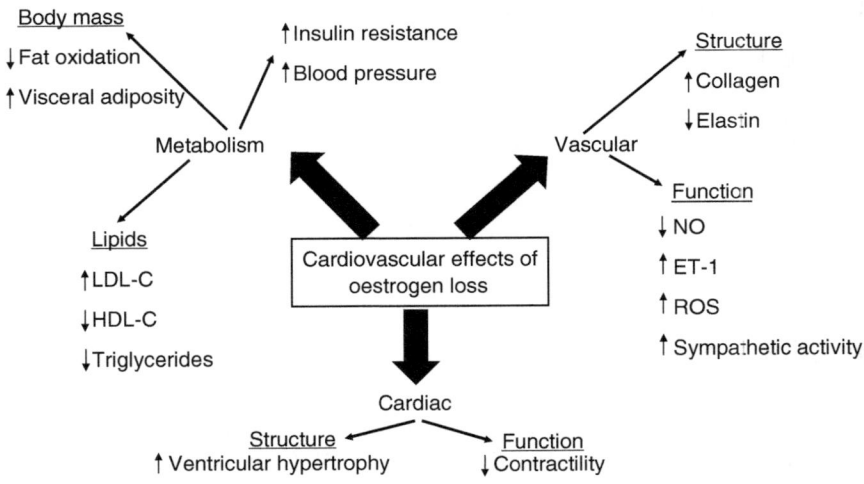

Figure 19.1 The effects of oestrogen loss, for example, after menopause, upon parameters of cardiovascular health.

Key
NO, nitric oxide; ET-1, endothelin-1; ROS, reactive oxygen species; LDL-C, low-density lipoprotein cholesterol; HDL-C, high-density lipoprotein cholesterol.

effect of menopausal hormone treatment in the early years of menopause, but that this impact decreased incrementally with time post menopause. Additionally, oral and transdermal routes of application and formulation of treatments affected outcomes (see Miller & Harman, 2017). Contiguously to the increased risk of CVD for the ageing female, it is known that 6–10 per cent of all global deaths from non-communicable diseases are attributed to physical inactivity (Lee et al., 2012). Currently, 34 per cent of females globally are judged to be physically inactive compared to 28 per cent of males (Hallal et al., 2012), while physical activity is associated with a 35 per cent reduction in cardiovascular mortality (Nocon et al., 2008). Notably, physically active postmenopausal females are at a lower risk of developing coronary heart disease in comparison to less physically active postmenopausal women (Manson et al., 2002). In this chapter, the cardioprotective effects of oestrogen are assessed, and the impact of exercise in hypo-oestrogenic conditions are considered. Details of hormonal contraception and menopausal hormone treatment have been discussed in more detail elsewhere in this book (Chapters 4 and 20, respectively).

Aims of the chapter

The aims of the chapter are as follows:

1   To understand the role of oestrogen in maintaining cardiovascular health.
2   To understand how the loss of oestrogen results in cardiovascular pathology.
3   To understand the role of exercise in restoring cardiovascular health when oestrogen is lost.

Oestrogen over the lifespan

While the risk of CVD in women over the lifespan may be impacted by physiological factors related to body size and/or sociological factors impacting both lifestyle and medical treatment, this chapter will focus upon the impact of fluctuations in key steroidal reproductive hormones. The process of steroidogenesis results in the production of oestrogen, progesterone, and testosterone from cholesterol. In premenopausal women the majority of oestrogen is produced in the granulosa cells of the follicle, with some and the majority of progesterone in the corpus luteum. Androgens are produced in the ovary and adrenal glands. The regulation of the production of these hormones via the hypothalamic pituitary axis varies across the lifespan. In the premenopausal years the major form of oestrogen is 17β-oestradiol, while following the menopause this becomes ovarian-produced oestrone. Oestrogen and progesterone drop to concentrations similar to those of men following the menopause, while testosterone concentration tends to be constant and lower than that of men throughout the lifespan.

The cardioprotective effects of oestrogen are regulated through its receptor complexes oestrogen receptor-alpha (ERα) and oestrogen receptor-beta (ERβ), while progesterone tends to act in opposition. These nuclear receptors are distributed broadly and allow genomic signalling by regulating the expression of target genes in the cell nucleus either directly via oestrogen response elements or indirectly by protein-protein tethering. Nongenomic oestrogen signalling is apparent in oestrogen receptors located in caveolea and lipid rafts of membranes, where interaction with other proteins mediates rapid intracellular signalling pathways. These nongenomic pathways include interactions with growth factor receptors, G proteins (including G protein-coupled oestrogen receptor: GPR30) and tyrosine kinases. It is thought that GPR30 plays a protective role in CVD (Feldman & Limbird, 2017). Thus, oestrogen exerts both rapid and long-term actions.

Oestrogen and metabolic risk

Moving into the postmenopausal status is associated with a decrease in fat oxidation and an increase in total body and visceral adiposity, without changes in energy intake. Longitudinal studies indicate a decrease in energy expenditure and an increase in intra-abdominal fat, independent of age and total fat mass across the menopausal transition (Lovejoy, Champagne, de Jonge, Xie, & Smith, 2008). These alterations are thought to be related to a loss in oestradiol activation of ERα in neurones of the ventromedial nucleus of the hypothalamus. This, in turn, impairs regulation of adipose distribution and activation of brown tissue thermogenesis (Xu et al., 2011). These changes and decreases in fat-free mass serve to alter glucose homeostasis. Decreased ERα action in skeletal muscle and the liver lead to increased oxidative stress, suppressed triglyceride deposition, and subsequent insulin resistance (Zhu et al., 2013). Decreased ERα and ERβ activity also impair β-cell survival and secretion, and thus insulin sensitivity. The EPIC-Interact study indicates an early menopause (<40 years) to be associated with a 32 per cent greater risk of type 2 diabetes compared with those occurring between 50 and 54 years (Brand et al., 2013), while an imbalance between ERα and ERβ expression in diabetes reduces the anti-inflammatory effects of oestrogen.

Oestrogen and arterial wall structure

Oestrogen contributes to arterial structure through regulation of the collagen and elastin fibre ratio. Females demonstrate higher arterial compliance than do males until the age of 50 after which arterial stiffness increases. Systolic blood pressure rises more steeply in ageing females versus males, which may be attributed to increases in arterial stiffness due to loss of oestrogen. Indeed, hypertension in older females is more prevalent compared to males and is associated with an increased incidence of stroke, left ventricular hypertrophy, and heart failure (Maas et al., 2011).

Oestrogen directly impacts cell proliferation and arterial remodelling by reducing collagen deposition and increasing elastin deposition. Natoli and colleagues (2005) indicated that all sex steroids reduced collagen deposition in human aortic smooth muscle cells. However, 17β-oestradiol and progesterone produced an 11-fold increase in the elastin: collagen ratio compared to testosterone and was associated with a decreased systemic vascular resistance. Postmenopausal women not taking hormone replacement therapy (HRT) are reported to have significantly reduced arterial compliance (0.26 ± 0.02 AU), compared to premenopausal women (0.57 ± 0.04 AU), and postmenopausal women taking HRT (0.43 ± 0.02 AU), suggesting greater arterial stiffness (Rajkumar et al., 1997). Indeed, withdrawal of HRT for 4 weeks significantly reduced systemic arterial compliance by 15 per cent, while resuming HRT for four weeks returned arterial compliance to prewithdrawal levels (Waddell et al., 1999).

Oestrogen and vascular function

Oestrogen exerts both nongenomic and genomic effects within the vasculature. Nongenomic effects include regulation of vasomotor tone and nitric oxide (NO) production within endothelial cells. Vascular control in premenopausal women is predominantly parasympathetic in nature, switching to greater sympathetic regulation following the menopause. Genomic effects include reduced incidence of atherosclerosis, reductions in vascular injury, increased endothelial cell growth, and decreased smooth muscle cell growth contributing to a healthy vascular environment.

Oestrogen promotes nitric oxide production

Endothelial cells maintain arterial wall impermeability, prevent atherosclerotic plaque formation, and control vasomotor tone, thus regulating pressure throughout the vascular system. An important vasodilator that contributes to platelet inhibition is NO. It is synthesised within endothelial cells before migrating to vascular smooth muscle cells, inducing relaxation, and thus contributing to maintenance of healthy vasculature function.

Oestrogen binds to ERα and ERβ on the endothelial surface. Oestrogen receptor-α is the primary receptor responsible for the atheroprotective effects that oestrogen exerts upon the endothelium. Expression of ERα is modulated by oestrogen status with low levels of ERα expression observed at lower oestrogen concentrations. In contrast, ERβ is required for normal vasodilation and regulation of blood pressure in both males and females. Binding of oestrogen to ERα at the plasma membrane induces a rapid signalling cascade, which stimulates the PI3K/Akt pathway. This results in increased modulation of endothelial nitric oxide synthase (eNOS) activity through rapid phosphorylation of eNOS at serine[1177] producing greater enzyme activity and upregulating NO, thus inducing vasodilation. Longer onset and duration of oestrogen action involves oestrogen binding to ERα and ERβ resulting in increased gene expression of eNOS messenger RNA (mRNA) and protein, resulting in enhanced NO bioavailability and improved vasodilatory capacity.

Oestrogen also plays a role in the regulation of cyclooxygenase within the endothelium. Cyclooxygenase is an enzyme responsible for the production of prostaglandins such as prostacyclin. Prostacyclin, an effective vasodilator, inhibits platelet activation and aggregation, thus promoting healthy vascular function. Oestradiol binds to ERα, which increases the expression of cyclooxygenase-1 and, in turn, upregulates prostacyclin production.

Loss of oestrogen, e.g., during menopause, removes inhibition of the production of the potent vasoconstrictor endothelin-1 (ET-1) at the mRNA level. Upregulation of ET-1, a direct antagonist to NO, impairs NO production and downregulates eNOS expression. Oestrogen treatment (phytoestrogen genistein) in postmenopausal females resulted in increases in endothelial function and decreases in ET-1 over 6 months of treatment (Squadrito et al., 2002). However, oestrogen replacement in older postmenopausal women (>80 years) or women with established CVD was less effective at maintaining endothelial function than in younger postmenopausal women free of CVD (Herrington et al., 2001).

Oestrogen counteracts reactive oxygen species production

Oxidative stress is a major cause of vascular damage, with ageing and disease contributing to greater inflammation. Oxidative stress is caused by production of reactive oxygen species (ROS) molecules, which include superoxide anions and peroxynitrite. In addition to being a potent vasodilator, NO acts as an anti-inflammatory molecule within the endothelium by scavenging ROS and decreasing leucocyte recruitment. Oestrogen further acts as an antioxidant through upregulation and activation of superoxide dismutase (SOD), contributing to clearance of superoxide anions within vascular smooth muscle cells.

It is difficult to delineate the effect of chronological ageing, which itself promotes inflammation, and the role of oestrogen loss upon changes in inflammatory pathways. Actions of SOD were not different between pre- and postmenopausal women (Bednarek-Tupikowska et al., 2006). However, menopausal declines in circulating oestrogen are associated with overproduction of pro-inflammatory cytokines such as interleukin-1β, interleukin-6 and tumour necrosis factor alpha (TNFα) (Chakrabarti, Lekontseva, & Davidge, 2008). Importantly, production of TNFα stimulates the synthesis and release of chemokines and adhesion molecules (e.g., ICAM-1 and E-selectin) leading to leucocyte recruitment (Korpelainen et al., 1993). TNFα further acts to activate nicotinamide adenine dinucleotide phosphate (NADPH), oxidase and downregulate eNOS (Chakrabarti et al., 2008). These actions culminate in inflammation of the endothelium, which may further contribute to vascular dysfunction and atherosclerotic risk in postmenopausal women.

Oestrogen and cardiac function

Oestrogen exerts both genomic and nongenomic effects on the myocardium by binding to receptors ERα and ERβ within cardiomyocytes. Nongenomic effects of oestrogen include increases in the contractile force of the heart and shortening of ventricular myocytes via oestrogen-mediated reductions in calcium current conductance. Long-term effects of oestrogen upon the myocardium involve increased expression of inducible NOS and eNOS.

Healthy women demonstrate greater cardiac contractility compared to age-matched males, with menopausal hormone treatment withdrawal leading to reduced cardiac contractility in females (Mendelsohn & Karas, 2005). Sex differences in contractility have been suggested to occur as a result of differences in intracellular calcium handling in cardiomyocytes. While left ventricular mass is smaller in females versus males, with age, myocardial mass is better preserved in women. This sex difference has been attributed to differences in cardiac expression of glycolytic and mitochondrial metabolic enzymes (Yan et al., 2004), prevention of cardiac fibrosis through ERβ pathways (Pedram, Razandi, O'Mahony, Lubahn, & Levin, 2010), and/ or effects of 17β-oestradiol on cardiomyocytes mediated by the ERα and PI3K/Akt pathways (Patten et al., 2004).

In addition to sex differences in cardiac structure and function, sex differences are also evident when examining the development of cardiac pathologies. Cardiac hypertrophy occurs in response to pressure or volume overload causing myocytes to lengthen. Oestrogen increases the expression of atrial natriuretic factor, which possesses anti-hypertrophic effects; indeed, following the menopause left ventricular hypertrophy becomes more prevalent (Hinderliter et al., 2002). Oestrogen deficiency facilitates, while oestrogen replacement prevents, the development of both right and left ventricular hypertrophy in rodent models of left ventricular hypertrophy, likely mediated by ERβ (Farhat et al., 1993). Ventricular hypertrophy contributes to heart failure of which at least 50 per cent of patients are female. Females with heart failure typically demonstrate preserved ejection fraction, suggesting diastolic heart failure, with the cause of heart failure attributed to hypertension (thus afterload) and diabetes. Indeed, females with heart failure tend to have smaller hearts with greater hypertrophy compared to those of males, which may be due to sex-specific gene expression, inducing different myocyte phenotypes (Maas et al., 2011). Chronic oestrogen administration in rats with sustained heart failure reduced total peripheral resistance and reduced left ventricular end-diastolic pressure (Nekooeian & Pang, 1998). Furthermore, 17β-oestradiol appears to increase the survival of cardiomyocytes following a myocardial infarction (Patten & Karas, 2006); indeed, oestrogen administration following a myocardial infarction in postmenopausal females has been associated with reduced mortality (Shlipak et al., 2001).

Exercise exerts a protective effect upon the cardiovascular system and can reverse declines in cardiovascular health

Physically active females have lower CVD risk

It is well known that physical activity reduces CVD-related morbidity and mortality. Notably, given the research that highlighted potentially adverse effects of menopausal hormone treatment, lifestyle factors including physical activity and exercise may play a significant role in reducing CVD risk in postmenopausal women. In females who are sedentary and who sit for long periods of time, a 63 per cent greater risk of CVD has been observed compared to physically active females who sit for shorter periods (Chomistek et al., 2013).

The Women's Health Study demonstrated that physically active females had lower weight and lower prevalence of CVD risk factors than inactive women. Lower levels of inflammatory and haemostatic biomarkers (e.g., C-reactive protein [CRP], fibrinogen, and ICAM-1) in more physically active women provided the greatest contribution in overall reduced CVD risk, followed by blood pressure, lipids (total, LDL-C, high-density lipoprotein cholesterol [HDL-C]), and body mass index (BMI), with a smaller contribution attributed to glucose (Mora, Cook, Buring, Ridker, & Lee, 2007).

Arterial stiffness is reduced in habitually endurance-trained, postmenopausal women compared to age-matched sedentary controls, with sedentary postmenopausal women demonstrating improvements in arterial stiffness following endurance exercise training (Moreau, Donato, Seals, DeSouza, & Tanaka, 2003). In contrast to males, lifelong exercise in females was not seen to be protective against age/menopausal associated decline in vascular function (Santos-Parker, Strahler, Vorwald, Pierce, & Seals, 2017). Endothelial function, measured via brachial artery flow-mediated dilation, was 34 per cent and 45 per cent lower in sedentary and active postmenopausal women, respectively, than it was in younger females (Santos-Parker et al., 2017). Interestingly, active postmenopausal women had lower circulating levels of CRP and oxidised LDL-C suggesting a favourable CVD risk profile; however, these factors were not correlated with flow-mediated dilation (Santos-Parker et al., 2017).

Exercise training modifies CVD risk factors in females

Implementation of an exercise training intervention can be used to prevent and/or reverse poor cardiovascular health in females. Aerobic exercise training for 12 weeks improved indices of cardiorespiratory fitness, decreased total cholesterol, increased apolipoprotein A-1, and surprisingly decreased HDL-C in both pre- and postmenopausal women, although no changes in LDL-C were observed. Only very small changes in body weight were observed (Blumenthal et al., 1991). When aerobic and resistance exercise training were combined for eight weeks of exercise training in postmenopausal women, there was a significant reduction in BMI and body fat compared to those who undertook aerobic exercise training only. Change in body composition was accompanied by reductions in CRP, TNFα, and total cholesterol (Lee, Kim, Seo, Kim, & Yoon, 2015). Resistance exercise for 16 weeks in postmenopausal women resulted in reductions in fasting blood glucose in addition to decreased body fat, but no changes in lipids (Conceição et al., 2013). Aerobic exercise training for six months has been shown to reduce resting glucose in postmenopausal women, with greater doses of exercise, as determined by higher energy expenditures, associated with the greatest reductions in resting glucose and systolic blood pressure (Earnest et al., 2013).

Following aerobic exercise training in postmenopausal women, Swift, Earnest, Blair, and Church (2011) indicated an improvement in endothelial function, although the greatest improvements occurred in individuals with pre-existing endothelial dysfunction. Reversal of endothelial dysfunction with exercise has also been shown in females following an eight-week aerobic exercise training intervention. Flow-mediated dilation increased significantly in the exercise group with no change in the age-matched inactive controls (Akazawa et al., 2012). During exercise there are increases in blood flow through arteries creating frictional force, or wall shear stress, along the endothelium. Increases in shear stress with exercise activates the PI3K/Akt pathway in endothelial cells, the same pathway activated by oestrogen and resulting in greater production of NO. Bioavailability of NO is improved through upregulation of eNOS gene expression, increased circulation of vascular endothelial growth factor (inducing angiogenesis and stimulating Akt-dependent eNOS phosphorylation), reduced NO inactivation, and an enhanced antioxidant system.

Moderate- and vigorous-intensity exercise for 12 weeks significantly reduced carotid artery stiffness by 27–29 per cent in postmenopausal women (Sugawara et al., 2006). Postmenopausal women, assigned to 12 weeks of combined aerobic and resistance exercise, demonstrated decreases in systolic and diastolic blood pressure accompanied by a decrease in peripheral arterial stiffness compared to a control group of sedentary postmenopausal women (Figueroa, Park, Seo, Sanchez-Gonzalez, & Baek, 2011). Exercise-induced changes in arterial structure may be due to a reduction in advanced glycation end-products, which are responsible for cross linking of collagen fibres and subsequent arterial stiffness (Bailey, 2001). Following an exercise training intervention in rats, there was a significant reduction in plasma advanced glycation end-products in exercise-trained versus sedentary rats (Boor et al., 2009). Additionally, Maeda and colleagues (2003) demonstrated significantly reduced blood pressure and plasma ET-1 concentrations in older, postmenopausal women following three months of cycling training. Exercise-induced reductions in ET-1 were associated with significant improvements in arterial compliance and significant reductions in systolic blood pressure (Maeda et al., 2009).

While peripheral adaptations appear to readily improve in response to exercise training, central adaptations, for example, changes in cardiac structure and function, are less apparent. Endurance exercise training for eight months in postmenopausal women increased resting left ventricular end-diastolic dimension and left ventricular ejection fraction compared to a control group (Morrison et al., 1986). However, in contrast to older males who demonstrate attenuation of age-related declines in left ventricular function following exercise, Spina, Ogawa, Miller, Kohrt, and Ehsani (1993) reported no change in left ventricular structure or function following 9–12 months of endurance exercise training in older females. Alterations in cardiac structure and function following exercise training are yet to be fully explored in relation to postmenopausal women and are, therefore, an important area for future research.

Practical recommendations based on research

Recommendations for using physical activity and exercise for primary and secondary prevention of CVD do not differ from exercise prescription guidelines. Maintenance/improvement of cardiovascular health can be achieved by:

- Increasing the volume of physical activity undertaken every day (walking, standing etc.).
- Taking part in higher-intensity exercise conducted in intervals of any duration.
- Taking part in low-intensity, high repetition weight training to improve insulin resistance.

Real-world example

In a Dunhill Medical Trust-funded training study of postmenopausal women not using menopausal hormone treatment in our laboratories, cycling exercise conducted in intervals at higher intensities resulted in positive changes in HDL-C, BMI, and arterial stiffness. Most importantly every woman in the study reported feeling stronger, experiencing better sleep, feeling more confident about exercise, and reported a perception of overall better health.

Summary

Oestrogen enhances cardiovascular structure and function. Reductions in oestrogen production through amenorrhoea or menopause result in elevated CVD risk. Exercise training and regular physical activity can be used as a tool to restore cardiovascular health.

References

Akazawa, N., Choi, Y., Miyaki, A., Tanabe, Y., Sugawara, J., Ajisaka, R., & Maeda, S. (2012). Curcumin ingestion and exercise training improve vascular endothelial function in postmenopausal women. *Nutrition Research, 32*(10), 795–799. https://doi.org/10.1016/j.nutres.2012.09.002.
Bailey, A. J. (2001). Molecular mechanisms of ageing in connective tissues. *Mechanisms of Ageing and Development, 122*(7), 735–755. https://doi.org/10.1016/S0047-6374(01)00225-1.
Bednarek-Tupikowska, G., Tworowska, U., Jedrychowska, I., Radomska, B., Tupikowski, K., Bidzinska-Speichert, B., & Milewicz, A. (2006). Effects of

oestradiol and oestroprogestin on erythrocyte antioxidative enzyme system activity in postmenopausal women. *Clinical Endocrinology, 64*(4), 463–468. https://doi.org/10.1111/j.1365-2265.2006.02494.x.

Blumenthal, J. A., Matthews, K., Fredrikson, M., Rifai, N., Schniebolk, S., German, D., ... Rodin, J. (1991). Effects of exercise training on cardiovascular function and plasma lipid, lipoprotein, and apolipoprotein concentrations in premenopausal and postmenopausal women. *Arteriosclerosis, Thrombosis, and Vascular Biology, 11*(4), 912–917. https://doi.org/10.1161/01.ATV.11.4.912.

Boor, P., Celec, P., Behuliak, M., Grančič, P., Kebis, A., Kukan, M., ... Šebeková, K. (2009). Regular moderate exercise reduces advanced glycation and ameliorates early diabetic nephropathy in obese Zucker rats. *Metabolism, 58*(11), 1669–1677. https://doi.org/10.1016/j.metabol.2009.05.025.

Brand, J. S. van der Schouw, Y. T., Onland-Moret, N. C., Sharp, S. J., Ong, K. K., Khaw, K.-T., ... The InterAct, C. (2013). Age at menopause, reproductive life span, and type 2 diabetes risk: Results from the EPIC-InterAct study. *Diabetes Care, 36*(4), 1012–1019. https://doi.org/10.2337/dc12-1020.

Chakrabarti, S., Lekontseva, O., & Davidge, S. T. (2008). Estrogen is a modulator of vascular inflammation. *IUBMB Life, 60*(6), 376–382. https://doi.org/10.1002/iub.48.

Chomistek, A. K., Manson, J. E., Stefanick, M. L., Lu, B., Sands-Lincoln, M., Going, S. B., ... Eaton, C. B. (2013). Relationship of sedentary behavior and physical activity to incident cardiovascular disease: Results from the women's health initiative. *Journal of the American College of Cardiology, 61*(23), 2346–2354. https://doi.org/10.1016/j.jacc.2013.03.031.

Conceição, M. S., Bonganha, V., Vechin, F. C., De Barros Berton, R. P., Lixandrão, M. E., Nogueira, F. R. D., ... Libardi, C. A. (2013). Sixteen weeks of resistance training can decrease the risk of metabolic syndrome in healthy postmenopausal women. *Clinical Interventions in Aging, 8*, 1221–1228. https://doi.org/10.2147/CIA.S44245.

Earnest, C. P., Johannsen, N. M., Swift, D. L., Lavie, C. J., Blair, S. N., & Church, T. S. (2013). Dose effect of cardiorespiratory exercise on metabolic syndrome in postmenopausal women. *American Journal of Cardiology, 111*(12), 1805–1811. https://doi.org/10.1016/j.amjcard.2013.02.037.

Farhat, M. Y., Chen, M. F., Bhatti, T., Iqbal, A., Cathapermal, S., & Ramwell, P. W. (1993). Protection by oestradiol against the development of cardiovascular changes associated with monocrotaline pulmonary hypertension in rats. *British Journal of Pharmacology, 110*(2), 719–723. https://doi.org/10.1111/j.1476-5381.1993.tb13871.x.

Feldman, R. D., & Limbird, L. E. (2017). GPER (GPR30): A nongenomic receptor (GPCR) for steroid hormones with implications for cardiovascular disease and cancer. *Annual Review of Pharmacology and Toxicology, 57*, 567–584. https://doi.org/10.1146/annurev-pharmtox-010716-104651.

Figueroa, A., Park, S. Y., Seo, D. Y., Sanchez-Gonzalez, M. A., & Baek, Y. H. (2011). Combined resistance and endurance exercise training improves arterial stiffness, blood pressure, and muscle strength in postmenopausal women. *Menopause, 18*(9), 980–984. https://doi.org/10.1097/gme.0b013e3182135442.

Hallal, P. C., Andersen, L. B., Bull, F. C., Guthold, R., Haskell, W., & Ekelund, U. (2012). Global physical activity levels: surveillance progress, pitfalls, and prospects. *The Lancet, 380*(9838), 247–257. https://doi.org/10.1016/S0140-6736(12)60646-1.

Hajar, R. (2016). Framingham contribution to cardiovascular disease. *Heart Views: The Official Journal of the Gulf Heart Association, 17*(2), 78–81. https://doi.org/10.4103/1995-705X.185130.

Herrington, D. M., Espeland, M. A., Crouse, J. R., Robertson, J., Riley, W. A., McBurnie, M. A., & Burke, G. L. (2001). Estrogen replacement and brachial artery flow-mediated vasodilation in older women. *Arteriosclerosis, Thrombosis, and Vascular Biology, 21*(12), 1955–1961. https://doi.org/10.1161/hq1201.100241.

Hinderliter, A. L., Sherwood, A., Blumenthal, J. A., Light, K. C., Girdler, S. S., McFetridge, J., … Waugh, R. (2002). Changes in hemodynamics and left ventricular structure after menopause. *American Journal of Cardiology, 89*(7), 830–833. https://doi.org/10.1016/S0002-9149(02)02193-8.

Korpelainen, E. I., Gamble, J. R., Smith, W. B., Goodall, G. J., Qiyu, S., Woodcock, J. M., … Lopez, A. F. (1993). The receptor for interleukin 3 is selectively induced in human endothelial cells by tumor necrosis factor alpha and potentiates interleukin 8 secretion and neutrophil transmigration. *Proceedings of the National Academy of Sciences of the United States of America, 90*(23), 11137–11141.

Lee, I. M., Shiroma, E. J., Lobelo, F., Puska, P., Blair, S. N., & Katzmarzyk, P. T. (2012). Effect of physical inactivity on major non-communicable diseases worldwide: an analysis of burden of disease and life expectancy. *The Lancet, 380*(9838), 219–229. https://doi.org/10.1016/S0140-6736(12)61031-9.

Lee, J. S., Kim, C. G., Seo, T. B., Kim, H. G., & Yoon, S. J. (2015). Effects of 8-week combined training on body composition, isokinetic strength, and cardiovascular disease risk factors in older women. *Aging Clinical and Experimental Research, 27*(2), 179–186. https://doi.org/10.1007/s40520-014-0257-4.

Lovejoy, J. C., Champagne, C. M., de Jonge, L., Xie, H., & Smith, S. R. (2008). Increased visceral fat and decreased energy expenditure during the menopausal transition. *International Journal of Obesity (2005), 32*(6), 949–958. https://doi.org/10.1038/ijo.2008.25.

Maas, A. H. E. M., & Appelman, Y. E. A. (2010). Gender differences in coronary heart disease. *Netherlands Heart Journal, 18*(12), 598–603. https://doi.org/10.1007/s12471-010-0841-y.

Maas, A. H. E. M., van der Schouw, Y. T., Regitz-Zagrosek, V., Swahn, E., Appelman, Y. E., Pasterkamp, G., … Stramba-Badiale, M. (2011). Red alert for women's heart: the urgent need for more research and knowledge on cardiovascular disease in women. Proceedings of the workshop held in Brussels on gender differences in cardiovascular disease, 29 September 2010. *European Heart Journal, 32*(11), 1362–1368. https://doi.org/10.1093/eurheartj/ehr048.

Maeda, S., Sugawara, J., Yoshizawa, M., Otsuki, T., Shimojo, N., Jesmin, S., … Tanaka, H. (2009). Involvement of endothelin-1 in habitual exercise-induced increase in arterial compliance. *Acta Physiologica, 196*(2), 223–229. https://doi.org/10.1111/j.1748-1716.2008.01909.x.

Maeda, S., Tanabe, T., Miyauchi, T., Otsuki, T., Sugawara, J., Iemitsu, M., … Matsuda, M. (2003). Aerobic exercise training reduces plasma endothelin-1 concentration in older women. *Journal of Applied Physiology, 95*(1), 336–341. https://doi.org/10.1152/japplphysiol.01016.2002.

Manson, J. E., Greenland, P., LaCroix, A. Z., Stefanick, M. L., Mouton, C. P., Oberman, A., … Siscovick, D. S. (2002). Walking compared with vigorous exercise for the prevention of cardiovascular events in women. *New England Journal of Medicine, 347*(10), 716–725. https://doi.org/10.1056/NEJMoa021067.

Mendelsohn, M. E., & Karas, R. H. (2005). Molecular and cellular basis of cardiovascular gender differences. *Science, 308*(5728), 1583–1587. https://doi.org/10.1125/science.1112062.

Miller, V. M., & Harman, S. M. (2017). An update on hormone therapy in postmenopausal women: mini-review for the basic scientist. *American Journal of Physiology-Heart and Circulatory Physiology, 313*(5), H1013–H1021. https://doi.org/10.1152/ajpheart.00383.2017.

Mora, S., Cook, N., Buring, J. E., Ridker, P. M., & Lee, I. -M. (2007). Physical activity and reduced risk of cardiovascular events. *Potential Mediating Mechanisms, 116*(19), 2110–2118. https://doi.org/10.1161/CIRCULATIONAHA.107.729939.

Moreau, K. L., Donato, A. J., Seals, D. R., DeSouza, C. A., & Tanaka, H. (2003). Regular exercise, hormone replacement therapy and the age-related decline in carotid arterial compliance in healthy women. *Cardiovascular Research, 57*(3), 861–868. https://doi.org/10.1016/S0008-6363(02)00777-0.

Morrison, D. A., Boyden, T. W., Pamenter, R. W., Freund, B. J., Stini, W. A., Harrington, R., & Wilmore, J. H. (1986). Effects of aerobic training on exercise tolerance and echocardiographic dimensions in untrained postmenopausal women. *American Heart Journal, 112*(3), 561–567. https://doi.org/10.1016/0002-8703(86)90522-3.

Natoli, A. K., Medley, T. L., Ahimastos, A. A., Drew, B. G., Thearle, D. J., Dilley, R. J., & Kingwell, B. A. (2005). Sex steroids modulate human aortic smooth muscle cell matrix protein deposition and matrix metalloproteinase expression. *Hypertension, 46*(5), 1129–1134. https://doi.org/10.1161/01.HYP.0000187016.06549.96.

Nekooeian, A. A., & Pang, C. C. (1998). Estrogen restores role of basal nitric oxide in control of vascular tone in rats with chronic heart failure. *American Journal of Physiology-Heart and Circulatory Physiology, 274*(6), H2094–H2099. https://doi.org/10.1152/ajpheart.1998.274.6.H2094.

Nocon, M., Hiemann, T., Müller-Riemenschneider, F., Thalau, F., Roll, S., & Willich, S. N. (2008). Association of physical activity with all-cause and cardiovascular mortality: a systematic review and meta-analysis. *European Journal of Cardiovascular Prevention & Rehabilitation, 15*(3), 239–246. https://doi.org/10.1097/HJR.0b013e3282f55e09.

Patten, R. D., & Karas, R. H. (2006). Estrogen replacement and cardiomyocyte protection. *Trends in Cardiovascular Medicine, 16*(3), 69–75. https://doi.org/10.1016/j.tcm.2006.01.002.

Patten, R. D., Pourati, I., Aronovitz, M. J., Baur, J., Celestin, F., Chen, X., ... Grohe, C. (2004). 17β-Estradiol reduces cardiomyocyte apoptosis in vivo and in vitro via activation of phospho-inositide-3 kinase/Akt signaling. *Circulation Research, 95*(7), 692–699. https://doi.org/10.1161/01.RES.0000144126.57786.89.

Pedram, A., Razandi, M., O'Mahony, F., Lubahn, D., & Levin, E. R. (2010). Estrogen receptor-β prevents cardiac fibrosis. *Molecular Endocrinology, 24*(11), 2152–2165. https://doi.org/10.1210/me.2010-0154.

Prescott, E., Hippe, M., Schnohr, P., Hein, H. O., & Vestbo, J. (1998). Smoking and risk of myocardial infarction in women and men: longitudinal population study. *British Medical Journal, 316*(7137), 1043. https://doi.org/10.1136/bmj.316.7137.1043.

Rajkumar, C., Kingwell, B. A., Cameron, J. D., Waddell, T., Mehra, R., Christophidis, N., ... Dart, A. M. (1997). Hormonal therapy increases arterial compliance in postmenopausal women. *Journal of the American College of Cardiology, 30*(2), 350–356. https://doi.org/10.1016/S0735-1097(97)00191-5.

Santos-Parker, J. R., Strahler, T. R., Vorwald, V. M., Pierce, G. L., & Seals, D. R. (2017). Habitual aerobic exercise does not protect against micro- or macrovascular endothelial dysfunction in healthy estrogen-deficient postmenopausal women. *Journal of Applied Physiology, 122*(1), 11–19. https://doi.org/10.1152/japplphysiol.00732.2016.

Shlipak, M. G., Angeja, B. G., Go, A. S., Frederick, P. D., Canto, J. G., & Grady, D. (2001). Hormone therapy and in-hospital survival after myocardial infarction in postmenopausal women. *Circulation, 104*(19), 2300–2304. https://doi.org/10.1161/hc4401.98414.

Spina, R. J., Ogawa, T., Miller, T. R., Kohrt, W. M., & Ehsani, A. A. (1993). Effect of exercise training on left ventricular performance in older women free of cardiopulmonary disease. *The American Journal of Cardiology, 71*(1), 99–104. https://doi.org/10.1016/0002-9149(93)90718-R.

Squadrito, F., Altavilla, D., Morabito, N., Crisafulli, A., D'Anna, R., Corrado, F., … Squadrito, G. (2002). The effect of the phytoestrogen genistein on plasma nitric oxide concentrations, endothelin-1 levels and endothelium dependent vasodilation in postmenopausal women. *Atherosclerosis, 163*(2), 339–347. https://doi.org/10.1016/S0021-9150(02)00013-8.

Staessen, J., van der Heijden-Spek, J., Safar, M., Den Hond, E., Gasowski, J., Fagard, R., … Van Bortel, L. (2001). Menopause and the characteristics of the large arteries in a population study. *Journal of Human Hhypertension, 15*(8), 511. https://doi.org/10.1038/sj.jhh.1001226.

Sugawara, J., Otsuki, T., Tanabe, T., Hayashi, K., Maeda, S., & Matsuda, M. (2006). Physical activity duration, intensity, and arterial stiffening in postmenopausal women. *American Journal of Hypertension, 19*(10), 1032–1036. https://doi.org/10.1016/j.amjhyper.2006.03.008.

Swift, D. L., Earnest, C. P., Blair, S. N., & Church, T. S. (2011). The effect of different doses of aerobic exercise training on endothelial function in postmenopausal women with elevated blood pressure: results from the DREW study. *British Journal of Sports Medicine, 46*(10), 753–758. https://doi.org/10.1136/bjsports-2011-090025.

Waddell, T. K., Rajkumar, C., Cameron, J. D., Jennings, G. L., Dart, A. M., & Kingwell, B. A. (1999). Withdrawal of hormonal therapy for 4 weeks decreases arterial compliance in postmenopausal women. *Journal of Hypertension, 17*(3), 413–418.

Xu, Y., Nedungadi, T. P., Zhu, L., Sobhani, N., Irani, B. G., Davis, K. E., … Clegg, D. J. (2011). Distinct hypothalamic neurons mediate estrogenic effects on energy homeostasis and reproduction. *Cell Metabolism, 14*(4), 453–465. https://doi.org/10.1016/j.cmet.2011.08.009.

Yan, L., Ge, H., Li, H., Lieber, S., Natividad, F., Resuello, R., … Loo, K. (2004). Gender-specific proteomic alterations in glycolytic and mitochondrial pathways in aging monkey hearts. *Journal of Molecular and Cellular Cardiology, 37*(5), 921–929. https://doi.org/10.1016/j.yjmcc.2004.06.012.

Zhu, L., Brown, W. C., Cai, Q., Krust, A., Chambon, P., McGuinness, O. P., & Stafford, J. M. (2013). Estrogen treatment after ovariectomy protects against fatty liver and may improve pathway-selective insulin resistance. *Diabetes, 62*(2), 424–434. https://doi.org/10.2337/db11-1718.

20 Menopause and the exercising female

Helen Jones, Madeleine France, and David A. Low

Introduction

The menopause is a significant life event characterised by a reduction in the hormone oestrogen (World Health Organization, 1996). Due to an increasing life expectancy, the number of females reaching menopausal age has increased and females spend a significant portion of their lifespan in the postmenopausal state. The menopausal transition (1–5 years) is associated with an increase in cardiovascular disease (CVD) risk and has significant side effects. The primary symptom of the menopause is hot flushes, which are also associated with increased CVD risk (Thurston et al., 2012).

Aims of the chapter

The aims of the chapter are as follows:

1   To present evidence of the positive effects of exercise on cardiovascular health during the menopausal transition and beyond.
2   To discuss how exercising during the menopausal transition can alleviate menopausal symptoms.
3   To make recommendations for females exercising during the menopausal transition.
4   To provide insight into the scientific issues that exercising, postmenopausal females may encounter.

Can exercise training in postmenopausal women enhance cardiorespiratory fitness?

Cardiorespiratory fitness is an important predictor of all-cause mortality (Blair et al., 1996) and morbidity (Fogelholm, 2010). Cardiorespiratory fitness declines with age with a notable decrease following the menopause; for example, cardiorespiratory fitness was $2.7\,\mathrm{ml.kg^{-1}.min^{-1}}$ lower in postmenopausal compared to premenopausal women of similar age (Nyberg

Table 20.1 Summary of cardiorespiratory fitness changes from exercise training studies performed in postmenopausal women

	Author	Exercise modality	Exercise frequency	Exercise duration (weeks)	Time since menopause (years)	Change in fitness (ml.kg^{-1}.min^{-1})
High-intensity	Egelund et al., 2017	Cycling	50 min 3×/week	12	1–8	3.1[2]
	Mandrup et al., 2017b	Cycling	1 hr 3×/week	12	>1	2.2[2]
	Nyberg et al., 2014	Indoor hockey	30 min 2×/week	12	1–3	1.6[2]
	Seidelin et al., 2017	Indoor hockey	1 hr 2×/week	12	1–3	1.4[2]
Moderate-intensity	Hodges et al., 2010b	Aerobic exercise	30 min 3×/week	12	N/A[1]	8.0[2]
	Black et al., 2009	Walking or cycling	30 min 3×/week	24	N/A[1]	7.0[2]
	Bailey et al., 2016b	Aerobic exercise	60 min 5×/week	16	1–4	4.5[2]
	Tanahashi et al., 2014	Walking or cycling	30–60 min 3×/week	12	N/A[1]	3.2[2]
	Swift et al., 2012	Walking or cycling	3 or 4×/week	24	N/A[1]	2.3[2]
Low-intensity	Asikainen et al., 2002	Walking	5×/week	24	2–10	2.9[2]
	Pierce et al., 2011	Walking	50 min 7×/week	8	>1	1.8
	Luoto et al., 2012	Aerobic exercise	50 min 4×/week	24	0.5–3	0.8[2]
	Moreau et al., 2013	Walking	45 min 7×/week	8	>1	-0.2
					Mean	3.0

Notes
1 N/A: not recorded.
2 Statistically significant change compared to baseline.

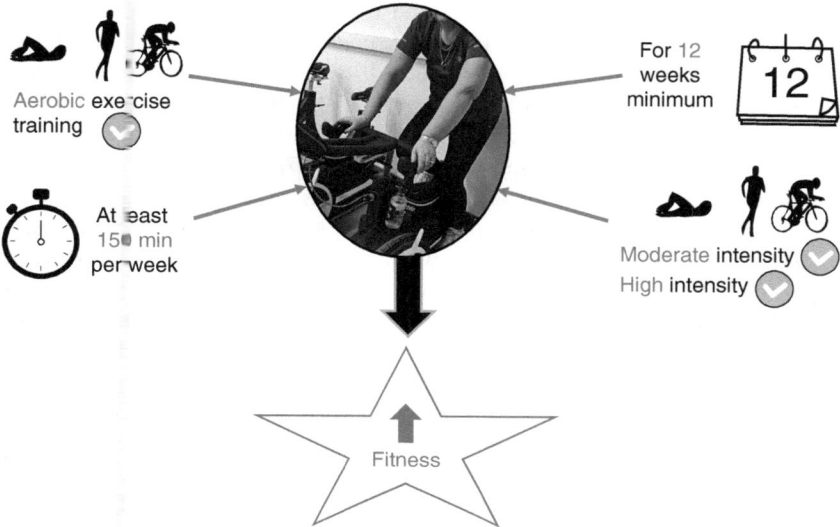

Figure 20.1 Practical recommendations for exercise training to increase cardiorespiratory fitness in postmenopausal women.

et al., 2014). Emerging evidence suggests that cardiorespiratory fitness can be improved during the menopause with exercise training (Table 20.1).

The few studies that have shown exercise training-mediated improvements in cardiorespiratory fitness in postmenopausal women employed aerobic exercise protocols. All but two studies showed a statistically significant improvement in cardiorespiratory fitness (Moreau, Stauffer, Kohrt, & Seals, 2013; Pierce, Eskurza, Walker, Fay, & Seals, 2011). The largest improvements in fitness were observed in studies employing moderate- and high-intensity exercise (see Table 20.1 for references) and/or had a stringent monitoring of individual exercise training sessions with supervision (Bailey et al., 2016a; Bailey et al., 2016b; Black et al., 2009; Hodges et al., 2010b; Tew et al., 2012). From a practical perspective, exercise training regimens, employing aerobic exercise at moderate-to-high intensities for a minimum of 12 weeks, mediate the greatest fitness benefits (Figure 20.1).

Exercise training in postmenopausal women can improve traditional cardiovascular risk factors

Hypertension and cholesterol

The increased CVD risk associated with the menopause is characterised by an increased incidence of hypertension and hypercholesterolaemia (Ben Ali et al., 2016). The menopause is associated with a 0.5 mmHg/year steeper rise in systolic blood pressure (SBP) compared to that of age-matched premeno-pausal women (Staessen, Bulpitt, Fagard, Lijnen, & Amery, 1994). Similarly, significant increases in total cholesterol and low-density lipoprotein choles-terol (LDL-C) levels are evident (Matthews et al., 2009). Exercise interven-tions that increase cardiorespiratory fitness in postmenopausal females also decrease CVD risk factors (Mandrup et al., 2017a; Nyberg et al., 2017; Nyberg et al., 2014). In an elegant attempt to separate the effect of the men-opause from the effect of ageing per se, the Copenhagen Women Study age-matched pre- and postmenopausal women (4.5-year difference between groups) (e.g., Nyberg et al., 2017). In support of elevated CVD risk associ-ated with the menopause, the postmenopausal women displayed higher SBP, total cholesterol, LDL-C, and high-density lipoprotein cholesterol (HDL-C) compared to premenopausal women (Egelund et al., 2017; Mandrup et al., 2017b). They also demonstrated that 12 weeks of high-intensity cycling exercise improved cardiorespiratory fitness and decreased diastolic blood pressure and total LDL-C in early postmenopausal women to a similar extent as it did in late premenopausal women (Mandrup et al., 2017b). Collec-tively, the research evidence suggests that exercise training during the men-opause can reduce CVD risk factors. A thorough overview of cardiovascular health, including that pertinent to postmenopausal women, is given in Chapter 19.

Body composition

Menopause negatively affects body composition, characterised by increased intra-abdominal and gluteo-femoral fat deposition, and reduced lean body mass (Seidelin et al., 2017; Trémollieres, Pouilles, & Ribot, 1996). The accumulation of intra-abdominal fat and loss in lean body mass is associated with an increased risk of type 2 diabetes mellitus (Kalyani, Corriere, & Ferrucci, 2014). Previous research has observed reductions in body fat and increased lean body mass in postmenopausal women (Sternfeld et al., 2004) with some showing similar changes to premenopausal women after exercise training (Mandrup et al., 2017b). Thus, exercise training is an effective method to decrease body fat percentage and attenuate the decline in lean body mass in postmenopausal women.

Metabolic syndrome

The menopausal transition is accompanied by adverse metabolic changes and an increased incidence of metabolic syndrome, defined as a clustering of CVD risk factors (Janssen, Powell, Crawford, Lasley, & Sutton-Tyrrell, 2008). There is a linear relationship between ageing and insulin resistance (DeNino et al., 2001), but this relationship is stronger during the menopause (Janssen et al., 2008). Little research has been conducted to determine how oestrogen affects the muscular insulin signalling cascade and adaptations to physical exercise. Nevertheless, insulin sensitivity in postmenopausal women is lower in comparison to premenopausal women matched for age and body composition (Mandrup et al., 2017a). Yet, with high-intensity exercise training, insulin sensitivity increased similarly in premenopausal and postmenopausal women (Mandrup et al., 2017a), indicating that insulin sensitivity in postmenopausal women can be reversed by exercise training.

Exercise training in the early menopausal period can have enhancements in cardiovascular function that have implications for CVD risk

Vascular function

Vascular dysfunction can precede and predict the future development of hypertension in postmenopausal women, independent of age (Rossi et al., 2004) and CVD risk. The bioavailability of endothelial-derived nitric oxide (NO) is increased via oestrogen (Mendelsohn & Karas, 1999). NO helps to maintain vascular wall health and regulate vasomotor function (Green, Maiorana, O'Driscoll, & Taylor, 2004). In females, the age-related decline in vascular function is exacerbated after the menopausal transition (Taddei et al., 1996) Postmenopausal women exhibit reduced flow-mediated dilation (a marker of large artery NO function) compared to males (Black et al., 2009) and possess higher levels of vascular inflammatory markers indicative of vascular dysfunction compared to premenopausal females of similar age (Nyberg et al., 2014). Exercise training has been proposed to increase the NO bioavailability due to repeated exposure to increased shear stress (Green et al., 2004).

Exercise training alone can elicit improvements in the vasculature of postmenopausal women (Bailey et al., 2016b). One recent study employed 12 weeks of exercise training (indoor hockey, 30 min, twice per week) and observed improved vascular function biomarkers and CVD risk profiles in both age-matched pre- and postmenopausal females (Nyberg et al., 2014). Nevertheless, in another study, postmenopausal females, receiving exogenous oestrogen treatment and exercise training, exhibited improved vascular function, but exercise training alone did not improve vascular function (Moreau et al., 2013). It is probable that oestrogen can enhance the exercise training response, but exercise training, which increases cardiorespiratory fitness, is required for improvements in vascular function during the menopause. Oestrogen's role in cardiovascular health is explored in Chapter 19.

Cardiac function

Aerobic exercise training causes positive adaptations in cardiac structure and function, which contribute to improvements in fitness (Hellsten & Nyberg, 2015). Cardiac adaptations in response to aerobic training appear to be smaller in premenopausal women than in men (Howden et al., 2015); while this could be explained by smaller body size and muscle mass, it has been argued that there is some contribution from oestrogen (Wernstedt et al., 2002). Therefore, hormonal changes after menopause may further reduce the ability of women to achieve cardiac adaptations with exercise training (Moreau, Hildreth, Meditz, Deane, & Kohrt, 2012; Pierce et al., 2011). Egelund and colleagues (2017) compared cardiac structure and function in age-matched pre- and postmenopausal women and assessed the effect of a 12-week, high-intensity exercise training programme. They found that cardiac dimensions and subclinical measures of cardiac function were similar in pre- and postmenopausal women and that exercise training induced similar beneficial adaptations in all women. While this finding suggests hormonal changes associated with the menopause have little impact on cardiac dimensions or functionality, existing literature suggests that oestrogen treatment, via hormone replacement therapy (HRT) during the menopause, improves diastolic function in postmenopausal women (Duygu et al., 2009). On balance, postmenopausal women have the capacity to achieve cardiovascular adaptations in response to exercise training.

The menopause may be an optimal time for exercise-induced improvements

The menopause may be an optimal time period to discuss the benefits of an active lifestyle with females (Gray et al., 2018). There is evidence of greater exercise-mediated changes in postmenopausal women. For example, 12 weeks of indoor hockey decreased body fat by 2.2 per cent in postmenopausal women, whereas there was no change in premenopausal women. A greater increase in lean body mass (1.5 kg compared to 0.7 kg) and an equivalent increase in leg lean mass (0.7 kg) was also observed in postmenopausal compared to premenopausal women (Seidelin et al., 2017). These studies show novel evidence that exercising during the menopausal transition provides physiological enhancements greater than those that occur prior to the menopause. More research separating the effect of menopause and ageing per se is warranted.

The impact of the menopausal transition

The menopause is associated with symptoms including hot flushes, vaginal dryness, reduced libido, sleep disturbance, anxiety, and depression (Bauld & Brown, 2009). Hot flushes are the most common menopausal symptom, experienced by ~70 per cent of women (Thurston, 2018). A hot flush is an extreme thermoregulatory event defined as the sudden and intense sensation of heat, causing skin reddening, flushing, and profuse sweating. Cutaneous vasodilatation increases by ~80 per cent and sweating increases ~5-fold during a hot flush (Bailey et al., 2016b; Low, Davis, Keller, Shibasaki, & Crandall, 2008). Hot flushes significantly impact quality of life by causing anxiety, embarrassment, and depression (Lindh-Åstrand, Nedstrand, Wyon, & Hammar, 2004). Standard effective treatment for hot flushes is HRT but uptake is poor due to concerns about increased risk of CVD (Manson et al., 2003), breast cancer (Murphy, Bartholomew, Carpentier, Bluethmann, & Vernon, 2012), and other contraindications. Guidelines for prescribing alternative emerging pharmacological treatment such as selective serotonin reuptake inhibitors or serotonin-noradrenaline reuptake inhibitors (Nelson et al., 2006) are sparse. Lifestyle interventions are a non-pharmacological alternative, short of the contraindications of HRT.

There is emerging research evidence that postmenopausal women who demonstrate vasomotor symptoms have a higher prevalence of CVD risk factors (Gray et al., 2018; Thurston et al., 2011). Intriguingly, women experiencing menopausal hot flushes and night sweats have increased carotid artery intima media thickness and decreased endothelial function, both risk factors for CVD (Gray et al., 2018; Thurston et al., 2012). The incidence of type 2 diabetes in 150,007 postmenopausal women in the USA was examined from 1993–2014 (Gray et al., 2018), and increased severity and duration of hot flushes were associated with an 18 per cent increase in risk of type 2 diabetes. This finding led to suggestions that hot flushes could be a biomarker of chronic disease in women (Franco et al., 2015). Therefore, targeting hot flushes in postmenopausal women will have dual benefits including improving quality of life and reducing CVD and risk of type 2 diabetes.

The impact of exercise training on menopausal symptoms

A small number of research studies have examined the impact of exercise training on menopausal symptoms (for references, see Table 20.2). Predominantly, the studies have utilised menopause-specific measurement tools, for example, the Menopause Quality of Life questionnaire (Hilditch et al., 1996), which provides subjective data. Generally, all of the exercise training studies show improvements in quality of life and subjective menopausal symptoms in postmenopausal women (Mansikkamaki et al., 2012). For example, studies have shown that exercise training improves psychological symptoms such as depression (Ağil, Abike, Daskapan, Alaca, & Tüzün, 2010), anxiety, and insomnia (Newton et al., 2014), while others have reported benefits in physical symptoms such as urogenital symptoms (Karacan, 2010). Importantly, and in line with the exercise training benefits on fitness, the magnitude of the intensity and duration of exercise training likely mediates the extent of benefits.

Hot flushes

Various studies have directly measured the impact of exercise training on subjective menopausal hot flushes and shown that exercise training decreases hot flush frequency in the range of 4 per cent (Luoto et al., 2012) to 64 per cent (Bailey et al., 2016b) and severity in the range of 5 per cent (Karacan, 2010) to 70 per cent (Bailey et al., 2016a) (Table 20.2). Bailey and colleagues (2016) compared the number of self-reported hot flushes per week between an exercise arm and no-intervention control arm. After adjusting for baseline hot flush frequency/severity, the mean frequency of hot flushes per week was 43 events (70 per cent) lower following the exercise intervention (mean: 18 events/week) versus following a same period of no-intervention control (mean: 60 events/week). Importantly, not all studies have reported a statistically significant reduction in hot flush frequency following exercise training compared with control (Daley et al., 2015; Newton et al., 2014; Sternfeld et al., 2014). Nevertheless, a number of these studies have not employed an exercise stimulus of high enough intensity or duration or with appropriate guidance to cause an increase in cardiorespiratory fitness; or, they did not even assess cardiorespiratory fitness. Overall, higher exercise intensity and longer duration as well as monitoring adherence generally mediated the largest improvements in hot flush frequency and severity (Table 20.2).

One of the major issues in interpreting the impact of exercise training on menopausal hot flushes is how much of a reduction is a meaningful change. In one study with an exercise guidance group and a group that received an educative DVD on the benefits of exercise, hot flush frequency was reduced by 8.9 events/week (22 per cent) more compared with control (Daley et al., 2015). Nevertheless, this change was lower than the authors' selected minimal clinically important difference of 50 per cent. The target reduction in hot flushes was rationalised based on hot flush responses to a drug trial, yet it is possible that a smaller reduction than 50 per cent may still be perceived as meaningful. Therefore, a meaningful reduction in hot flushes combined with the knowledge that exercise training does not incur any of the longer-term side effects that HRT incurs, further support the argument for exercising during the menopausal transition.

Taken together, all of the exercise training studies performed prior to 2015 (Table 20.2) were included in the recommendations for the National Institute for Health and Care Excellence and North American Menopause Society guidelines on menopausal treatment (Carpenter et al., 2015; Sarri, Davies, & Lumsden, 2015). These guidelines included systematic reviews on exercise and menopausal symptoms, and reported that the data on exercise training were inconclusive due to a lack of controlled studies ($n = 5$ included)

Table 20.2 The exercise training-mediated changes in hot flush frequency and severity measured using subjective rating scales

Author	Exercise modality	Exercise frequency	Exercise duration (weeks)	Time since menopause (years)	Scale	Change in frequency (%)	Change in severity (%)
Bailey et al., 2016b	Aerobic exercise	60 min 5×/week	16	1–4	Sloan	64[2]	72[2]
Lindh-Åstrand et al., 2004	Aerobic exercise	60 min 3×/week	36	N/A[1]	Kupperman's Index	50	39
Newton et al., 2014	Yoga	4×/week	12	N/A[1]	Daily diaries	35	15
Sternfeld et al., 2014	Aerobic exercise	60 min 3×/week	12	N/A[1]	Daily diaries	33	17
Daley et al., 2015	Aerobic exercise	30 min 5×/week	24	N/A[1]	Hot flush rating scale	22	N/A[1]
Luoto et al., 2012	Aerobic exercise	50 min 3×/week	12	0.5–2	Women's Health Questionnaire	4[2]	17
Reed et al., 2014	Aerobic exercise	60 min 3×/week	12	<5	Menopausal Quality of Life	N/A[1]	22[2]
Reed et al., 2014	Yoga	1×/week + 20 min practice daily	12	<5	Menopausal Quality of Life	N/A[1]	23[2]
Karacan, 2010	Aerobic exercise	55 min 3×/week	24	N/A[1]	Menopause Rating Scale	N/A[1]	5[2]
Moilanen et al., 2012	Aerobic exercise	50 min 4×/week	24	0.5–3	Women's Health Questionnaire[3]	–	–

Notes
1 N/A: not recorded.
2 Statistically significant change compared to baseline.
3 Unable to determine values.

(Daley, Stokes-Lampard, & Macarthur, 2011, 2009). Nevertheless, one focus of these systematic reviews was a comparison of exercise training interventions to HRT. While it is well established that hot flushes are alleviated by HRT, any lifestyle intervention will be different from HRT mechanistically, given that it does not involve oestrogen, with fewer side effects. The systematic review data, along with the studies reporting subjective changes in menopausal hot flushes, led to exercise not being recommended for menopause management or included in these guideline documents. Yet, the research studies that have been published since (Ağil et al., 2010; Bailey et al., 2016a, 2016b; Egelund et al., 2017; Mandrup et al., 2017a, 2017b; Moilanen et al., 2012; Nyberg et al., 2017, 2014; Seidelin et al., 2017) suggest positive benefits of exercising in the menopausal transition. In a study examining the impact of exercise training on objective menopausal hot flushes for the first time, participants completed a 16-week moderate-intensity exercise training intervention; physiological measurements of core body temperature, sweat rate, skin and cerebral blood flow were recorded (Bailey et al., 2016a). The researchers found that exercise training reduced the sweating and skin blood flow response typically observed during a hot flush episode as well as finding that there was an attenuated decrease in cerebral blood flow (Bailey et al., 2016a). The physiological changes also related to reductions in the subjective description of sweating, skin reddening, and feeling faint/light headed, respectively, thus providing direct evidence that exercise training reduces the physiological severity of menopausal hot flushes through the improvement of thermoregulatory and systemic vascular responses during a hot flush.

Exercise training can improve menopausal hot flushes

Only one study to date has examined the potential physiological mechanisms of how exercise training can improve menopausal hot flushes. The cardiovascular and thermoregulatory control systems are the logical physiological targets for alleviating hot flush outcomes. Both these physiological systems become dysfunctional during the menopause and are implicated in the causal pathway for menopausal hot flushes (Deecher & Dorries, 2007).

Endothelial function

The severity of hot flushes is linked to vascular (endothelial) dysfunction in postmenopausal women (Bechlioulis et al., 2010). Endothelial dysfunction is associated with increased CVD risk and is important in the pathophysiology of hot flushes via the release of NO (Green et al., 2004; Hubing et al., 2010). During exercise, the endothelium releases NO in response to episodic increases in blood flow, and subsequently causes shear stress along the artery wall. Exercise training, as performed in the study by Bailey and colleagues

(2016b), induced regular, episodic increases in vascular shear stress, which likely caused NO release during exercise sessions. Following the exercise training intervention, endothelial function increased compared to control.

Thermoregulation

The thermoregulatory system is implicated in the causal pathway of hot flushes. The efficiency of the thermoregulatory system is reduced following the menopause (Bailey et al., 2016b). An increase in cardiorespiratory fitness is key to improving thermoregulatory function (Bailey et al., 2016a, 2016b). Bailey and colleagues (2016a) showed that 16 weeks of exercise training that improved fitness, improved thermoregulatory efficiency in symptomatic postmenopausal women by reducing the body temperature threshold for sweating and cutaneous vasodilation (Bailey et al., 2016b). The improvements coincided with reductions in frequency and severity of hot flushes in postmenopausal women and could provide a mechanistic explanation for the alleviation of hot flushes.

Real-world example

The real-world example originates from a participant who took part in our study where we examined the effect of exercise training on the frequency of menopausal hot flushes (e.g., Bailey et al., 2016a, 2016b). The participant, who was in the early stages of the postmenopausal period, reported volunteering for the study as she was interested to know if there were any alternative approaches to managing the hot flushes she was experiencing, which disrupted her day-to-day life, and her sleep patterns. She also expressed concern over the side effects of HRT, which she suspected increased her mother's risk of developing cancer.

Table 20.3 summarises this participant's increased level of fitness and weight loss after 16 weeks of aerobic exercise under supervision (Bailey et al., 2016b) The exercise training had decreased CVD risk by enhancing blood vessel function and alleviating the participant's perception of hot flush severity.

Summary

Based on the research evidence presented in this chapter, exercise during the menopause has important health benefits. We have provided a summary of guidelines for postmenopausal women exercising during the menopause in Figure 20.1. In addition, we have shown a real-world example of one woman who exercised early in the postmenopausal period as part of a study from our laboratory (Table 20.3).

Table 20.3 Participant characteristics and menopausal systems prior to (pre) and following (post) 16 weeks of moderate-intensity supervised exercise

	Pre[1]	Post[1]	Change
Traditional CVD risk factors			
Weight (kg)	77.3	74.3	↓
BMI (kg/m^2)	28.4	27.3	↓
Blood pressure (mmHg)	132/70	134/64	↓
Fitness			
Resting HR[2] (beats/min)	79	68	↓
$\dot{V}O_2$max (ml.kg^{-1}.min^{-1})	21.7	24.9	↑
Vascular function			
Function (FMD[3] %)	5.0	7.6	↑
Resting brain blood flow (cm/s)	56	56	~
Hot flush characteristics			
Hot flush frequency (per week)	63	20	↓
Hot flush severity	91	25	↓

Source: Bailey et al., 2016b.

Notes

1 Data are presented as mean.
2 HR: heart rate.
3 FMD: flow-mediated dilation.
4 $\dot{V}O_2$max: maximal oxygen consumption.
5 BMI: body mass index.

References

Ağil, A., Abike, F., Daskapan, A., Alaca, R., & Tüzün, H. (2010). Short-term exercise approaches on menopausal symptoms, psychological health, and quality of life in postmenopausal women. *Obstetrics and Gynecology International, 2010,* 1–7. https://doi.org/10.1155/2010/274261.

Bailey, T. G., Cable, N. T., Aziz, N., Atkinson, G., Cuthbertson, D. J., Low, D. A., & Jones, H. (2016a). Exercise training reduces the acute physiological severity of post-menopausal hot flushes. *The Journal of Physiology, 594*(3), 657–667. https://doi.org/10.1113/JP271456.

Bailey, T. G., Cable, N. T., Aziz, N., Dobson, R., Sprung, V. S., Low, D. A., & Jones, H. (2016b). Exercise training reduces the frequency of menopausal hot flushes by improving thermoregulatory control. *Menopause, 23*(7), 708–718. https://doi.org/10.1097/gme.0000000000000625.

Bauld, R., & Brown, R. F. (2009). Stress, psychological distress, psychosocial factors, menopause symptoms and physical health in women. *Maturitas, 62*(2), 160–165. https://doi.org/10.1016/j.maturitas.2008.12.004.

Bechlioulis, A., Kalantaridou, S. N., Naka, K. K., Chatzikyriakidou, A., Calis, K. A., Makrigiannakis, A., … Michalis, L. K. (2010). Endothelial function, but not carotid intima-media thickness, is affected early in menopause and is associated with severity of hot flushes. *The Journal of Clinical Endocrinology & Metabolism, 95*(3), 1199–1206. https://doi.org/10.1210/jc.2009-2262.

Ben Ali, S., Belfki-Benali, H., Ahmed, D. B., Haddad, N., Jmal, A., Abdennebi, M., & Romdhane, H. B. (2016). Postmenopausal hypertension, abdominal obesity, apolipoprotein and insulin resistance. *Clinical and Experimental Hypertension, 38*(4), 370–374. https://doi.org/10.3109/10641963.2015.1131286.

Black, M. A., Cable, N. T., Thijssen, D. H., & Green, D. J. (2009). Impact of age, sex, and exercise on brachial artery flow-mediated dilatation. *American Journal of Physiology-Heart and Circulatory Physiology, 297*(3), H1109-H1116. https://doi.org/10.1152/ajpheart.00226.2009.

Blair, S. N., Kampert, J. B., Kohl, H. W., Barlow, C. E., Macera, C. A., Paffenbarger, R. S., & Gibbons, L. W. (1996). Influences of cardiorespiratory fitness and other precursors on cardiovascular disease and all-cause mortality in men and women. *Journal of the American Medical Association, 276*(3), 205–210.

Carpenter, J., Gass, M. L., Maki, P. M., Newton, K. M., Pinkerton, J. V., Taylor, M., ... Shapiro, M. (2015). Nonhormonal management of menopause-associated vasomotor symptoms: 2015 position statement of The North American Menopause Society. *Menopause, 22*(11), 1155–1174. https://doi.org/10.1097/GME.0000000000000546.

Daley, A., Stokes-Lampard, H., & Macarthur, C. (2011). Exercise for vasomotor menopausal symptoms. *Cochrane Database of Systematic Reviews,* (11), CD006108. https://doi.org/10.1002/14651858.CD006108.pub3.

Daley, A. J., Stokes-Lampard, H. J., & Macarthur, C. (2009). Exercise to reduce vasomotor and other menopausal symptoms: A review. *Maturitas, 63*(3), 176–180. https://doi.org/10.1016/j.maturitas.2009.02.004.

Daley, A. J., Thomas, A., Roalfe, A. K., Stokes-Lampard, H., Coleman, S., Rees, M., ... MacArthur, C. (2015). The effectiveness of exercise as treatment for vasomotor menopausal symptoms: Randomised controlled trial. *BJOG: An International Journal of Obsetrics & Gynaecology, 122*(4), 565–575. https://doi.org/10.1111/1471-0528.13193.

Deecher, D. C., & Dorries, K. (2007). Understanding the pathophysiology of vasomotor symptoms (hot flushes and night sweats) that occur in perimenopause, menopause, and postmenopause life stages. *Archives of Women's Mental Health, 10*(6), 247–257. https://doi.org/10.1007/s00737-007-0209-5.

DeNino, W. F., Tchernof, A., Dionne, I. J., Toth, M. J., Ades, P. A., Sites, C. K., & Poehlman, E. T. (2001). Contribution of abdominal adiposity to age-related differences in insulin sensitivity and plasma lipids in healthy nonobese women. *Diabetes Care, 24*(5), 925–932. https://doi.org/10.2337/diacare.24.5.925.

Duygu, H., Akman, L., Ozerkan, F., Akercan, F., Zoghi, M., Nalbantgil, S., ... Akin, M. (2009). Comparison of the effects of new and conventional hormone replacement therapies on left ventricular diastolic function in healthy postmenopausal women: A Doppler and ultrasonic backscatter study. *The International Journal of Cardiovascular Imaging, 25*(4), 387–396. https://doi.org/10.1007/s10554-009-9429-2.

Egelund, J., Jørgensen, P. G., Mandrup, C. M., Fritz-Hansen, T., Stallknecht, B., Bangsbo, J., ... Hellsten, Y. (2017). Cardiac adaptations to high-intensity aerobic training in premenopausal and recent postmenopausal women: The Copenhagen Women Study. *Journal of the American Heart Association, 6*(8). https://doi.org/10.1161/jaha.117.005469.

Fogelholm, M. (2010). Physical activity, fitness and fatness: relations to mortality, morbidity and disease risk factors. A systematic review. *Obesity Reviews, 11*(3), 202–221. https://doi.org/10.1111/j.1467-789X.2009.00653.x.

Franco, O. H., Muka, T., Colpani, V., Kunutsor, S., Chowdhury, S., Chowdhury, R., & Kavousi, M. (2015). Vasomotor symptoms in women and cardiovascular risk markers: Systematic review and meta-analysis. *Maturitas, 81*(3), 353–361. https://doi.org/10.1016/j.maturitas.2015.04.016.

Gray, K. E., Katon, J. G., LeBlanc, E. S., Woods, N. F., Bastian, L. A., Reiber, G. E., ... LaCroix, A. Z. (2018). Vasomotor symptom characteristics: Are they risk factors for incident diabetes? *Menopause*. 4 December. https://doi.org/10.1097/GME.0000000000001033.

Green, D. J., Maiorana, A., O'Driscoll, G., & Taylor, R. (2004). Effect of exercise training on endothelium-derived nitric oxide function in humans. *The Journal of Physiology, 561*(Pt 1), 1–25. https://doi.org/10.1113/jphysiol.2004.068197.

Hellsten, Y., & Nyberg, M. (2015). Cardiovascular adaptations to exercise training. *Comprehensive Physiology, 6*(1), 1–32. https://doi.org/10.1002/cphy.c140080.

Hilditch, J. R., Lewis, J., Peter, A., van Maris, B., Ross, A., Franssen, E., ... Dunn, E. (1996). A menopause-specific quality of life questionnaire: Development and psychometric properties. *Maturitas, 24*(3), 161–175.

Hodges, G. J., Sharp, L., Stephenson, C., Patwala, A. Y., George, K. P., Goldspink, D. F., & Cable, N. T. (2010b). The effect of 48 weeks of aerobic exercise training on cutaneous vasodilator function in post-menopausal females. *European Journal of Applied Physiology, 108*(6), 1259–1267. https://doi.org/10.1007/s00421-009-1330-0.

Howden, E. J., Perhonen, M., Peshock, R. M., Zhang, R., Arbab-Zadeh, A., Adams-Huet, B., & Levine, B. D. (2015). Females have a blunted cardiovascular response to one year of intensive supervised endurance training. *Journal of Applied Physiology, 119*(1), 37–46. https://doi.org/10.1152/japplphysiol.00092.2015.

Hubing, K. A., Wingo, J. E., Brothers, R. M., Del Coso, J., Low, D. A., & Crandall, C. G. (2010). Nitric oxide synthase inhibition attenuates cutaneous vasodilation during the post-menopausal hot flash. *Menopause, 17*(5), 978–982. https://doi.org/10.1097/gme.0b013e3181d674d6.

Janssen, I., Powell, L. H., Crawford, S., Lasley, B., & Sutton-Tyrrell, K. (2008). Menopause and the metabolic syndrome: The Study of Women's Health Across the Nation. *Archives of Internal Medicine, 168*(14), 1568–1575. https://doi.org/10.1001/archinte.168.14.1568.

Johnell, O., & Kanis, J. (2006). An estimate of the worldwide prevalence and disability associated with osteoporotic fractures. *Osteoporosis International, 17*(12), 1726–1733. https://doi.org/10.1007/s00198-006-0172-4.

Kalyani, R. R., Corriere, M., & Ferrucci, L. (2014). Age-related and disease-related muscle loss: The effect of diabetes, obesity, and other diseases. *The Lancet Diabetes & Endocrinology, 2*(10), 819–829. https://doi.org/10.1016/S2213-8587(14)70034-8.

Karacan, S. (2010). Effects of long-term aerobic exercise on physical fitness and postmenopausal symptoms with menopausal rating scale. *Science & Sports, 25*(1), 39–46. https://doi.org/10.1016/j.scispo.2009.07.004.

Lindh-Åstrand, L., Nedstrand, E., Wyon, Y., & Hammar, M. (2004). Vasomotor symptoms and quality of life in previously sedentary postmenopausal women randomised to physical activity or estrogen therapy. *Maturitas, 48*(2), 97–105. https://doi.org/10.1016/s0378-5122(03)00187-7.

Low, D. A., Davis, S. L., Keller, D. M., Shibasaki, M., & Crandall, C. G. (2008). Cutaneous and hemodynamic responses during hot flashes in symptomatic postmenopausal women. *Menopause, 15*(2), 290–295. https://doi.org/10.1097/gme.0b013e3180ca7cfa.

Luoto, R., Moilanen, J., Heinonen, R., Mikkola, T., Raitanen, J., Tomas, E., ... Nygard, C. H. (2012). Effect of aerobic training on hot flushes and quality of life – A randomized controlled trial. *Annals of Medicine, 44*(6), 616–626. https://doi.org/10.3109/07853890.2011.583674.

Mandrup, C. M., Egelund, J., Nyberg, M., Enevoldsen, L. H., Kjaer, A., Clemmensen, A. E., ... Stallknecht, B. M. (2017a). Effects of menopause and high-intensity training on insulin sensitivity and muscle metabolism. *Menopause.* https://doi.org/10.1097/gme.0000000000000981.

Mandrup, C. M., Egelund, J., Nyberg, M., Lundberg Slingsby, M. H., Andersen, C. B., Logstrup, S., ... Hellsten, Y. (2017b). Effects of high-intensity training on cardiovascular risk factors in premenopausal and postmenopausal women. *American Journal of Obstetrics & Gynecology, 216*(4), 384.e381–384.e311. https://doi.org/10.1016/j.ajog.2016.12.017.

Mansikkamäki, K., Raitanen, J., Nygård, C. H., Heinonen, R., Mikkola, T., Tomás. E., & Luoto, R. (2012). Sleep quality and aerobic training among menopausal women – a randomized controlled trial. *Maturitas, 72*(4), 339–345. https://doi.org/10.1016/j.maturitas.2012.05.003.

Manson, J. E., Hsia, J., Johnson, K. C., Rossouw, J. E., Assaf, A. R., Lasser, N. L., ... Detrano, R. (2003). Estrogen plus progestin and the risk of coronary heart disease. *The New England Journal of Medicine, 349*(6), 523–534. https://doi.org/10.1056/NEJMoa030808.

Matthews, K. A., Crawford, S. L., Chae, C. U., Everson-Rose, S. A., Sowers, M. F., Sternfeld, B., & Sutton-Tyrrell, K. (2009). Are changes in cardiovascular disease risk factors in midlife women due to chronological aging or to the menopausal transition? *Journal of the American College of Cardiology, 54*(25), 2366–2373. https://doi.org/10.1016/j.jacc.2009.10.009.

Mendelsohn M. E., & Karas, R. H. (1999). The protective effects of estrogen on the cardiovascular system. *New England Journal of Medicine, 340*(23), 1801–1811. https://doi.org/10.1056/NEJM199906103402306.

Moilanen, J. M., Mikkola, T. S., Raitanen, J. A., Heinonen, R. H., Tomas, E. I., Nygård, C. H., & Luoto, R. M. (2012). Effect of aerobic training on menopausal symptoms – A randomized controlled trial. *Menopause, 19*(6), 691–696. https://doi.org/10.1097/gme.0b013e31823cc5f7.

Moreau, K. L., Hildreth, K. L., Meditz, A. L., Deane, K. D., & Kohrt, W. M. (2012). Endothelial function is impaired across the stages of the menopause transition in healthy women. *The Journal of Clinical Endocrinology & Metabolism, 97*(12), 4692–4700. https://doi.org/10.1210/jc.2012-2244.

Moreau, K. L., Stauffer, B. L., Kohrt, W. M., & Seals, D. R. (2013). Essential role of estrogen for improvements in vascular endothelial function with endurance exercise in postmenopausal women. *The Journal of Clinical Endocrinology & Metabolism, 98*(11), 4507–4515. https://doi.org/10.1210/jc.2013-2183.

Murphy, C. C., Bartholomew, L. K., Carpentier, M. Y., Bluethmann, S. M., & Vernon, S. W. (2012). Adherence to adjuvant hormonal therapy among breast cancer survivors in clinical practice: A systematic review. *Breast Cancer Research and Treatment, 134*(2), 459–478. https://doi.org/10.1007/s10549-012-2114-5.

Nelson, H. D., Vesco, K. K., Haney, E., Fu, R., Nedrow, A., Miller, J., ... Humphrey, L. (2006). Nonhormonal therapies for menopausal hot flashes: Systematic review and meta-analysis. *Journal of the American Medical Association,* *295*(17), 2057–2071.

Newton, K. M., Reed, S. D., Guthrie, K. A., Sherman, K. J., Booth-LaForce, C., Caan, B., ... LaCroix, A. Z. (2014). Efficacy of yoga for vasomotor symptoms: A randomized controlled trial. *Menopause, 21*(4), 339–346. https://doi.org/10.1097/GME.0b013e31829e4baa.

Nyberg, M., Egelund, J., Mandrup, C. M., Andersen, C. B., Hansen, K., Hergel, I. F., ... Hellsten, Y. (2017). Leg vascular and skeletal muscle mitochondrial adaptations to aerobic high-intensity exercise training are enhanced in the early postmenopausal phase. *The Journal of Physiology, 595*(9), 2969–2983. https://doi.org/10.1113/jp273871.

Nyberg, M., Seidelin, K., Andersen, T. R., Overby, N. N., Hellsten, Y. & Bangsbo, J. (2014). Biomarkers of vascular function in premenopausal and recent postmenopausal women of similar age: Effect of exercise training. *American Journal of Physiology Regulatory, Integratvie and Comparative Physiology, 306*(7), R510–R517. https://doi.org/10.1152/ajpregu.00539.2013.

Pierce, G. L., Eskurza, I., Walker, A. E., Fay, T. N., & Seals, D. R. (2011). Sex-specific effects of habitual aerobic exercise on brachial artery flow-mediated dilation in middle-aged and older adults. *Clinical Science (London), 120*(1), 13–23. https://doi.org/10.1042/cs20100174.

Rossi, R., Chiurlia, E., Nuzzo, A., Cioni, E., Origliani, G., & Modena, M. G. (2004). Flow-mediated vasodilation and the risk of developing hypertension in healthy postmenopausal women. *Journal of the American College of Cardiology, 44*(8), 1636–1640. https://doi.org/10.1016/j.jacc.2004.07.027.

Sarri, G., Davies, M., & Lumsden, M. A. (2015). Diagnosis and management of menopause: Summary of NICE guidance. *BMJ: British Medical Journal (Online), 351.* https://doi.org/10.1136/bmj.h5746.

Seidelin, K., Nyberg, M., Piil, P., Jørgensen, N. R., Hellsten, Y., & Bangsbo, J. (2017). Adaptations with intermittent exercise training in post-and premenopausal women. *Medicine and Science in Sports and Exercise, 49*(1), 96–105.

Staessen, J. A., Bulpitt, C. J., Fagard, R., Lijnen, P., & Amery, A. (1994). The influence of menopause on blood pressure. *Hypertension in Postmenopausal Women,* 15–26. https://doi.org/10.1007/978-3-642-79077-5_3.

Sternfeld, B., Guthrie, K. A., Ensrud, K. E., LaCroix, A. Z., Larson, J. C., Dunn, A. L., ... Caan, B. J. (2014). Efficacy of exercise for menopausal symptoms: A randomized controlled trial. *Menopause, 21*(4), 330–338. https://doi.org/10.1097/GME.0b013e31829e4089.

Sternfeld, B., Wang, H., Quesenberry Jr, C. P., Abrams, B., Everson-Rose, S. A., Greendale, G. A., ... Sowers, M. (2004). Physical activity and changes in weight and waist circumference in midlife women: Findings from the Study of Women's Health Across the Nation. *American Journal of Epidemiology, 160*(9), 912–922.

Taddei, S., Virdis, A., Ghiadoni, L., Mattei, P., Sudano, I., Bernini, G. ... Salvetti, A. (1996). Menopause is associated with endothelial dysfunction in women. *Hypertension, 28*(4), 576–582.

Tanahashi, K., Akazawa, N., Miyaki, A., Choi, Y., Ra, S.-G., Matsubara, T., ... Maeda, S. (2014). Aerobic exercise training decreases plasma asymmetric dimethylarginine concentrations with increase in arterial compliance in postmenopausal women. *American Journal of Hypertension, 27*(3), 415–421. https://doi.org/10.1093/ajh/hpt217.

Tew, G. A., George, K. P., Cable, N. T., & Hodges, G. J. (2012). Endurance exercise training enhances cutaneous microvascular reactivity in post-menopausal women. *Microvascular Research, 83*(2), 223–228. https://doi.org/10.1016/j.mvr.2011.09.002.

Thurston, E. C. (2018). Vasomotor symptoms: natural history, physiology, and links with cardiovascular health. *Climacteric*, 1–5. https://doi.org/10.1080/13697137.2018.1430131.

Thurston, R. C., El Khoudary, S. R., Sutton-Tyrrell, K., Crandall, C. J., Gold, E., Sternfeld, B., ... Matthews, K. A. (2012). Vasomotor symptoms and lipid profiles in women transitioning through menopause. *Obstetrics & Gynecology, 119*(4), 753. https://doi.org/10.1097/AOG.0b013e31824a09ec.

Thurston, R. C., Sutton-Tyrrell, K., Everson-Rose, S. A., Hess, R., Powell, L. H., & Matthews, K. A. (2011). Hot flashes and carotid intima media thickness among midlife women. *Menopause, 18*(4), 352–358. https://doi.org/10.1097/gme.0b013e3181fa27fd.

Trémollieres, F. A., Pouilles, J.-M., & Ribot, C. A. (1996). Relative influence of age and menopause on total and regional body composition changes in postmenopausal women. *American Journal of Obstetrics & Gynecology, 175*(6), 1594–1600. https://doi.org/10.1016/S0002-9378(96)70111-4.

Wernstedt, P., Sjöstedt, C., Ekman, I., Du, H., Thuomas, K. Å., Areskog, N. H., & Nylander E. (2002). Adaptation of cardiac morphology and function to endurance and strength training. *Scandinavian Journal of Medicine & Science in Sports, 12*(1), 17–25. https://doi.org/10.1034/j.1600-0838.2002.120104.x.

World Health Organization. (1996). *Research on the menopause in the 1990s: Report of a WHO scientific group*. Ottawa: Public Health Agency of Canada.

Index

Page numbers in **bold** denote tables, those in *italics* denote figures.